USMLE Step 2 Triage

USMLE Step 2 Triage

An Effective, No-nonsense Review of Clinical Knowledge

Kevin Schwechten, MD

Teaching Faculty and Staff Physician
Magnolia Regional Health Center
Magnolia Regional Health Center Residency Program
Corinth, Mississippi

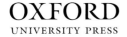

OXFORD
UNIVERSITY PRESS

2011

Oxford University Press, Inc., publishes works that further
Oxford University's objective of excellence
in research, scholarship, and education.

Oxford New York
Auckland Cape Town Dar es Salaam Hong Kong Karachi
Kuala Lumpur Madrid Melbourne Mexico City Nairobi
New Delhi Shanghai Taipei Toronto

With offices in
Argentina Austria Brazil Chile Czech Republic France Greece
Guatemala Hungary Italy Japan Poland Portugal Singapore
South Korea Switzerland Thailand Turkey Ukraine Vietnam

Published by Oxford University Press, Inc.
198 Madison Avenue, New York, New York 10016

www.oup.com

Oxford is a registered trademark of Oxford University Press.

Library of Congress Cataloging-in-Publication Data

Schwechten, Kevin.
USMLE step 2 triage : an effective no-nonsense review of clinical knowledge / Kevin Schwechten.
p. ; cm.
Includes index.
ISBN 978-0-19-538327-0
1. Medicine—Examinations, questions, etc. 2. Medicine—Outlines, syllabi, etc. 3. Physicians—Licenses—United States—Examinations—Study guides.
I. Title. [DNLM: 1. Clinical Medicine—Outlines. 2. Licensure, Medical—Outlines. WB 18.2 S412ua 2011]
R834.5.S385 2011
610.76—dc22
2010003468

9 8 7 6 5 4 3 2 1

Printed in China
on acid-free paper

Contents

To my amazing family: Dawn, my wife, whose support has meant everything, and to my children, Ariel and Tristan, who gave me the great gifts of motivation, inspiration, and hope.

Also, to the soldiers, medics, and officers of the US Army's 2-4 Infantry battalion, 10th Mountain Division (2008), who did a truly professional job in Iraq and made it possible for all of us to come home.

Preface

Step 2 Clinical Knowledge is designed to test your ability to apply advanced medical principles in the patient care environment. It's not just another test and it's certainly not Step 1. Background knowledge is crucial, but just as crucial is your ability to apply that knowledge. Because this test is given before residency, it's very important you demonstrate adeptness of knowledge application to showcase your skill. However, don't be fooled into thinking the more background the better. The application of knowledge you've already learned is the key factor, not learning minutiae you don't need. That application of retained medical knowledge will be the bane of your career no matter what you specialize in, thus, is the focus of Step 2 CK. To add a third component to the exam, time is a strict restraint. So to succeed you need to prepare efficiently and effectively. The information in this book is prioritized with emphasis on commonly tested medical material and gives a focused overview to those areas less tested. Its emphasis is on diagnosis and treatment. Its detail is purposely controlled to provide efficient review. And its format is designed for quick assimilation. Used properly, this book provides all the review you'll need to kill this exam!

How to Use This Book

USMLE Step 2 Triage is designed to simply be the most efficient and complete resource for increasing and broadening background knowledge for Step 2 Clinical Knowledge. When studying it, note those areas with greater emphasis and quoted authoritative group recommendations, as these are the most highly tested areas on the test. Master the information in all sections completely and review any areas you have trouble with over and over. This will fill in knowledge gaps where you need it. Take many notes in the margins and look up in other resources any information needing clarification or enhancement. Highlight areas of importance and memorize important diagnosis or treatment aspects according to the text. In all, this book should look thoroughly used and abused by the time the test comes. Using this book, coupled with your medical school training, will get you the background knowledge needed for this extensive exam.

However, don't be fooled into thinking you're done. You also need to practice. And practice constantly. This should be done by using the USMLE practice test materials (questions) and practice material sold by the National Board of Medical Examiners (NBME). These practice questions are of the highest quality available and you should spend significant time not only testing yourself but also trying to infer the question-writers' intent and motives. Then, as these "gold standard" resources are finite, use other commercial resources for practice. As there are many practice questions available commercially, note the difference in quality and accuracy; however, the practice and not the absolute answers are what's important. Finally, master answering these questions within the time constraints provided. During the actual test, you'll have an average of 1–1.3 minutes per question, thus, this should be the average time for each test question in your practice. Timing needs repetition and training even for the most experienced test taker.

Logistics

Test Registration

Registration for this test is similar to that of Step 1 in that it can be accomplished online. If you're a graduate of an American or Canadian medical school, go to www.nbme.org and navigate to the registration section of the site and proceed as instructed. If you're a graduate of a different foreign medical school, go to www.ecfmg.org and do the same. Both should be straightforward. Plan on enough time to register, pay your dues, receive the scheduling permit in the mail, then schedule your test date. Don't expect to be able to schedule a test date for anytime close to the time you register. Also, a note on payment: this is not the time for experimenting with a new debit charge card or trying out a new credit line. Be prepared to use a major charge card which you know is worthy of accepting the substantial charge of this test. If you risk the charge being declined, you risk the chance for a smooth registration for this important test.

After you register, an orange scheduling permit will be mailed to your listed address. This permit has a number (CIN) which allows you then to call the Prometric testing center (at 800-633-3926) or schedule your test online at www.prometric.com. The scheduling permit will allow you to request a test day within a 3 month eligibility period which you choose. That is, you may pick the May-June-July eligibility period which then allows you to request a test day within those months. If, for some reason, you need to move your test day, you may only do so within those three months without an additional fee. When calling or scheduling online, be prepared to request several different testing days since these test centers fill up quickly and you might not be granted your first preference.

Question Format

Step 2 is made up of 370 multiple choice questions taken in eight 60-minute blocks. The testing day is actually 9 hours long and includes 45 to 60 minutes of break time, including an initial, optional, 15 minute computerized tutorial at the beginning of the testing day. If you're familiar with the testing format, skip the tutorial and add that time to your breaks. It's highly recommended you become familiar with the test delivery software before attempting the exam. Breaks may be taken after and between testing blocks, not during. If, for absolutely any reason, you need to take a break during a block, the testing clock will keep running. Within each block, as time permits, you may answer any question in any order, review previous questions or answers, and change any answers you feel you need to. After time expires for any block, you may not return to it for any reason. If you finish with a block early, you may technically end the block manually and add the remaining time in that block to your break time. However, it's highly recommended instead of taking this extra time for break, you review your answers to those questions you found difficult and correct any answers you feel unsure about.

Questions are formatted to be multiple choice. These include single best answer, matching, and multiple question vignettes. Answer choices for each question may be chosen from four to ten different choices. Commonly, multiple question vignettes include 2, 3, or 4 different questions associated with them. You should use the practice software and cases to become familiar with the format of the testing software. There are several useful tools including highlighting, annotations, and strikethrough, as well as navigation buttons and a status bar containing timing of your test session. Make sure you're a wizard at the software before you walk into the testing center!

Organization

Step 2 CK contains questions relating to all major areas of medicine including pediatrics, internal medicine, surgery, obstetrics, etc. Questions in these areas relate to specific areas including immunologic disorders, cardiovascular disorders, nutritional and digestive disorders, etc. Questions will require you to answer based on several tasks. These are finding the diagnosis or prognosis, indicating the underlying mechanism of disease, finding the next step in care, or establishing the best choice of preventive medicine or health maintenance measure. Emphasis is divided according to this rough estimate:

15%–20% Promoting preventive medicine and health maintenance

20%–35% Understanding mechanisms of disease

25%–40% Establishing a diagnosis

15%–25% Applying principles of management

You're encouraged to examine the areas of emphasis on the USMLE website at www.usmle.org.

Passing the Exam

Step 2 CK is reported in three different score formats: pass/fail report, 3-digit score, and 2-digit score. The minimum requirements for passing Step 2 are a 3-digit score of 184 which corresponds to a 2-digit score of 75. Scores above these receive a pass report and denote success. Scores below these must be retaken to pass the exam. Average 3-digit scores for LCME accredited institutions in the U.S. are between 200-220, which correspond to a historic pass rate between 93% and 95%. Score reports should arrive by mail within 8 weeks of your test date, although 4-5 weeks is more typical. If you haven't received your score by eight weeks after taking the exam, you should contact the USMLE.

Remember, this test is the last major standardized exam before you graduate medical school and are officially made a doctor. It represents standardization and a common hurdle for all those graduating medical school with the eventual goal of practicing in the U.S. It has been a long road and is soon to be over. My advice is to work hard, study hard, know your profession, and kill this exam. Good luck on this test and thereafter.

Kevin Schwechten, MD

1 General Principles, Ethics, and Statistics

House Officer Issues

These issues are commonly encountered by the new house officer and are skills that will be followed throughout residency. These are guidelines for survival on the wards or on an inpatient rotation, not rules, since every residency has its own procedures.

The List

The list is most often a census of patients who are still on the inpatient service and need work and rounds completed on during the day; this is most commonly kept by residents or interns. This continually updated list keeps everyone organized and serves as both scratch paper and as a working, living document. Your technique for organization may vary, but consider using a "box and check" system of listing tasks needing to be done on each patient. This list is then updated and printed out for the oncoming night shift when the evening handoff is done.

Handoffs

A handoff is simply the transfer of care from one physician to another; these commonly occur during shift change or emergency room consultations. The handoff should include a separate presentation for each patient as well as any tasks that still need to be done on each patient. Good handoffs often include tasks to complete care of the patient. These undone tasks should not be viewed as sloppy work since taking care of the patient is everyone's responsibility! Elements of the handoff vary but should include the name, age, leading diagnosis, brief hospital course, brief oral presentation (see below), and outstanding tasks. Presentations are customarily shortened if the oncoming team is familiar with the patient.

A popular method follows the pneumonic SBAR:

S—Situation
Identify the patient and sum up their current situation including most relevant diagnosis, current treatments, etc.

B—Background
State the relevant history, physical assessment, relevant lab data, recent treatments, clinical course, and any recent changes. Identify relevant consultation services.

A—Assessment
Offer your conclusions about the present situation. Explain anticipated changes in the patient's condition or treatment.

R—Recommendations
Explain what you think needs to be done for the patient, his/her code status (DNR/DNI status), and what to watch for. Emphasize important pending results.

Due to the nature of medicine, the attendings are not commonly present during the handoffs. Thus, police yourselves or further oversight can make this process more painful than necessary.

The Oral Presentation

The practical, non-ICU presentation should be mastered as soon as possible in the clinical years of med school. Consider the context in which you're presenting, as focused presentations are a valued thing in almost every setting. Internists and pediatricians like long, orderly presentations; ER docs and surgeons love short ones. However, the skill to develop concise and relevant presentations is one that evolves throughout residency and is often far from innate.

Order of Elements

Subjective
Start with the leading diagnosis. This is not the chief complaint but "flags" what you're saying!

History of Present Illness
Include any relevant piece of information about the patient. Include duration of illness, precipitating factors, timing, hospital/ER course, relieving factors, outpatient course, and severity. Risk factors for major diseases are always appreciated.

Past Medical History
Include relevant PMH that relates to the present condition in any way. Make this concise since, in practicality, many attendings do not want to hear about former eye conditions in the intestinal obstruction patient. Include smoking, EtOH use, drug history, and current and prior medications as appropriate.

Past Surgical History
Include rough timing of surgery, complications, and effects if appropriate.

Social History
Often not needed in the oral presentation unless relevant.

Objective
Vital Signs
If changes are relevant, include these. If an ongoing inpatient, give ranges over the last 24 hours for BP, HR, RR, O_2 sats, and pain scale. For temperature, give the "T_{max}" or maximum temperature over the last 24 hours. Do not forget to note if supplemental oxygen is used when reporting the O_2 sats.

Physical Exam
Focus on the systems that relate to the patient's main problem. When psychiatric or neurologic systems are affected, expand on these.

Laboratories
Have these ready to read off at this point of the presentation.

Imaging
Either have the radiology report available or your own succinct impressions.

ECG
Do not blindly relate the "computer read" of the ECG. Make your own assessment.

Assessment
This is where the thinking is done. Several techniques exist. Consider using a numbered list with a separate A/P for each diagnosis. Regardless, make a diagnosis, then support it with pieces of information from the S/O. Discussion should not be rambling, but supported with cited elements from the S/O portion. Mention the differential diagnosis list in the discussion but order it in descending order of likelihood for the patient's presentation.

Plan

Make the plan relevant to the diagnosis. Include the disposition plan for the patient including the expected date of d/c. For extra brownie points, mention smoking cessation or social support as a last point.

Take Home Points

- Never, ever ask questions of anyone during the presentation.
- Have written lab results or imaging results with you when presenting.
- Make eye contact, at least from time to time.
- Many attendings frown on "reading a presentation," but notes are generally accepted.
- Be prepared for interruptions, questions, and clarifications from others.

Human Development

The various stages and characteristics of childhood development are discussed in the table on page 5.

Common Developmental Challenges

The common developmental challenges are discussed in the table on page 6.

Normal Puberty

Puberty is a normal stage in pediatric development when an accelerated growth and sexual maturation stage interrupts linear growth. This stage is dominated by sexual maturation and development in sexual organs, body hair amount and distribution, body fat content, and in boys, spermatogenesis, in girls, onset of menarche. Presumably, after the completion of this time of rapid physiologic change, the body is prepared and capable of reproduction.

Girls

In females, the first secondary sexual characteristic to emerge is thelarche (breast/areola development) beginning on average at age 11 years. This is followed closely by the onset of a growth spurt seen most dramatically in height increase. The next stage is pubarche, or the development of pubic hair. Menarche then follows, on average, 2.5 years after the onset of thelarche, marking the last stage of development. The individual duration and peak velocity of these stages is dependent on several factors which commonly relate to each individual patient.

Boys

The first secondary sexual characteristic in males is increase in testicular size (from < 3 mL to about 30 mL in adults), followed closely by the onset of the pubertal growth spurt (seen in boys as both height and muscular development). The penis then lengthens and frequent erections commonly occur. Development of pubic hair, pubarche, occurs next and is preceded by the development of axillary and facial hair by approximately 2–2.5 years after the onset of puberty. At a variable time in each boy's life, the first ejaculation generally occurs between 12.5 and 14.5 years. During male development, other changes including voice deepening and heightened libido will be noted.

A staged scale of physical development called the Tanner stages (discussed in table on page 6) outlines development of various physical features in both boys and girls. The scale relays a spectrum according to five discrete stages detailing development of the breasts, male external genitalia, and pubic hair distribution. Stage 1 is noted as prepubertal, and stage 5 is adult.

TABLE 1.1 Childhood Development

Age	Social	Emotional	Cognitive	Language	Motor
3 months	• Social smile • Imitates facial expressions	• Enjoys play with others • Facial expressions	• Immature • Localizes sound	• Smiles at the sound of voice • Babbles • Sound imitation	• Raises head when prone • Starts coordinating hands/eyes
7 months	• Enjoys social play • Interested in mirror images	• Responds to people's emotions and expressions • Appears joyful often	• Explores with hands and mouth • Struggles to get objects that are out of reach	• Responds to own name • Begins to respond to "no" • Babbles chains of sounds	• Rolls both ways • Uses hands to rake objects • Supports whole weight on legs
1 year	• Stranger anxiety • Cries with parent separation • Tests parental response to behavior	• May be fearful in unfamiliar situations • Extends extremity for help when getting dressed • Shows preferences	• Explores objects in different ways • Looks at correct picture when image is named • Imitates gestures	• Responds to simple verbal requests • Says "dada" and "mama" • Uses simple gestures such as shaking head for "no"	• Uses pincer grasp • Walks alone • Lets objects go voluntarily
2 years	• Imitates behaviors of others • More excited about company of peers	• Demonstrates independence development • Begins to be defiant at times	• Finds hidden objects well • Begins imaginary play • Begins to sort by shape and color	• Recognizes names of familiar people, objects, body parts • Uses 2–4 word sentences • Follows simple instructions	• Climbs up/down stairs alone • Kicks a ball • Begins to run • Scribbles on their own
3 years	• Imitates adults and playmates • Can take turns in games • Shows affection toward playmates	• Expresses range of emotion • Separates without anxiety from parents • Objects to routine changes	• Makes mechanical toys work • Completes puzzles with 3 or 4 pieces • Plays make believe with dolls, animals, people	• Follows a 2- or 3-part command • Understands most sentences • Uses 4–5 word sentences • Uses pronouns	• Climbs well • Pedals tricycle • Turns book pages one at a time • Turns rotating handles
4 years	• Interested in new experiences • Dresses and undresses self • Plays "mom" and "dad"	• Imagines "monsters" • Self aware • May not be able to tell the difference between fantasy and reality	• Understands counting and may know some numbers • Recalls parts of a story • Tells stories from memory or imagination	• Has mastered some basic rules of grammar • Speaks in short sentences • Speech is clear enough for strangers to understand	• Often catches bounced ball • Copies square shapes • Hops and stands on one foot • Throws ball overhand
5 years	• Wants to please friends • Likes to sing, dance, act	• Aware of gender • Able to distinguish fantasy/reality	• Can count 10 or more objects • Understands the concept of time • Names at least 4 colors	• Speaks sentences relatively fluidly • Uses future tense	• Hops, somersaults • Skips • Draws person with body • Uses fork/spoon

TABLE 1.2 Developmental Challenges

Age of Presentation	Issue
1–3 months	Colic
1–4 months	Night feeding
9 months	Stranger anxiety
12 months	Exploratory behavior
18 months	Common temper tantrums
24 months	Toilet training
24–36 months	New sibling rivalry
>36 months	Nightmares and preference to sleep with parents

TABLE 1.3 Tanner Pubertal Hair Development

Stage 1	Prepubertal
Stage 2	Sparse growth of long and mildly pigmented hair, straight or curled. First occurring at the base of the penis or along labia.
Stage 3	Darker, coarser hair, spreading sparsely outward in the pubic region.
Stage 4	Hair becomes adult in type including color and coarseness although covering a smaller area than adult hair. No hair has yet reached the thighs.
Stage 5	Adult in type and quantity including spread to the thighs.

Take Home Points

- Puberty occurs at different times for all kids; however, reasons for delayed or absent puberty include hormonal imbalance, genetic disorder, anatomical disorder, medication influence, lack of energy calorie intake, or failure to thrive.
- Tanner stages are commonly used to classify puberty.
- Consider the patient's anxiety about this time of life.

Childhood Failure to Thrive

Failure to thrive (FTT) does not have a universal definition; however, many experts regard this condition as having the following features:

- Weight below the 3rd percentile for gestation corrected age and sex on more than one occasion.
- Weight < 80 percent of ideal body weight for age, using standard growth charts. Ideal body weight = weight matched to the corresponding percentile of length.
- Depressed weight/length (<10th percentile).
- A rate of weight gain that causes a crossing of **two or more major percentile lines** over time.

- A rate of daily weight gain less than that expected for age:
  - 26 to 31 g/day for those 0 to 3 months
  - 17 to 18 g/day for those 3 to 6 months
  - 12 to 13 g/day for those 6 to 9 months
  - 9 to 13 g/day for those 9 to 12 months
  - 7 to 9 g/day for those 1 to 3 years

Causes of FTT are numerous and commonly divided into two categories: organic and nonorganic. Organic causes are those diseases that affect nutrient utilization and may further be categorized as: decreased nutrient intake, malabsorption, impaired metabolism, increased excretion, or increased energy requirements. Nonorganic causes include denial of available calories, which may be due to family poverty, neglect, food unavailability, or child abuse.

Diagnosis

History is essential in elucidating a cause of FTT. A very detailed history must be taken in which the following elements are discussed with the primary caregiver: growth chart review, diet history, assessment of the child's elimination pattern, medical history, family history, and social history.

Labs: Limited screening laboratories should be done. The best strategy is to let the history and clinical presentation dictate labs. However, some screening labs may include: CBC, urinalysis, BUN/creatinine, electrolytes, lead level, albumin, and stool studies including reducing substances, ova and parasite screen. Other tests perhaps indicated by a directed history are sweat chloride testing, genetic analysis, TSH, alkaline phosphatase, etc.

Treatment

Addition of dietary calories is the treatment of choice for nonorganic causes.

If the etiology is organic, treatment varies, which makes accurate diagnosis essential. Hospitalization and direct observation and feeding may be needed in those cases when discerning etiology, despite investigation, is still necessary.

Take Home Points

- FTT has several implications for growth and growth velocity. However, there is no universal and absolute definition.
- Classify causes of FTT as organic or nonorganic.
- Thorough investigation for physiologic causes should be undertaken. FTT is a diagnosis of exclusion.

Child Abuse

Child abuse comprises several different types, including: sexual, physical (nonaccidental trauma), psychological, emotional, and neglect. Estimates of abuse victims' mortality are as high as 1/2000 deaths per year. Risk factors include: poverty, parental substance abuse, lower educational status of parents, maternal history of abuse, negative attitude of mother toward pregnancy, prior abuse in parents, parental isolation, and discord or abuse amongst parents.

Symptoms

All too commonly, child abuse is outwardly asymptomatic. Children innately attempt to deny to investigators that there is anything wrong. As well, victims are often sworn to secrecy by the abuser by threat of consequence or harm to themselves or other family members. Symptoms, however, may include social isolation, depression, sexually-themed play, self destructive play, emotional distancing, disproportionate fear of quick hand motions from authority figures ("hand shyness"), sleep disturbance, bedwetting, anxiety issues, bruising, pain in strange places, or pain in the genital region.

Diagnosis

Physical exam: Bruising may be found anywhere on the body; however, look for bruises on the anterior/posterior rib cage, on the back, neck, and especially buttocks. Striking a child hard enough in punishment to create a bruise is often considered abuse. Other skin findings may be electrical cord markings, object impressions such as coat hangers etc, stocking or glove burns from emersion in scalding water, cigarette burns/scars, or belt marks.

Ophthalmologic exam may show retinal hemorrhages or rarely, retinal detachment. Sexual abuse and genital/anal trauma should be evaluated by a qualified physician trained in recognizing typical features. These features include bruising, circumferential edema (tire sign), excoriations, fissures, bleeding, or significant tissue damage.

Labs: Sexual abuse may warrant wet mount for motile sperm or cytopathology for sperm, gonorrhea/chlamydia testing, β-hCG, RPR or VDRL for syphilis, hepatitis panel, or HIV testing. Investigate neglect with CBC for anemia, stool exam, PPD for TB, albumin, and lead level.

Imaging: X-ray bone survey: Bone pathology including fractures or calluses may be seen. Typical locations are anterior/posterior ribcage, chip fractures or "bucket-handle" fractures, spiral fractures of the long bones, fracture of the femur, cervical spine fracture, or facial fractures. CT or MRI should be used if head trauma is suspected. Bone scan may be of use to illicit existence of old fractures.

Treatment

Suspected abuse should be reported to an authoritative agency. These include Child Protective Services (CPS), local police, or a governmental social worker. It is important to realize the initial encounter with the suspected abuse victim is not meant to determine if abuse is present, only if suspicion exists. Thus, referral to these services is critical if child abuse is a possibility to explain the child's injuries or emotional state, in fact, it is mandated in many states. The physician cannot be prosecuted for reporting suspected child abuse in any state.

Consider hospitalization of the child if there is a risk of further abuse or flight of the family.

Take Home Points

- Severe abuse may have very subtle signs.
- Children won't volunteer information or report abuse.
- It is not the responsibility of the physician to determine if abuse is present; only if reasonable suspicion of abuse exists.

Ethics

Withdrawal of Care

The withdrawal or stoppage of medical care upon the request or presumed will of the patient. The person holding health care power of attorney may make this decision for the patient.

Euthanasia

The active administration of lethal means to end the patient's life, usually in the attempt to end suffering or prolonged illness. Euthanasia is done in the presumed best interest of the patient.

Physician Assisted Suicide

The assistance of the physician to commit active suicide by the patient. PAS is completed at the express request of the patient.

Advance Directive

A document reviewed and signed by the patient to direct their end-of-life decisions. These vary in details but consist of a written document stating the limitations of desired interventions during a life threatening event or situation. These include "Do Not Resuscitate" and "Do Not Intubate" orders.

Health Care Power of Attorney

A designated or defaulted representative who is trusted by the patient to make competent end-of-life decisions on the patient's behalf. This is usually specifically designated in a legal document. However, upon the patient's incapacitation, is often defaulted to the next of kin (spouse, children, etc). If an advanced directive doesn't exist, the holder of the health care power of attorney is legally able to make end-of-life decisions.

Restraints

Use of chemical or physical restraints may be employed by the physician (usually attending only) based on the patient's physical danger to themselves or others. A written "restraint note" detailing the indication, use, limitations of use, and time of expiration is required to be placed on the medical record on a daily basis in most states. Details and timing vary by state.

Involuntary Hold

The involuntary admission or committal of an adult patient due to the physician's belief that the patient is in danger of harming themselves or others. The laws regarding IH vary by state; however, hold without court involvement is usually allowed for 48–72 hours. After this period, a court hearing must be convened to further hold the adult patient against their will.

Competence

A judgment or legal distinction regarding a patient's comprehension and ability to understand their current health care situation. This also implies ability to make sound, rational decisions in their own best interest. The physician is often called upon to judge competence, which should be done by interview regarding both general issues as well as the patient's current situation. The extreme classic case is that a depressed, suicidal patient should not be considered competent to choose if they should be allowed to die or not.

Informed Consent

The relaying of information from the physician to the patient regarding their health care. This has several aspects, which include: diagnosis, prognosis without treatment, prognosis with treatment, detailed proposed treatment, alternative treatments, and risks/benefits of the proposed treatment. Informed consent may only be granted if the patient is deemed competent, otherwise it must be discussed with the holder of the patient's health care power of attorney.

Health Care of Minors (Age <18 years)

Minors may give informed consent and be treated as adults in specific situations, although laws on this vary by state. These situations include: pregnancy, birth control, and treatment of STDs; or if the patient is married, legally emancipated from their guardians, raising children, living independently, or serving in the Armed Forces. Never delay emergent care of a minor for lack of parental consent.

Statistics

TABLE 1.4 Two × Two Table of Outcomes Based on Disease Presence and Results of Test

	Disease	No disease
Positive test	A	B
Negative test	C	D

Sensitivity

The probability that a person with a certain disease will have a positive test result. Basically, sensitivity is a measure of how well a test will show a positive result when the disease is present. High sensitivity is desirable for a screening test.

$$\text{Sensitivity} = a/(a+c).$$

Specificity

The probability that a person without the disease will have a negative test result. Basically, specificity is the measure of how well a test will show a negative result when the disease is not present. High specificity is desirable for a confirmatory test.

$$\text{Specificity} = d/(b+d).$$

Positive Predictive Value (PPV)

The probability that a person with a positive test result has the disease. Basically, PPV is a measure of how much you can rely on a positive result to actually be positive.

$$\text{PPV} = a/(a+b).$$

Negative Predictive Value (NPV)

The probability that a person with a negative test result does not have the disease. Basically, NPV is a measure of how much you can rely on a negative result to actually be negative.

$$\text{NPV} = d/(c+d).$$

Incidence

The number of new cases of disease per specified number of a general population per specified unit of time. Thus, a new disease may have an incidence of 1/100,000 people per year.

Prevalence

The number of cases, new or old, present in a population at one (usually now) point in time. Thus, a disease may have a prevalence of 2.5/100,000 people in the U.S.

TABLE 1.5 Two × Two Table of Outcomes Based on Exposure and Disease Development

	Disease develops	No disease
Exposure	A	B
No exposure	C	D

Relative Risk (RR)

Compares the chance of a given disease in the group exposed to the particular risk factor with the chance of disease in those not exposed to the risk factor. Seen in prospective or experimental studies.

$$RR = \frac{a/(a+b)}{c/(c+d)}$$

Odds Ratio (OR)

Describes the odds of exposure to a given risk factor in individuals with the disease compared to those without the disease. Used in retrospective studies.

$$OR = ad/bc$$

Absolute Risk Reduction (ARR)

A measure of risk reduction in the treated group as compared to the placebo group. Basically, the change in risk in the treated group as measured on the same scale as the untreated group. Used in randomized control trials.

$$ARR = \text{untreated group risk} - \text{treated group risk}$$

Relative Risk Reduction (RRR)

A measure of risk reduction in the treated group as a percentage of the untreated group risk. Used in randomized control trials.

$$RRR = (\text{untreated group risk} - \text{treated group risk})/\text{untreated group risk}$$

ARR versus RRR Example

A population of breast cancer survivors is enrolled in a large study to measure the effect of a new cancer-preventing medication on the incidence of recurrent breast cancer. This population is followed for a total of 5 years during which time other identifiable risk factors are controlled. The placebo group is given a sugar pill and the treatment group is given the investigative drug. The experimental groups are followed throughout the study period and the placebo group was found to have developed breast cancer at a rate of 5%. The treated group was found to have developed cancer at a rate of 3%. The absolute risk reduction of the experimental medication is 5–3 = 2%. The relative risk reduction is 2/5 = 0.4 = 40%. For obvious reasons, many pharmaceutical companies express results of their trials in relative risk reductions!

Number Needed to Treat (NNT)

Number of individuals needed to treat in order to save one life.

$$NNT = 1/ARR$$

P-value

Expression of the chance that an observed outcome is the product of random chance alone. A p-value of <0.05 (accepted value for statistical significance) means that the observed outcome has a <5% chance that it was a random occurrence.

Confidence Interval (CI)

CI expresses the certainty that the result of the study is real or random chance. The percentage is the reciprocal of the p-value. Used with RR or OR, the CI states the percent chance the observed RR or OR is within the interval stated.

Error Types

Type 1 error: Rejection of the null hypothesis when it is true. An arrogant error.

Type 2 error: Acceptance of the null hypothesis when it is not true. A humble error.

Study Design

Cohort

Selects a large population and divides it into groups based on exposure to a given risk factor. Generally, this population is observed **prospectively** and development of disease is recorded. May be retrospective in some cases. RR is calculated. Disadvantages include cost and time.

Case Control

Selects a population with a particular disease and looks **retrospectively** to evaluate presence or absence of a given risk factor. OR is calculated. Good for rare diseases but must be retrospective.

Cross Sectional Prevalence Survey

Looks at a given population for presence of disease and risk factors. A causative link can not be established for disease and risk factors. Takes place at one point in time.

Randomized Control Trial

A study in which subjects are randomly assigned to placebo or treatment groups, intervention is given over a specified time interval, and effects are recorded. The gold standard amongst study designs. Double blinded refers to a situation where both experimenter and subject are unaware to which group, placebo or treatment, the subjects belong (of course a key does exist). Single blind refers to blinding of only the subjects. Disadvantages include cost, time, and risks to subjects.

Meta-analysis

Analysis of past studies in regard to a particular clinical question. Basically, the pooling of much research on a particular subject in an attempt to consolidate a higher N-number and derive an answer closer to actual truth. A study of studies.

Health Maintenance

Vaccinations

Current recommendations include vaccination for the following diseases: Hep A and B, diphtheria, tetanus, pertussis, H flu type B (Hib), polio, measles, mumps, rubella, varicella, herpes zoster, *Meningococcus, Pneumonococcus,* rotavirus, and HPV. Individual safety and allergy contraindications vary. Requirements for children upon entry to school vary by state. Immunocompromised patients should never receive a live virus vaccine. Pregnant patients should not receive MMR, varicella, or HPV vaccine.

See www.cdc.gov/vaccines for more information.

An outline of vaccines and times for vaccination is shown in the table below.

TABLE 1.6 Recommended Vaccination Schedule

Vaccine	Recommended Schedule
Hep B	Birth, 1–2, 6–18 months
Diphtheria-tetanus-accellular pertussis (DTaP)	2, 4, 6, 15–18 months, 4–6 years
Rotavirus*	2, 4, 6 months
H. influenza type B (Hib)	2, 4, 6, 12–18 months
Inactivated poliovirus (IPV)	2, 4, 6–18 months, 4–6 years
Pneumonicoccal conjugate vaccine (PCV)	2, 4, 6, 12–15 months
Measles-mumps-rubella (MMR)*	12–15 months, 4–6 years
Varicella*	12–15 months, 4–6 years
Hep A	12–23, 18–41 months
Influenza	>6 months
Meningococcal conjugate	11–12 years
Human papillomavirus (HPV)	11–12 years (+2 months, then +6 months)
Herpes zoster	60 years
Pneumonococcal polysaccharide vaccine (PPV)	≥65 years

* Live virus vaccines

Smoking Cessation

Smoking cessation includes several stages. Treatment may be tailored to the individual stage. These include:

Pre-contemplative—Inquire if the patient would like to quit smoking. If not, remind them of the health effects and offer literature on assistance.

Contemplative—Patient agrees or wants to quit, but not within a specified time table. Counsel them further on benefits of quitting and reassure of techniques to quit, pharmacologic and social support.

Action—Plan on date of last cigarette/chew, and provide counseling, group classes, or behavioral therapies to assist. Assess suitability for pharmacologic assistance. This includes:

Nicotine replacement techniques—Gum, patch, lozenges, inhaler, etc. These techniques encourage the patient to get used to an alternate form of delivery of the same addiction. Then, a slow taper off will provide the end nicotine. Do not underdose, especially in the beginning.

Bupropion (Zyban)—Reduces the urge to continue smoking. Initially, it is harder to quit with this technique, but after the acute phase the bupropion suppresses the urge to smoke.

Combination therapy may be effective in those with strong addictions.

Varenicline (Chantix) is another option and consists of a partial nicotine agonist effect.

Maintenance—Close follow-up and/or social support groups have shown higher success rates in this stage. Consider addition or dosage elevation if needed.

Relapse—Identify trigger barriers, assess strategies, and formulate another plan for quitting.

Cancer Screening Summary

Cervical Cancer

Different groups have slightly different recommendations on when/how often to begin screening. The American College of Obstetrics and Gynecology (ACOG) recommends starting at age 21 and then every 2 years until age 30. After age 30, screen every 3 years if the patient has had three consecutive negative paps (and if risk factors are minimal). The United States Preventative Services Task Force (USPSTF) recommends screening at least every three years and makes no distinction after age 30. The American Cancer Society (ACS) recommends starting within 3 years of sexual activity or age 21 and annually until age 30 if using the conventional pap or every 2 years if with cytologic based technique. After age 30, every 2–3 years if the patient has had three negative paps.

Breast Cancer

Screening: Different recommending bodies differ on recommendations for screening, especially under the age of 50. The American Medical Association (AMA), the American College of Radiology (ACR), and the American Cancer Society (ACS) all support screening with mammography and clinical breast exam (CBE) beginning at age 40. The American College of Obstetricians and Gynecologists (ACOG) supports screening with mammography beginning at age 40 and CBE beginning at age 19. The American Academy of Family Physicians (AAFP) recommends beginning mammography for average-risk women at age 50 with mammography in high-risk women beginning at age 40. The AAFP also recommends that all women aged 40–49 be counseled about the risks and benefits of mammography before making decisions about screening.

Organizations also differ on their recommendations for the appropriate interval for mammography. Annual mammography is recommended by AMA, ACR, and ACS. Mammography every 1–2 years is recommended by the AAFP. And finally, ACOG recommends mammography every 1–2 years for women aged 40–49 and annually for women aged 50 and older.

Prostate Cancer

Screening is a controversial subject in the general population. The United States Preventive Services Task Force (USPSTF), American Academy of Family Physicians (AAFP), American College of Preventive Medicine (ACPM), and American College of Physicians (ACP) recommendations state that there is, to date, no evidence strong enough to recommend routine population screening for prostate cancer. The American Cancer Society (ACS), however, states that since PSA and digital rectal exam (DRE) have proven useful in cancer detection, yearly screening should start at age 50 (or age 45 in high risk individuals). Thus, there is apparent disagreement among authoritative groups with the consensus siding to not routinely screen for prostate cancer (although providing the patient with information is highly encouraged).

Colorectal Cancer

The American Cancer Society recommends screening average risk patients for colorectal cancer beginning at age 50 years by one of the following:

- Fecal occult blood testing (FOBT) annually.
- Flexible sigmoidoscopy every 5 years.
- Annual FOBT plus flexible sigmoidoscopy every 5 years.
- Double-contrast barium enema every 5 years.
- Colonoscopy every 10 years.

Performed on 2–3 consecutive stools at home. In office single FBOT inadequate.

These recommendations are supported by the USPSTF and the AAFP.

Increased risk and high risk patients generally should obtain colonoscopy every 1–3 years.

2 Psychiatry and Behavioral Medicine

Schizophrenia

A major psychiatric thought disorder affecting behavior, thought processes, speech, social interaction, appearance, and perception.

Types of disease:

1. Paranoid type
2. Disorganized type
3. Catatonic type
4. Undifferentiated type
5. Residual type

History often reveals males > females in their teenage to young twenties, lower socio-economic status, smoking, and family history. The suicide rate is as high as 10%.

Symptoms/Diagnosis

Criteria and Key Features

1. Psychotic symptoms present for at least **1 month** including at least 2 of the following:
   - Hallucinations
   - Delusions
   - Disorganized speech
   - Disorganized or catatonic behavior
   - Negative symptoms

Plus

2. Impairment of social or occupational functioning.
3. Symptoms not primarily due to a mood disorder or schizoaffective disorder.
4. Symptoms not due to a medical, neurological, or substance-induced disorder.
5. Continuous signs of illness lasting ≥ **6 months.**

TABLE 2.1 Symptom Classification of Schizophrenia

Positive Symptoms*	Negative Symptoms†
Delusions	Flat affect
Hallucinations (often auditory)	Decreased speech
Bizarre behavior	Apathy
Thought disorder	Anhedonia
Poor attention	

*Better prognosis and better response to therapy.
†Worse prognosis and less response to therapy.

Treatment/Side Effects

Admit to the hospital if the patient is a threat to self or others. Generally, this may be done legally, with a 48–72 hour "involuntary hold." This may be extended with a court order but the case must be brought to court.

Neuroleptics (antipsychotics) are the drug class of choice. Divide starting dose until steady state is reached, about 4–5 days depending on half-life.

Atypical neuroleptics—Risperidone (Risperdal), olanzapine (Zyprexa), quetiapine (Seroquil), and ziprasidone (Zeldox, Geodon). These are first line for schizophrenia largely due to better side effect profile than typical agents. They have a decreased incidence of extrapyramidal symptoms and anticholinergic effects, although they do have higher incidence of weight gain, DM type II, and QT prolongation.

Typical neuroleptics examples:

High potency—Haloperidol (Haldol) and fluphenazine (Prolixin).

Low potency—Chlorpromazine (Thorazine) and thioridazine (Mellaril).

Side effects of neuroleptics are especially important and very often tested. See below.

TABLE 2.2 Extrapyramidal Side Effects

Effect	Typical Time Course	Signs/Symptoms	Treatment
Acute dystonia	10–14 days	Torticollis (writhing of neck), oculogyric movements, unusual tongue or facial muscle movements.	Consider change to low potency agent or decrease current dose. Add benztropine (Cogentin) or trihexyphenidyl (Artane).
Akathisia	10–14 days	Feelings of extreme restlessness. Walking or pacing.	Addition of benztropine, antihistamines, anticholinergics, or β-blocker. Benzodiazepines such as diazepam if refractory.
Drug-induced Parkinsonism	Months	Cogwheel stiffness in muscles, drooling, mask-like facies, shuffling gait.	Anticholinergics such as benztropine (Cogentin), trihexyphenidyl (Artane), antihistamine, or lower the dose of current treatment.
Tardive dyskinesia	Years	Involuntary movements of tongue, lips (lip smacking), sucking, eye blinking, and grimacing.	Discontinue the neuroleptics! Otherwise, no treatment.

Neuroleptic malignant syndrome—May occur at anytime during therapy. May be life threatening. Characterized by severe muscle rigidity, **fever**, altered mental status, and autonomic instability. Labs show elevated WBC, CPK, and AST/ALT. Treatment involves admission (possibly to ICU), supportive care, discontinuing neuroleptics, administering dantrolene (Dantrium), amantadine (Symmetrel), or bromocritine (Parlodel).

Anticholinergic side effects—Dry mouth, dry eyes, urinary retention, and constipation.

Other common side effects include sedation, weight gain, orthostatic hypotension, cardiac effects, retinitis pigmentosa, photosensitivity, and cholestatic jaundice, as well as signs of increased prolactin such as gynecomastia, lactation, impotence, menstrual dysfunction, and libido change.

Clozapine (Clozaril)—Unique atypical agent reserved for refractory cases. Unique side effect profile with low or no excess prolactin, extrapyramidal, or neuroleptic malignant syndrome problems. Side effects include agranulocytosis, eosinophilia, leukopenia, and seizures. These make **frequent CBCs** mandatory.

Take Home Points

- Schizophrenia shows symptoms for ≥6 months.
- Both positive and negative symptoms are considered when making the diagnosis.
- Neuroleptic medications have a group of well known and often tested side effects.

Psychotic Disorders

TABLE 2.3 Psychotic Disorders

Disorder	Time Course	Signs/Diagnosis	Treatment
Brief psychotic disorder	1 day–1 month	Criteria for schizophrenia are met except for time course. Often preceded by emotional event/stress. Patient returns to normal after event ends.	Admit if harm to self or others; brief course of neuroleptic may help; Lorazepam (Ativan) or short acting benzodiazepine as indicated.
Schizophreniform disorder	1–6 months	Criteria for schizophrenia are met except for time course.	Admit if harm to self or others; start course of neuroleptic; treat mood disturbances as needed.
Schizoaffective disorder	≥ 6 months	Symptoms meet criteria for schizophrenia *and* mood disorder. Mood symptoms must be present for significant portion of the illness (although psychotic symptoms are present without them).	Admit if harm to self or others; start course of neuroleptic for psychotic symptoms. Start antidepressant (SSRI, TCA, etc.) for mood symptoms. Start mood stabilizer if bipolar symptoms are present.

Panic Attacks

An acute and unpredictable onset of intense anxiety causing marked interference with the patient's life. Attacks often lead to fear of additional episodes, causing the victim to change their lifestyle or behavior.

Symptoms/Diagnosis

Recurrent, unexpected attacks with peak intensity within 10 minutes and ≥ 4 of the following symptoms: palpitations, sweating, trembling, shortness of breath, feeling of choking, chest pain, nausea, dizziness or lightheadedness, depersonalization, fear of losing control or going crazy, fear of dying, parasthesias, or chills/hot flashes. Panic attacks are often accompanied by agoraphobia. The patient often adapts by avoiding situations of anticipated attack triggers. Inter-attack anxiety of the next attack is classic and often prominent.

Treatment

Cognitive behavioral therapy, relaxation, and breathing techniques can be very effective.

Propanolol (Inderal) may be used as "Dumbo's feather" and may be taken 30–45 minutes before anticipated situation leading to attack (e.g. public speaking).

Selective serotonin reuptake inhibitors (SSRIs) (paroxetine, sertraline, etc), tricyclic anti-depressants (TCAs) (imipramine, amitriptyline), or rarely monoamine oxidase inhibitors (MAOIs) are first line although they must be scheduled and not taken PRN.

Benzodiazepines may be useful as scheduled (alprazolam (Xanax), clonazepam (Klonopin)) or PRN (lorazepam (Ativan)) medication. However, they are addictive and may over sedate if used improperly.

Buspirone (BuSpar) is *not* effective for panic disorder.

Take Home Points

- Panic disorder causes intense fear of additional attacks, causing the patient to alter their lifestyle.
- β-blockers, antidepressants, antianxiety medications, and benzodiazepines may be used for treatment.

Generalized Anxiety Disorder

The clinical syndrome of excessive worry and anxiety that is difficult to control and causes significant distress and impairment. This may be accompanied by somatic disturbances such as increased muscle tone, autonomic hyperactivity, or hypervigilance.

Symptoms/Diagnosis

Criteria include:

Excessive anxiety or worry most days during at least a **six month** period accompanied by at least three of the following:

- restlessness
- easy fatigability
- difficulty concentrating
- irritability
- muscle tension
- sleep disturbance

Treatment

Combine medications with psychotherapy (including cognitive behavioral therapy and insight oriented psychotherapy) for best results.

Venlafaxine (Effexor) and buspirone (BuSpar) are first line but both take weeks to work.

Other SSRIs may also be tried and are first line. Time course to action is 2–4 weeks.

Benzodiazepines are faster but considered second line due to side effects and addictive potential. If used, plan to taper after several weeks of therapy; this is commonly done while awaiting efficacy of one of the above agents.

Kava kava is an alternative therapy proposed for treatment of GAD but research has not shown benefit and concerns of hepatotoxicity have cast recent doubt on its safety.

Take Home Points

- Patients with generalized anxiety disorder commonly have other comorbid psychiatric disturbances.
- Venlafaxine (Effexor) and buspirone (BuSpar) are first line for GAD.
- Benzodiazepines such as alprazolam (Xanax) and clonazepam (Klonopin) are second line.

Phobias

An unreasonable fear of a situation or object that goes beyond an uncomfortable feeling and causes avoidance and alteration of lifestyle such that it significantly impacts quality of life. Types of phobias are: specific, social, and agoraphobia.

Symptoms/Diagnosis

Unreasonable and excessive anxiety most commonly leads to behavioral changes but somatic symptoms such as flushing, sweating, and tachycardia are often present. Response or anticipation of response may provoke a panic attack. This response, or anticipation of response, interferes significantly with the individual's life. Duration of symptoms ≥ **6 months**.

Treatment

Cognitive behavioral therapy (CBT) is the mainstay of treatment for simple phobias and includes exposure and desensitization combined with relaxation and deep breathing techniques.

β-blockers and benzodiazepines may be effective adjuncts to CBT.

Social phobias may be treated with exposure-type therapy, although SSRIs (but not TCAs) are also effective. MAOIs are second line and are to be used in refractory cases.

Agoraphobia, which often has comorbid anxiety or panic disorder, may be treated with cognitive behavioral therapy, SSRIs, or TCAs.

Take Home Points

- Types of phobias include specific, social, and agoraphobia.
- Treatment combines psychotherapy and, possibly, medications.

Obsessive-Compulsive Disorder (OCD)

Recurrent, persistent, intrusive but conscious compulsions or obsessions that negatively impact quality of life. Overall lifetime prevalence of OCD is 2.5%.

Symptoms/Diagnosis

Symptoms consist of thoughts, images, impulses, or bizarre behaviors that the patient experiences without apparent reason. Repetitive behavior is common and may range from fairly logical, such as hand washing, to bizarre, such as touching a wall a certain way before leaving the room. The patient recognizes them as intrusive and negative and a function of their own mind and may try to compensate and suppress them. Behaviors often take a significant amount of time, typically > 1 hour/day.

Treatment

Combination of medication and cognitive behavioral therapy is most effective.
CBT should consist of thought stopping, desensitization, or flooding techniques.
Medications include clomipramine (Anafranil) and SSRIs (may require high dosage).

Take Home Points

- OCD behaviors can be significantly time consuming.
- The patient often recognizes the disability of the behaviors.
- Treatment consists of combination of psychotherapy and medications.

Post Traumatic Stress Disorder (PTSD)

A psychological disorder developed after exposure to an overly traumatic event involving persistent re-experiencing of the event as well as other debilitating psychological symptoms. Traumatic events vary in severity but often involve war, natural disaster, or threat to the patient's life.

Symptoms/Diagnosis

Symptoms including feelings of guilt, poor impulse control, aggression, personality change, and depression occur after a significantly stressful event such as combat, rape, etc. The patient persistently re-experiences the event through intrusive thoughts, nightmares, "daymares," and flashbacks. Persistent feelings of detachment, anhedonia, amnesia; restricted or blunted affect; and feelings of avoidance of similar or related events are present. A general state of increased arousal persists after the event and may contribute to other symptoms such as insomnia and exaggerated startle response. Symptoms collectively cause impaired occupational and social functioning which significantly impacts the patient's life. For PTSD, by definition, symptoms occur ≥ **1 month** after the event.

Acute Stress Disorder

The above features of PTSD with onset < **1 month** from the time of the event and lasting for 2 days–4 weeks.

Treatment

Psychotherapy, behavioral therapy, support groups, and family therapy are effective and should be used with medications.

SSRIs such as sertraline (Zoloft), paroxetine (Paxil) etc, are first line medications. SNRIs such as venlafaxine (Effexor) are also very effective. TCAs and MAOIs may be used as alternatives.

Propanolol, lithium, prazosin (Minipress), anticonvulsants, and buspirone (BuSpar) may be effective if antidepressants fail.

Consider referral to psychiatry especially if patient has suicidal or homicidal ideation.

Take Home Points

- PTSD occurs > 1 month after an unusually traumatic event.
- Acute stress disorder is essentially PTSD lasting < 1 month and is often self limited.
- Treat with a combination of psychotherapy and pharmacotherapy for best results.

Adjustment Disorder

The development of emotional or behavioral symptoms in response to an identifiable stressor that is out of proportion to what might normally be expected for such a stressor. These symptoms significantly impact the patient's life.

Symptoms/Diagnosis

Symptoms similar to depression, including thoughts of hopelessness, depressed mood, anhedonia, sleep disturbance, eating disturbance, amotivation, possible thoughts of suicide, and temporary obsession with triggering event or stressor. Symptoms occur within **3 months** of the onset of a particular stressor but don't last longer than **6 months** from the termination of the stressor.

Treatment

Psychotherapy and talk therapy are first line. In most patients, expressing feelings surrounding inciting event begins them on the road to recovery.

Medications: SSRIs are classically effective but take 3–4 weeks to show effect. TCAs are second line due to possible toxicity and side effects; thought also to be less effective.

Electroconvulsive therapy (ECT) is not indicated for adjustment disorder.

Take Home Points

- Adjustment disorder occurs in relation to a traumatic stressor/event.
- Symptoms occur within 3 months onset of the stressor but last no longer than 6 months after the termination of the stressor.
- Exclude other psychological disorders such as bereavement, depression, PTSD, before diagnosing adjustment disorder.

Bereavement

The state of experiencing grief and emotional distress in connection to the death of someone close to the patient. Mourning is the psychological process in which the patient undoes the emotional bonds they had with the deceased.

Symptoms/Diagnosis

Associated most commonly with death or significant loss of a loved one. Symptoms tend to be classified into several stages.

The classic five stages of grief are:

1. Denial
2. Anger
3. Bargaining
4. Depression
5. Acceptance

Some sources organize these into stages that include shock, preoccupation, and resolution. These begin within 2 months and may last over 1 year. Despite the time course, this is a temporary condition.

Treatment

Psychotherapy and talk therapy are first line. In most patients, expressing feelings surrounding their loved one (or their death) starts them on the road to recovery.

Medications: SSRIs are classically effective but take 3–4 weeks to show effect. TCAs are second line due to possible toxicity and side effects.

Electroconvulsive therapy is not indicated for bereavement.

Take Home Points

- Bereavement is the psychological process of dealing with the death of a loved one.
- Grief classically has five stages: denial, anger, bargaining, depression, and acceptance.

Major Depressive Episodes/Disorder

A primary mood disorder involving one or more major depressive episodes and which requires the presence of five or more depressive features *including* either depressed mood or anhedonia (lack of interest in pleasurable activities). Depression is thought to have a pathophysiology rooted in neurotransmitter imbalance involving mainly serotonin and norepinephrine, although dopamine likely plays a role. Lifetime prevalence is as high as 20%–25% of the general population and death from suicide in those who are depressed is thought to be as high as 15%.

Symptoms/Diagnosis

Characterized by symptoms reported by the patient or someone close to them, including those in Table 2.4 below. Several clinical tools exist to aide in diagnosis including a well-known pneumonic:

SIGECAPS Sleep, Interest, Guilt, Energy, Concentration, Appetite, Psychomotor status, Suicidal ideation.

These symptoms occur for more than **2 weeks** and can't be associated with bereavement, mixed mood disorder, bipolar, or other medical reason for the syndrome.

TABLE 2.4 DSM-IV Features for Major Depressive Episode

Features
Depressed mood.
Diminished interest in previously pleasurable activities (anhedonia).
Change in appetite. This may lead to change in weight when no purposeful diet change is attempted.
Insomnia or hypersomnia.
Psychomotor agitation or retardation.
Fatigue or loss of energy.
Guilt or feelings of worthlessness.
Concentration disturbance or trouble thinking or making decisions.
Recurrent thoughts of death or suicide.

Major depressive episode includes 5 or more of the above features with one or more being depressed mood and anhedonia.
Symptoms above may be self-reported or reported by person close to the patient. Symptoms occur most of the day, nearly every day.

Variants exist and are listed in the table below:

TABLE 2.5 Variants of Major Depressive Episode

Variant	Distinguishing Feature
Psychotic features	Hallucinations, delusions
Chronic	Lasting 2 years and more severe than dysthymia
Catatonic features	At least two of the following: 1. Motor immobility or stupor 2. Excessive purposeless movement 3. Extreme negativism or mutism 4. Bizarre posturing, stereotyped movement, or grimacing 5. Echolalia or echopraxia
Melancholic features	Excessive anhedonia and at least three of the following: 1. Depressed mood 2. Worse in the AM 3. Early AM wakening 4. Psychomotor slowing 5. Significant weight loss 6. Excessive guilt
Atypical features	At least two of the following: 1. Significant weight gain from excessive diet 2. Hypersomnia 3. "Heavy" feeling in extremities 4. Chronic fear of rejection with resultant social isolationism
Postpartum	Onset within 4 weeks of delivery
Seasonal pattern	Recurrence during darker (late fall, winter, early spring) months. Over 2 years, symptoms have occurred twice.

Dysthymia is very similar but is a milder form of mood disorder. It may include less intense symptoms and be present more often than not over a period of **2 years**.

Treatment

Screen for suicidal or homicidal ideation. If present, have patient "contract for safety" and write it down. Admit if necessary.

Psychotherapy should be tried before medications and may be very helpful especially in patients with extrinsic reasons for depression. This stepwise approach should not be used for patients with suicidal or homicidal ideations (SI or HI) or risk factors for either.

Medications: SSRIs are first line therapy but generally take 3–4 weeks for effect. None have been shown superior to any other in efficacy but selection is based on coexisting symptoms. For example, sertraline (Zoloft) is used more widely for depressive symptoms, paroxetine (Paxil) for anxiety. Common side effects include insomnia, sexual dysfunction, GI upset, and agitation.

TCAs are second line and also take 3–4 weeks for effect. Side effects are generally worse in the first month and include anticholinergic effects, sedation, and **cardiovascular effects** in overdose. Thought to be a poor choice for potentially suicidal patients given toxic CV effects in overdose.

MAOIs are rarely used. Side effects can be severe and include orthostatic hypotension and hypertensive "tyramine crisis" if patient does not strictly follow accompanying diet of low tyramine foods.

Atypical agents include bupropion (Wellbutrin), venlafaxine (Effexor), nefazodone (Serzone), and mirtazapine (Remeron). These agents may be better in refractory cases or pregnancy but also have unique side effects.

Phototherapy may be effective for seasonal affective disorder.

Use of medication with counseling is often more effective than either alone.

Electroconvulsive therapy (ECT) has shown good response in depression and should be considered in refractory cases.

Take Home Points

- Major depression consists of a syndrome of repeated major depressive episodes that last at least 2 weeks.

- DSM-IV supports the presence of 5 or more of 9 clinical features with the presence of either or both depressed mood and anhedonia.

- Treatment should consist of a stepwise approach (in absence of SI/HI) starting with psychotherapy then adding medications.

Bipolar Disorder

A major mood disorder characterized by repeated cycles of depressed mood alternating with mood elevation. Extremes of periods of mood elevation classify the two major types of disease as bipolar I and II.

Symptoms/Diagnosis

Bipolar I—Major depressive episodes mixed with periods of mania. Classically presents as patient that spends money excessively, is hypersexual, has grandiose thoughts/schemes, and doesn't sleep.

Bipolar II—Major depressive episodes mixed with hypomanic periods.

Mania—Mood disturbance involving irritability, inflated self esteem/grandiosity, decreased sleep, talkativeness, flight of ideas, distractibility, increased goal-directed behavior, and excessive involvement in pleasurable activities with a high potential for harm (e.g. sexual indiscretion).

Hypomania—The same basic elements of mood as mania but less intense and for a lesser period of time.

Treatment

Screen for suicidal or homicidal ideation. If present, have patient "contract for safety" and write it down. Admit to the hospital if necessary.

Cognitive behavioral therapy in combination with medications is most effective.

SSRIs may be used, but do so in conjunction with a mood stabilizer to avoid precipitation of manic episodes.

Mood stabilizers:

Lithium (Eskalith, Lithonate) is first line but toxic levels may easily be reached. Before beginning, check TSH, BUN/creatinine, electrolytes, blood glucose level, and ECG. Then monitor lithium levels weekly for 2 months and every month thereafter. Signs of toxicity include tremor, polyuria, thirst (diabetes insipidus), edema, weight gain, nausea, diarrhea, hypothyroidism, rash, elevated WBC, and T-wave flattening on ECG. Interactions include: NSAIDs, ACE inhibitors, and diuretics. Hemodialyize if toxic levels are reached.

Carbamazepine (Tegretol) is used as second line. Pretreatment evaluation includes LFTs, ECG, CBC, electrolytes, and BUN/creatinine. Monitor levels for first month. Side effects include agranulocytosis, aplastic anemia, leukopenia, hepatitis, Stevens-Johnson syndrome, ataxia, confusion, and tremor.

Valproic acid (Depakene) is quickly becoming a favorite secondary to low side effect and toxicity profile. More effective for "**rapid cyclers**" than either lithium or carbamazepine. Check CBC, platelets, PT/PTT for the first month of therapy. Side effects include: GI distress including nausea/vomiting, sedation, mild elevations of LFTs, thrombocytopenia, and elevation of ammonia.

Gabapentin (Neurontin) is a newer agent used for both neuropathic pain syndromes and mood stabilization. Little pretreatment evaluation is needed and only includes renal function (BUN/creatinine). Side effects include somnolence, fatigue, ataxia, nausea/vomiting, dizziness, and weight change.

Other newer agents include: Lamotrigine (Lamictal), topiramate (Topamax), tiagabine (Gabitril), and oxcarbazepine (Trileptal). These agents have all been used widely for other disorders such as seizures or pain syndromes and have recently been added to mood stabilization regimens. Side effects have been lower than traditional mood stabilizers but efficacy is less proven.

ECT is effective but used only after mood stabilizers and other therapies have failed.

Take Home Points

- Bipolar disorder has two types (bipolar I and II) which differ on degree of manic episodes.
- When treating bipolar disorder, antidepressants are useful, but a mood stabilizer should be given concomitantly to avoid undue manic or hypomanic episodes.

Somatoform and Factitious Disorders

Somatoform disorders are largely unconsciously created, while factitious disorders are not (see table below).

TABLE 2.6 Somatoform and Factitious Disorders

Disorder	Key Elements	Treatment
Somatization disorder	Onset before age 30 Many varied physical complaints Not explained by organic disease or severity of illness All of the following are present at any time during the course of illness: 　Four pain symptoms, 　Two GI tract symptoms, 　One sexual symptom, and 　One pseudoneurologic symptom	Psychotherapy to address emotional issues underlying problem Regular doctor visits
Conversion disorder	Symptoms of neurologic or muscular origin (e.g., blindness, seizure) Not intentionally produced Not organic in origin Related to stressful event	Symptoms typically remit on their own after weeks/months Insight-oriented or behavioral therapy Anxiolytics and relaxation techniques may help
Hypochondriasis	Preoccupation with fear of having a serious medical condition Not reassured by negative test results Duration > 6 months	Group therapy Regular doctor visits
Body dysmorphic disorder	Preoccupation with imagined defect in body appearance	Individual or group counseling, CBT, or SSRIs and clomipramine (Anafranil) are effective

(continued)

TABLE 2.6 Continued

Disorder	Key Elements	Treatment
Factitious disorder	Intentional production of physical or psychological symptoms to assume the sick role Munchausen syndrome- symptoms in self Munchausen by-proxy syndrome—symptoms/signs in patient's child	Try to recognize early No specific treatment exists
Malingering	Staging of symptoms for secondary gain (e.g., money, time off work, etc.)	No specific treatment exists Criminal prosecution if indicated

CBT=Cognitive Behavioral Therapy

Anorexia Nervosa

An eating disorder with two subtypes: restrictive type and binge eating/purging type. Restrictive type involves limiting intake of calories while binge eating/purging type involves food binging accompanied by purging activities such as self-induced vomiting or laxative use.

Symptoms/Diagnosis

Usually female patient with distorted sense of self appearance in regard to weight and body fat. Often **refuses to maintain weight above 85% of ideal body weight** and feels intense fear of gaining weight. Denial of seriousness of current low weight and desires to lose more. **Amenorrhea for at least three cycles** in menstruating women is often seen. Classically, this disorder presents in the female student of higher socioeconomic status with good grades and exceptional will to excel.

Treatment

Psychotherapies including psychodynamic psychotherapy, family therapy, behavioral therapy, and group therapy.

Since major depression is common, SSRIs may be appropriate.

Bupropion (Wellbutrin) is contraindicated due to risk of seizures.

Inpatient admission is indicated for seriously emaciated patients or those with severe, acute weight loss.

Close monitoring, possibly inpatient, of oral calorie intake.

Replace electrolytes as needed.

Take Home Points

- Anorexia involves patients intentionally losing weight below 85% ideal body weight accompanied by dysmorphic sense of body image and/or menstrual irregularity.

- Consider admission to the hospital in severe cases.

- Cognitive behavioral therapy with or without addition of antidepressants is most effective.

Bulimia Nervosa

An eating disorder commonly occurring in patients at or above average weight. Two types exist: purging type, involving self induced vomiting and laxative use; or non-purging type, which involves excessive fasting periods or episodes of exercise to compensate for caloric intake.

Symptoms/Diagnosis

The patient engages in binging/purging cycles characterized as excessive eating then vomiting or heavy laxative use. Use of compensatory behavior for calorie intake is common and may include laxative use, excessive exercise, diuretic use, or vomiting. These episodes occur an average of **twice per week for at least three months**. Lack of control of these episodes is a central theme. Unlike anorexia patients, bulimia patients tend to be average or above average weight. Physical exam findings include poor dentition or finger/finger nail abnormalities due to acid effect from vomitis.

Treatment

Cognitive behavioral therapy is most helpful.

SSRIs, particularly fluoxetine (Prozac), are effective.

TCAs are also used, including imipramine (Tofranil) and desipramine (Norpramin).

Bupropion (Wellbutrin) is contraindicated due to risk of seizures.

Take Home Points

- Bulimia differs from anorexia of the binge eating/purging type in that bulimia patients are generally average or above average weight and lack other somatic symptoms such as menstrual irregularity.

- Cognitive behavioral therapy with or without addition of antidepressants is most effective.

Behavioral Disorders in Children

TABLE 2.7 Childhood Behavioral Disorders

Disorder	Symptoms/Diagnosis	Treatment
Conduct disorder	Child who is severely defiant and almost constantly in trouble. Displays **cruelty to animals, lack of remorse, and enjoys destroying property.** Often lies and violates the law. The adult form is termed **antisocial personality disorder.**	Cognitive behavioral therapy, individual therapy, group and family counseling. Intense behavioral modification techniques are needed. Various mood stabilizers, antidepressants, propanolol (Inderal), neuroleptics, and atypical antidepressants have been tried with varied success.
Oppositional-defiant disorder	Milder form of behavioral disorder which includes behavior that is stubborn, negativistic, provocative, and at times hostile. However, these kids are not lying, cheating criminals.	Behavioral modification techniques such as token economies and reward systems. Generally, medication is not needed unless other disorders exist.

Attention Deficit/Attention Deficit Hyperactivity Disorder

Two closely related disorders involving impairment of attention and/or hyperactivity leading to significantly affected cognitive, academic, behavioral, emotional, and social functioning. Prevalence in school-aged children ranges between 3% and 5%.

Symptoms/Diagnosis

ADD and ADHD are two separate diagnoses.

Attention deficit (ADD) has at least 6 of the following characteristics:

- carelessness
- inattention
- does not listen
- lack of task completion
- disorganized
- dislike for goal-oriented tasks and homework
- often loses things
- distractibility
- forgetfulness

Add to these at least 6 of the following hyperactive symptoms for ADHD:

- fidgeting in seat
- often unable to stay seated
- often runs or climbs at inappropriate times
- difficulty with quiet play
- often "on the go"
- talkativeness
- often answers questions before they are complete
- difficulty waiting their turn
- often interrupts or intrudes on others

These symptoms must be present in **2 or more settings** (i.e. school and home) and some degree of these symptoms is present **before age 7 years**. There also must be clear evidence of social, academic, or occupational impairment.

Adult ADD/ADHD is basically the existence of many of the symptoms seen in children, although many may be replaced by adult equivalents. For example, the feeling of "on the go" in adults may manifest as restlessness or inability to relax. Also, there must be a historic link to these symptoms existing in early childhood (before age 7 years).

Treatment

ADD/ADHD patients tend to do better in a structured, consistent environment. It is essential for everyone in an authority role to use the same set of rules so the child learns boundaries.

Token economies have shown good efficacy.

Medications: Stimulant medications are the most effective class. These include methylphenidate (Ritalin, Ritalin SR, Concerta, Metadate, Daytrana), dexmethylphenidate (Focalin), dextroamphetamine (Dexedrine), lisdexamfetamine (Vyvanse), and amphetamine-dextroamphetamine (Adderall). Start with methylphenidate and titrate dosage to effect. Only short-acting amphetamine-dextroamphetamine is approved for children under 6 years. Adverse effects include insomnia, decreased appetite, stomach pain, headache, **emergence or worsening of tics**, **decreased growth velocity** (although end growth appears unaffected), tachycardia, blood pressure elevation, rebound or deterioration of ADHD behaviors when medication wears off, emotional lability, irritability, social withdrawal and flattened affect. Stimulant medications should not be used in children with known heart conditions due to evidence of exacerbation and worsening of condition.

Atomoxetine (Strattera) is a non-stimulant medication that selectively inhibits norepinephrine reuptake and has shown good efficacy.

Consider "drug holidays" on the weekends or during the summer school break.

Other medications can be used, such as bupropion (Wellbutrin), but should only be done so in consult with psychiatry.

Consider that these are controlled, addictive substances. Look for secondary gain motives in parents who are asking to increase dose/obtain more of these meds.

Take Home Points

- Diagnosis requires symptoms in 2 or more settings with some degree present before 7 years of age.
- Treatment consists of structured environment, token economy, and either stimulant or non-stimulant medications.
- Stimulant medications have a "paradoxical" effect in those with ADHD, wherein lies their efficacy.

Autistic Disorder

An idiopathic developmental disorder which begins in early childhood and is characterized by social and communicative delays accompanied by repetitive and non-purposeful actions.

Symptoms/Diagnosis

Definitive diagnosis is best done by a professional trained in evaluation of autistic spectrum disorders (ASD).

A disorder characterized by otherwise typical children seeming to "shut down" and stop communicating. Characteristics include three groups of impairment:

1. Impairment in social interaction including failure to use nonverbal gestures, failure to develop peer relationships, lack of seeking to share enjoyment or achievements, and lack of social reciprocity.
2. Qualitative impairment in communication: delay or lack of development of spoken language; in individuals with adequate speech a marked impairment of initiating or sustaining conversation; repetitive use of language; lack of varied, spontaneous imaginative play or social imitative behavior.
3. Restricted repetitive and stereotyped patterns of behavior: preoccupation of stereotyped behavior in intensity or focus; inflexible adherence to specific, nonfunctional routines; repetitive motor mannerisms; preoccupation with parts of objects.

Add to these, before **age 3 years,** delays or abnormal functioning in social interaction, language as used in communication, or symbolic or imaginative play. Also, the disorder must not be better accounted for by two rare psychologic disorders: Rett syndrome or childhood disintegrative disorder (CDD).

Various autism clinical scales exist including: Autism Behavioral Checklist (ABC), Gilliam Autism Rating Scale (GARS), Autism Diagnostic Interview-Revised (ADI-R), Childhood Autism Rating Scale (CARS), as well as others which may be useful and used in evaluation.

Asperger syndrome is clinically similar to autism and constitutes an autism-related disorder (ASD). Asperger patients' disorder seems to revolve around qualitative impairment in social interaction and restricted repetitive behaviors or actions. These cause significant impairment of social, occupational, or other areas of life. However, language and cognitive development (other than social interaction) are commonly spared.

Treatment

There is no cure for autism. However, specialized school programs and behavioral programs do exist and have shown good efficacy, especially if begun early. Responsive patients may eventually compensate very well for their disorder and become very high functioning.

Medications: Various classes, including SSRIs, TCAs, stimulants, bupropion, etc., have been used with varied success to target symptoms. These medications are basically only for specific symptoms and do not treat the underlying autism disorder.

Take Home Points

- There exists three areas of impairment in autism: social interaction, qualitative language development, and the presence of restricted repetitive behaviors.
- Asperger syndrome is a less severe autism spectrum disorder (ASD).
- Begin treatment early!

Dementia

Dementia is the gradual decline of global mental and cognitive functioning. Onset is usually insidious but may be stepwise (vascular); sudden; related to other medical conditions, drug effects/abuse, or other brain disease (Parkinson, Pick, Alzheimer); or may be idiopathic. The most common cause remains Alzheimer disease (see Chapter 3: Diseases of the Nervous System for complete section).

Symptoms/Diagnosis

Symptoms always include some degree of memory impairment along with aphasia (language disturbance), apraxia (motor impairment), agnosia (identification disturbance), or executive brain functioning problems. Delirium must be ruled out. Patients are often unaware of these declines and they may be confused about their current situation.

Several clinical dementia scales exist but most common is the Mini Mental Status Exam, which includes cognitive function testing. A score > 24 is generally considered normal, but take education level into account.

Labs/Imaging: CBC with diff, Basic chemistry, hepatic function panel, TSH, UA, drug screen, vitamin B12/folate levels, and RPR or VDRL. Consider obtaining heavy metal screen, lumbar puncture, EKG, chest X-ray, EEG, and MRI for possible infarcts. These will eliminate possibility of delirium.

Treatment

Make sure patient is not experiencing delirium; if so, treat it.

Minimize medications that may contribute to anticholinergic effects.

See Chapter 3: Diseases of the Nervous System for treatment of Alzheimer type dementia. Medications include donepezil (Aricept), rivastigmine (Exelon), and memantine (Namenda).

If vascular dementia suspected, control blood pressure, give aspirin, and control risk factors (consider CVA).

For agitation:

Acute therapy includes haloperidol (Haldol) and lorazepam (Ativan). These are quick-acting but dose appropriately for renal function and age. Sedative effects often last much longer in the elderly.

Additional options include buspirone (BuSpar), trazodone (Desyrel), risperidone (Risperdal), olanzapine (Zyprexa), and divalproex (Depakote).

SSRIs may be used for concurrent depression but TCAs are avoided due to anticholinergic effects.

Social support for the family is essential and often involves assigning medical power of attorney to a relative, utilizing support groups, and close monitoring.

Ensure the patient's home safety.

Take Home Points

- Dementia is a common manifestation of neurologic or other derangements in the elderly.
- Eliminate delirium as a possibility.
- Many types of dementia may respond to pharmacotherapy that is effective for Alzheimer disease.

Post-concussive Syndrome

A continued presence of neurologic symptoms associated with concussion or traumatic brain injury (TBI). The pathophysiology is yet unknown, but is the subject of much speculation including theories of lasting structural, biochemical, and psychogenic alteration. The range of affected patients with TBI and concussion is wide and between 30%–80%.

Symptoms/Diagnosis

Symptoms may include headache, dizziness, fatigue, irritability, anxiety, insomnia, loss of concentration and memory, and noise sensitivity. These are non-specific and many exist in some background prevalence in the general population—hence the controversy on this topic. If post-concussive syndrome (PCS) is the etiology of symptoms, mild concussion or traumatic brain injury (TBI) must have occurred in the recent past. Symptoms may last up to 3 months in some patients but true time course maximum is yet unknown. CT/MRI should have been done at time of TBI evaluation but if not previously done, order an MRI for better images of the brain. Neuropsychological testing has only shown a very small difference in PCS patients and is not considered clinically useful. Seizures and vomiting are *not* a part of PCS and should be evaluated.

Treatment

Exclude structural brain injury.

Reassure the patient and provide education.

Treat symptoms such as headaches and insomnia.

Take Home Points

- PCS is a syndrome with ill-defined symptoms but is nonetheless a well recognized consequence of brain injury.
- Exclude structural brain injury.

Alcohol Withdrawal

Symptoms/Diagnosis

TABLE 2.8 Features of Alcohol Withdrawal

Syndrome	Clinical Symptoms	Onset After Last Drink	Duration
Minor withdrawal	Tremulousness, mild anxiety, headache, diaphoresis, palpitations, anorexia, GI upset, tachycardia	6–36 hours	Up to 2 weeks
Seizures	Generalized, tonic-clonic seizures, rarely status epilepticus	6–48 hours	Usually seconds to minutes
Alcoholic hallucinosis	Auditory > visual, tactile	12–48 hours	< 6 days
Delirium tremens (DTs)	Delirium, tachycardia, hypertension, agitation, fever, diaphoresis	2–5 days	< 3 days

Treatment

Patients should be assessed for risk of serious withdrawal. If high risk or unknown, patient should be placed in the ICU for close monitoring.

A clinical assessment tool such as the CIWA (Clinical Institute Withdrawal Assessment for Alcohol Scale) scale should be used for routine objective monitoring. The same person should judge this score each time evaluation is done.

IV fluids should be started with replacement of likely fluid deficit. Multivitamins and electrolyte replacement should be started concurrently. Classically, **thiamine** is the vitamin most needing replacement in alcoholics. **Always give thiamine before glucose** to prevent eliciting Wernicke encephalopathy or Korsakoff syndrome. Often a "banana bag" can suffice for repletion.

Medications: Benzodiazepines: For acute control, lorazepam (Ativan) is most effective because of rapid onset in IV/IM form and short half-life. Diazepam (Valium) may also be given acutely but has a somewhat longer half-life. For prophylactic administration in the high risk (non-vomiting) patient, chlordiazepoxide (Librium) or oxazepam (Serax) may be scheduled PO.

Barbiturates (Phenobarbital) or propofol (Diprivan) may be used if patient refractory to high dose benzodiazepines. If these are necessary, prepare for intubation.

Haloperidol (Haldol) and other antipsychotics are not recommended due to their tendency to lower the seizure threshold as well as their lack of cross-tolerance with alcohol.

Schedule an alcohol cessation program at the end of treatment.

Take Home Points

- Look for EtOH withdrawal syndrome as a reason for unexplained symptoms in those admitted to the hospital with an unrelated illness.
- Thiamine repletion is important in chronic alcoholics.
- Benzodiazepines can be used for aid in withdrawal.

Chemical/Drug Abuse/Dependence

TABLE 2.9 Features of Common Illicit Drugs

Illicit Drug	Intoxication	Withdrawal Syndrome	Intoxication Treatment
Opioids (heroin, RX pain meds)	CNS depression, pupillary constriction, respiratory depression, constipation	Yes	Naloxone (Narcan) acutely
Amphetamines (crystal meth, speed, crank)	Psychomotor agitation, tachycardia, pupillary dilation, paranoia, sudden death	Yes	Haloperidol (Haldol) or other antipsychotics. Benzodiazepines acutely as needed
Phencyclidine hydrochloride (PCP)	Belligerence, psychosis, violence, vertical/horizontal nystagmus	Yes	Benzodiazepines acutely. Haloperidol may be useful to calm patient
LSD	Hallucinations, delusions, pupillary dilation	No	Benzodiazepines acutely
Marijuana	Euphoria, impaired judgment, dry mouth, increased appetite, conjunctival injection, paranoia	No	Isolation from drug
Cocaine	Euphoria, insomnia, impulsive behavior, arrhythmia, cerebral infarct, paranoid ideation, weight loss	Yes	Benzodiazepines and antipsychotics acutely. Clonidine, amantadine (Symmetrel), or carbamazepine (Tegretol) may decrease cravings.

Personality Disorders

TABLE 2.10 Cluster A Personality Disorders (Weird)

Type	Features	Treatment
Paranoid	Suspiciousness, fear of exploitation, harm, bearer of grudges, reactionary	Psychotherapy
Schizoid	Social detachment, restricted affect, solitary by choice, lack of friends. Similar to negative symptoms usually linked to schizophrenia.	Individual psychotherapy
Schizotypal	Odd beliefs and magical thinking, paranoia, suspiciousness. Strange behavior. Similar to positive symptoms usually linked to schizophrenia.	Psychotherapy. Antipsychotics may be useful for excessive delusional states.

TABLE 2.11 Cluster B Personality Disorders (Wild)

Type	Features	Treatment
Antisocial	Deceitfulness, criminality, exhibits disregard for and violation of others' rights. Lack of remorse for behavior. Associated with **conduct d/o** as a child.	Inpatient group therapy if available.
Borderline	Fear of abandonment, intense personal relationships, imagined traumatic behavior, splitting, self mutilation.	Psychotherapy. SSRIs for depressive, anxiety symptoms.
Histrionic	Excessive emotionality and attention seeking. Need to be center of attention. Often hypersexual behavior.	Insight-oriented psychotherapy.
Narcissistic	Egotistical, delusions of grandeur, sense of entitlement, lacks empathy. Superiority complex.	Psychotherapy.

TABLE 2.12 Cluster C Personality Disorders (Whacky)

Type	Features	Treatment
Avoidant	Social inhibition, excessively sensitive to criticism, feelings of inadequacy prevail. Inferiority complex.	Individual or group psychotherapy, assertiveness training, desensitization training. SSRIs are often helpful.
Dependent	Submissive, clinging behavior. Pervasive need to be cared for. Difficulty making decisions.	Insight-oriented psychotherapy, group and behavioral therapies. Family therapy.
Obsessive-Compulsive	Preoccupation with orderliness, cleanliness, perfectionism. Reluctance to delegate tasks. Rigid.	Long-term individual therapy.

Mental Retardation

The state of intellectual functioning that is persistently below average coupled with adaptive functioning deficit or impairment. These two characteristics must be present before age 18 years. Many varied causes may lead to mental retardation (MR) and are generally classified into prenatal, perinatal, and postnatal groups.

Symptoms

Sub-average mental functioning. Mild cases are sometimes overlooked until later in schooling. Commonly discovered by poor academic performance and inability to keep up with peer group. Moderate to severe cases are often found soon after birth and may exhibit other genetic abnormalities that lead to the diagnosis.

Diagnosis

Often low cognitive function coupled with low adaptive skills in two or more of the following areas: communication, self-care, home living, social skills, community interaction, self-direction, health and safety, and functional academics.

Several well known standardized intelligence tests exist and are used to determine IQ score. These include: Stanford-Binet Intelligence Scale, Wechsler Preschool and Primary Scale of Intelligence (WPPSI), Kaufman Assessment Battery for Children, and others.

TABLE 2.13 MR Classification by IQ

Severity	IQ Range
Mild	55–69
Moderate	40–54
Severe	25–39
Profound	0–24

Etiology is often idiopathic, but look for preventable causes such as transient hypoxia, phenylketoneuria. Do genetic testing for common syndromes such as Down syndrome and fragile X. This may be useful for parents in planning future pregnancies.

Treatment

If preventable, prevent it. This may be eliminating phenylalanine in the diet in PKU (must be done early). In nonpreventable, supportive care is the standard. Often caregiver counseling and training must be done to adjust to living with patient. If severe or profound, parents may elect to place child in an assisted living facility. Educational needs should be addressed, as many patients benefit from special education tailored to their level of function. This is required by law in public school systems.

Take Home Points

- Mental retardation has many etiologies, thus cause should be explored for possible treatment.
- IQ is always sub-average but range determines classification.
- Special education of some degree is almost always needed.

3　　Diseases of the Nervous System

Infectious Diseases of the CNS

Tetanus

Infection of the neurologic system by *C. tetani* causing blockage of synaptic inhibitory neurotransmitters leading to skeletal muscle tonic spasm. Disease involves several clinical presentations that are variations of muscular spasm: generalized, localized, cephalic, and neonatal. Incubation period from suspected wound infection can be extremely variable from a few days to months.

Symptoms

Classically presents with trismus (lock-jaw). Fever, malaise, or signs of local infection are common. History of disease entry is often present such as recent injury. As the disease progresses, many muscular and neurologic signs may evolve including: convulsions, drooling, dysphagia, arrhythmias, hydrophobia, muscular spasticity/rigidity, nuchal rigidity, risus sardonicus (fixed smile), or sudden cardiac death.

Diagnosis

This is a clinical diagnosis made by presentation with muscle spasm, history of wound (usually), and no history of immunization.

Labs: CBC for possible leukocytosis. Wound culture may grow *C. tetani* but infection is very possible even with negative culture.

ECG to evaluate for and track possible arrhythmias.

TABLE 3.1 Tetanus Prophylaxis in Wounds

	Clean Wound	Dirty Wound
History of adequate vaccination with tetanus toxoid	Give toxoid if last dose of booster is > 10 years ago	Give toxoid if last dose of booster is > 5 years ago
Unknown or inadequate vaccination with toxoid	Start primary series of 3 toxoid doses.*	Give tetanus immunoglobulin (250 units IM) **plus** start primary series of 3 toxoid doses.*

American College of Physicians' Task Force on Adult Immunization and Infectious Diseases Society of America. *Guide for Adult Immunizations*. Philadelphia: American College of Physicians, 1994.
*Primary series = One dose toxoid now, repeat in one month, and repeat in one year. Adequate vaccination consists of completion of primary toxoid series.

Treatment

Debridement of wound is essential to minimize the release of further toxin.

Give **penicillin G or doxycycline**. Metronidazole if pen allergic.

Give **tetanus immunoglobulin** to neutralize unbound toxin.

Give **tetanus/diphtheria toxoid** for active immunization (since not conferred after disease).

Supportive care is commonly needed and may include long term intubation, trachiostomy, and ICU admission. Death by respiratory failure must be guarded against.

Adjunctive treatment:

Consider sedation with **benzodiazepines** or propofol for muscle spasms. Place patient in dark, quiet room.

Consider muscle relaxants, classically, **pancuronium** if sedatives are inadequate.

Labetolol may be used to control autonomic dysfunction since alpha and beta activity is so high. Avoid other beta blockers. May also consider clonidine or atropine for greater control.

Take Home Points

- Prevention is by far the best strategy for disease control. Any patient with a wound should have evaluation for tetanus prophylaxis.

- Death may occur from arrhythmia, meningitis, or respiratory compromise.

- Recovery is often complete after the conclusion of disease.

Poliomyelitis

An enterovirus infection with subsequent neurologic involvement. Types include bulbar (cranial nerves), encephalopathic, and spinal (arms/legs). The second phase, which occurs years later, termed post-polio syndrome (PPS), can involve pain, weakness, fatigue, and decreased concentration. PPS always occurs in the same nerves and muscles involved in the original infection. Polio infection may also evolve to post-poliomyelitis progressive muscular atrophy (PPMA) which produces marked atrophy of muscles innervated by affected nerves.

Symptoms

Acute infection may show symptoms of aseptic meningitis including fever, tachycardia, headache, vomiting, neck stiffness, or unilateral tremor. This may progress to a paralytic stage involving myalgias, lower motor neuron signs, then to respiratory failure.

Uncommonly, this is a biphasic disease with acute illness in childhood then a second phase usually > 35 years later. Ninety-five percent of overall cases are asymptomatic. The rest may acutely present as aseptic meningitis or encephalopathy. May progress to lasting neurological disease involving paralysis or muscle atrophy.

Diagnosis

Viral culture of pharynx or stool may demonstrate virus. CSF viral culture is the diagnostic gold standard but is rarely performed. CSF analysis shows increased WBCs and elevated protein. Serum levels of antibodies are increased and classically **4 fold** normal.

PPS can be evaluated with electromyography and muscle biopsy but results are nonspecific and show effects of denervation.

Treatment

Prevention with vaccination is the most effective strategy.

In acute phase, supportive care is needed. Intubation and ICU admission is warranted in a small proportion of patients. Multidisciplinary team approach needed for any symptomatic acute infection. No specific treatment is proven effective.

Second phase is also treated symptomatically. Non-narcotic analgesics and physical therapy are the mainstay.

Take Home Points

- Polio is an enterovirus infection of which 95% is asymptomatic.
- Types include bulbar, encephalopathic, and spinal.
- Diagnose with viral culture from CSF, throat, or stool.
- Prevent with universal vaccination.

Creutzfeldt-Jakob Disease

Caused by a prion (PrPSc) infection which is often linked to ingestion or exposure to infected animal tissue (historically found in British beef). The bovine form is termed "mad cow" disease or bovine spongiform encephalopathy. Almost all instrument cleaning techniques are ineffective in combating the organism, including autoclave.

Symptoms

Progressive mental deterioration and myoclonus are main features of disease. Variants exist which also may involve almost any other neurologic signs. Focal defect involving brain stem and cerebellar regions are more common. Dementia as well as mood changes are also often observed.

Diagnosis

Clinical features typical of CJD are observed as above but it is very difficult to make a definitive diagnosis while the patient is alive. Typical EEG with CSF assay indicative of prion disease may be found. History of rare exposure, presence in certain geologic areas, and lack of other suggested etiology point toward this disease.

Definitive diagnosis includes typical specialized histopathologic staining and genetic analysis of brain tissue derived by biopsy or autopsy specimen. These are generally only done at tertiary care laboratory centers.

Imaging: MRI with FLAIR (fluid-attenuated inversion recovery) imaging studies recognize changes in typical brain areas and are helpful when paired with typical features of disease.

Treatment

Purely supportive until death, which is usually under one year.

Take Home Points

- CJD is caused by a very fastidious organism called a prion.
- Believed to have crossed over from cattle to humans by consumption of muscle and nerve tissue of infected animals.
- Definitive diagnosis is only available on autopsy of brain tissue.
- Treatment is supportive until inevitable early death.

Rabies

A rapidly progressive viral disease of the central nervous system that is almost universally fatal. This disease has become rare in developed nations since implementation of standard post-exposure prophylaxis measures; however, it still does affect a small number of people in developing countries.

Symptoms

Strong history of prior bite from a wild animal or infected domestic animal. Once symptoms occur, no treatment is effective. Symptoms include aphasia, **throat spasm leading to hydrophobia,** lack of coordination, fever, salivation, dysphasia, paresis, and paralysis. Progression of disease to point of coma, DIC, cardiac arrhythmias, and cardiac arrest is practically assured.

Diagnosis

Since disease is often manifest before antibody formation and thus detection, prophylaxis is important before lab diagnosis. Refer to the table below for guidelines regarding animal diagnosis and treatment. After symptoms occur, viral assay may be helpful in confirming diagnosis of disease.

TABLE 3.2 Rabies Prophylaxis

Animal	Evaluation Consideration	Treatment
Domestic dogs and cats	Caught and observed × 10 days	If asymptomatic, no vaccination is necessary
	Escaped	Full vaccination and RIG course
Wild animals including: Bats, foxes, raccoons, wolves, woodchucks	Caught and sacrificed→ brain tissue examined	If positive, full vaccination and RIG course
	Escaped	Full vaccination and RIG course
Livestock, wild rodents, squirrels, hamsters, chipmunks, rats	Wild or domesticated	Consult local health department but rabies is rare in these animals. Remember: there is no such thing as a rabid rabbit!

Treatment

Clean and debride the wound as much as possible.

Active and passive prophylaxis:

Active: Vaccination with one of three available cell cultured vaccines (HDCV). 1.0 mL IM at days 0, 3, 7, 14, and 28. If patient has previously been vaccinated, repeat vaccination at days 0 and 3 only.

Passive: Rabies immune globulin (RIG) 20 IU/kg injected around site of bite (as much as anatomically possible) then the rest given IM.

Rabies itself has no treatment or cure.

Take Home Points

- Throat spasm and hydrophobia are classic symptoms for rabies.
- Postexposure vaccination must be both active and passive.
- Give rabies IG into and around injury site, then the rest IM.
- Rabies itself is almost universally fatal.

Meningitis

Inflammation of the meninges and surrounding CSF fluid commonly due to infection. Causes include bacteria, virus, and fungi/yeast infection. Risk factors include: recent neurological or abdominal surgery, sinusitis/otitis media, exposure to infected patient, or immunocompromised status.

Symptoms

Global CNS symptoms such as headache, fever, photophobia, confusion, irritability, decreased consciousness, and lethargy. Rash may be reported.

Diagnosis

Physical exam: Nuchal rigidity, positive Kernig and Brudzinski signs (meningeal irritation), mental status change, and fever. Classic skin rash is more common when causative organism is *N meningitidis*. Rash is petechial or purpuric and blanching but presentations vary. Check retinas for possible signs of increased ICP.

Imaging: CT to rule out mass effect from some other cause then proceed to lumbar puncture (LP).

Labs: Obtain LP, evaluating for opening pressure (rarely done in practicality); glucose levels, protein levels, gram stain, antigenic testing (wellcogens), smear, and culture.

TABLE 3.3 Typical CSF Analysis in Suspected Meningitis

	Viral	Bacterial	Fungal
Glucose	Normal	Less than 2/3 serum glucose	Normal-low
Protein	Normal-elevated	Elevated	Elevated
Predominant cell type	Lymphocytes	PMNs	Lymphocytes

Also obtain CBC, CRP, coagulation profile, blood cultures, CMP, and serum glucose levels.

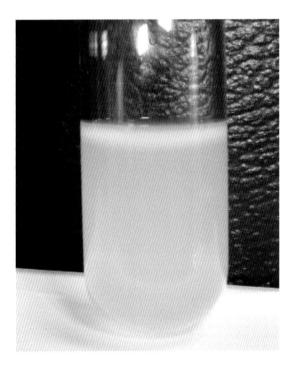

FIGURE 3.1 CSF from a bacterial meningitis patient is commonly cloudy or "turbid." Reprinted with permission from Humphreys H, Irving WL. *Problem-Oriented Clinical Microbiology and Infection*, 2nd edition. 2004, Oxford University Press.

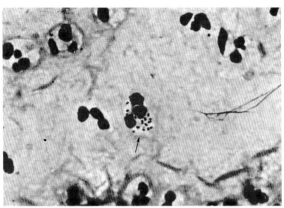

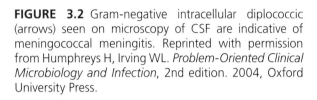

FIGURE 3.2 Gram-negative intracellular diplococcic (arrows) seen on microscopy of CSF are indicative of meningococcal meningitis. Reprinted with permission from Humphreys H, Irving WL. *Problem-Oriented Clinical Microbiology and Infection*, 2nd edition. 2004, Oxford University Press.

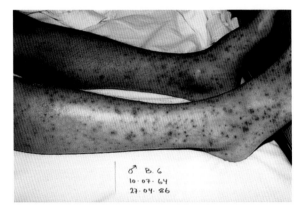

FIGURE 3.3 Macular hemorrhagic lesions on the legs of a 21-year-old man with meningococcemia caused by *N meningitides*. Reprinted with permission from Warrell DA, Cox TM, et al. *Oxford Textbook of Medicine*, 4th edition. 2003, Oxford University Press.

Treatment

If viral meningitis, treatment is generally supportive (unless HSV suspected) and full recovery is often expected. Outpatient treatment may be appropriate.

For bacterial or fungal cause, give steroids (**dexamethasone**) to lower morbidity early on, preferably before or with antibiotics. Then give multiple IV antibiotic regimen, empirically.

Regimens differ depending on age and clinical presentation. However, should be started before culture results (or other CSF analysis) is complete.

Adults: Include third generation cephalosporin **ceftriaxone (Rocephin) or cefotaxime**, plus **vancomycin** and **acyclovir** (if HSV is suspected), consider adding **ampicillin** if patient is > 55 years old (to cover *Listeria*).

Pediatrics: **Ampicillin plus cefotaxime or gentamicin**. Add acyclovir if HSV suspected.

Tailor regimen based on CSF analysis and eventually culture.

Provide supportive care, pain management, and antiemetics as needed. ICU admission is usually indicated.

Take Home Points

- Consider meningitis in all patients with headache and fever.
- Kernig and Brudzinski signs are classic for meningeal irritation.
- LP is the test of choice although do not wait for culture results to treat if other findings are typical.
- Viral meningitis may be treated with low acuity, while bacterial meningitis is a neurologic emergency.
- Don't forget to give dexamethasone concomitantly or before the first dose of antibiotics.

Viral Encephalitis

Inflammation of the brain and surrounding meninges and spinal cord due to viral infection. Specific types of viruses are numerous but the most common include HSV, Epstein-Barr, varicella-zoster, and arboviruses (St. Louis, Japanese, Eastern and Western equine, etc).

Symptoms

Viral prodrome is common but progresses to involve global neurologic dysfunction such as lethargy, slurred speech, confusion, headaches, photophobia, seizures, and meningeal signs. May also involve focal neurologic deficit including paralysis, hearing loss, cranial nerve involvement, and gustatory/olfactory hallucinations.

Diagnosis

Labs: CSF analysis is essential and will be similar to viral meningitis: normal to elevated protein, normal glucose, and lymphocytic predominance on microscopic analysis. **HSV PCR** is diagnostic for HSV encephalitis. Viral culture is also useful but will take much too long to be practical before therapy. ELISA antibody testing in serum and CSF is important with some causes but may only be useful in retrospect.

Imaging: Brain CT is helpful in eliminating other causes and looking for evidence of increased ICP. Brain **MRI** is the best imaging technique in detecting likely HSV by characteristic appearance of temporal lobes.

Brain biopsy may be helpful and definitive but is limited by practicality and benefit.

EEG: If inflammation is from HSV encephalitis, EEG shows characteristic pattern termed periodic lateralized epileptic form discharges (PLEDs).

Treatment

Start acyclovir if viral etiology possible. Then give corticosteroid such as dexamethasone and anticonvulsants.

Add broad spectrum antibiotics if bacterial cause possible.

Remember to watch for signs of SIADH and treat as appropriate. Otherwise, treatment is supportive and sedation may be an option to guide patient through difficult disease course.

Take Home Points

- Encephalitis may be preceded by a nonspecific viral prodrome.
- Treatment consists of antiviral medication and IV steroids if the etiology is viral or HSV related. Have a low threshold for adding antibiotics to this regimen.

Brain Abscess

A single or multiple abscesses in brain tissue. Disease often starts as a focal cerebritis that becomes necrotic and then encapsulated. Concurrent systemic or distant disease is commonly present acting to "seed" the abscess. Specific organisms include *Staph*, *Strep*, enteric gram negatives, and those harbored by immunocompromised hosts (*Toxoplasma gondii* and *Nocardia*).

Symptoms

Mental status changes, seizures, headache, or focal neurologic deficits are common. History may be positive for immunocompromised status (toxo or fungal ball), post surgery (dental), dental infection, skull fracture, recent otitis infection, sinusitis, or distant infection.

Diagnosis

Physical exam: Look for cranial nerve deficits (III, VI) and papilledema indicating increased intracerebral pressure.

Labs: CBC for elevated WBCs. ESR/CRP elevated. Check electrolytes and BMP for SIADH. CSF analysis may be dangerous due to increased ICP. If obtained, findings may range from normal to those indicative of bacterial meningitis.

Imaging: Contrast enhanced CT is classic for **ring enhancing lesions**. MRI is more sensitive but takes longer.

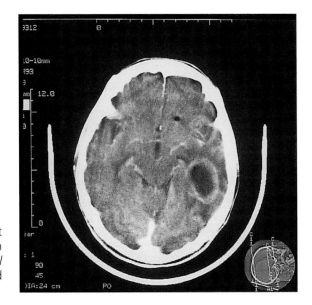

FIGURE 3.4 CT scan showing brain abscess in left temporal lobe. Reprinted with permission from Humphreys H, Irving WL. *Problem-Oriented Clinical Microbiology and Infection*, 2nd edition. 2004, Oxford University Press.

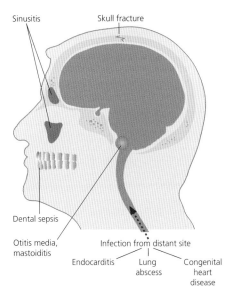

FIGURE 3.5 Predisposing factors in brain abscess. Reprinted with permission from Humphreys H, Irving WL. *Problem-Oriented Clinical Microbiology and Infection*, 2nd edition. 2004, Oxford University Press.

Treatment

Consult **neurosurgery** ASAP for likely drainage.

   Give **dexamethasone** to reduce brain edema and ICP.

Antibiotics: prolonged course of 6–8 weeks. Different regimens exist so culture and sensitivity should be used to guide treatment. Ceftriaxone (Rocephin) *plus* metronidazole (Flagyl) are common.

Give anticonvulsants during clinical course as is warranted to prevent/treat seizures.

Take Home Points

- Brain abscess may form after a brief attack of cerebritis or distant seeding of typical organism.
- Look for a characteristic ring enhanced lesion on CT scan.
- Admit to the hospital and consult neurosurgery.

Alzheimer Disease (AD)

Characterized by progressive intellectual deterioration and dementia, this common disorder involves neurofibrillary tangles of β-amyloid protein, cerebral senile plaque development, and loss of acetylcholine in the forebrain. Risk factors include age, smoking history, family history of AD, Down syndrome, history of head trauma, and low education level. Inheritance of the E4 allele of apolipoprotein E gene on chromosome 19 is strongly linked to AD, but a causative relationship has not been established.

Symptoms

Progressive, insidious memory loss is the hallmark of this disease. It commonly starts with misplacing objects, then time disorientation and getting lost, which progresses to inability to recognize relatives; aphasia, apraxia, and dementia follow over the course of years.

Diagnosis

Generally a clinical diagnosis but may be supported by eliminating other causes of dementia and imaging. Mini mental status exam is useful in tracking progression. Clinically assess for depression.

Labs: Obtain CBC, CMP, Vit B12/folate, syphilis testing, TSH, HIV, and ESR/CRP. E4 allele of apolipoprotein E gene is available for prognostic and family testing but accuracy and practicality is not yet established.

Imaging: CT may support diagnosis but MRI shows cerebral atrophy and decreased hippocampal volume more accurately.

Gross exam of brain (at autopsy) shows neuritic plaques and neurofibrillary tangles.

(a) 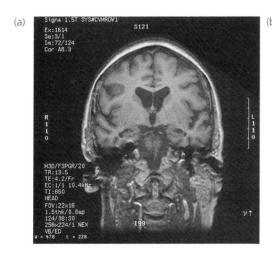 (b)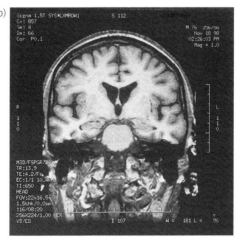

FIGURE 3.6 Coronal T1-weighted MRI scan of a patient with early Alzheimer disease showing bilateral early hippocampal atrophy (a). Compare with normal subject (b). Reprinted with permission from Warrell DA, Cox TM, et al. *Oxford Textbook of Medicine*, 4th edition. 2003, Oxford University Press.

Treatment

Manage symptoms such as depression, psychosis, and sleep disturbance medically as indicated.

Anticholinesterase inhibitors are the mainstay: Start with donepezil (Aricept), rivastigmine (Exelon), galantamine (Reminyl, Razadyne), or tacrine (Cognex). Others in the new NMDA receptor antagonist class such as memantine (Namenda) have recently been found to be very effective.

Remember to look for social aspects such as elder abuse and social support from family or friends (these are very popular questions on standardized tests!).

Take Home Points

- Pathologic hallmarks include: neurofibrillary tangles of β-amyloid protein, cerebral senile plaques, and loss of acetylcholine in the forebrain.
- Alzheimer disease remains a clinical diagnosis although testing may suggest presence of disease.
- Specific therapies include anticholinesterase inhibitors and NMDA receptor antagonists.

Normal Pressure Hydrocephalus

The neurologic disease state of pathologically-increased ventricular size and normal CSF pressure. Etiology may be idiopathic or secondary to disease, causing an imbalance of CSF production by the choroid plexus and absorption by the arachnoid villi in the sagital sinus. Commonly implicated are occult subarachnoid hemorrhages and chronic meningitis.

Symptoms

Classic clinical triad of **gait disturbance, urinary incontinence, and dementia** although other diffuse signs of dementia may be present.

Diagnosis

Labs: Lumbar puncture is prudent to eliminate other causes of symptoms. Protein, glucose, cell count, gram stain, and culture should be normal in NPH.
Imaging: CT and MRI can both be helpful showing hydrocephalus. Widened ventricles are seen.
Special testing: Miller Fisher test (also called intermittent high volume tap) involves removal of 30–60 mL CSF and objectively measuring improvement of gait symptoms. May correlate with prognosis to ventriculoperitoneal (VP) shunting.

Treatment

Ventriculoperitoneal shunting is the mainstay of therapy. Good response is usually achieved fairly quickly with long term efficacy.

No known medical therapy has shown good efficacy.

Take Home Points

- Look for the clinical triad of gait disturbance, urinary incontinence, and dementia.
- Removal of a small amount of CSF fluid and monitoring for clinical improvement (Miller Fisher test) is the test of choice for NPH.
- Treat with placement of a VP shunt.

Parkinson Disease

A progressive neurodegenerative disease involving the loss of dopaminergic neurons in the substantia nigra at an increased rate. Etiologies are unclear and point to no definitive cause although some studies suggest possible toxin or viral effect. Age of onset is rare before 60 years.

Symptoms

Progressive bradykinesia, muscular rigidity, tremor, and later onset postural instability are the cardinal symptoms of this disease. Others include shuffling gait, dementia, insomnia, micrographia, and masked (expressionless) facies are also commonly seen. Consistent history in a young person may be from illicit heroin use (the process of making synthetic street heroin sometimes makes MPTP, a neurotoxic byproduct).

Diagnosis

Physical exam: "Cogwheel" rigidity of arms and legs, clonus, shuffling gait, and resting "pill rolling" tremor.
Imaging: None specifically
Gross microscopic: Lewy bodies in the substantia nigra on autopsy exam.

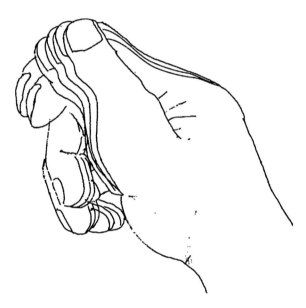

FIGURE 3.7 Typical "pill rolling" tremor of Parkinson disease. Reprinted with permission from Cox NLT, Roper TA. *Clinical Skills*. 2005, Oxford University Press.

Treatment

Therapies are aimed at replacing or blocking degradation of dopamine to relevant pathways. **Levodopa-carbadopa (Sinemet)** is first line. Add dopamine agonists such as bromocriptine (Parlodel), pergolide (Permax), ropinirole (Requip), and pramipexole (Mirapex) as disease progresses. MAOIs like selegiline (Eldepryl) may be neuroprotective and thus should be started early. Anticholinergics, amantidine (Symmetrel), COMT inhibitors, and SSRIs can be started to lessen symptoms as disease progresses. Side effects of these medications are the development of hyperkinesias, tics, and exaggerated movements which can also be debilitating.

Multiple surgical approaches have been tried but limited success reported. Fetal midbrain substantia nigra neuronal transplant (illegal in U.S.) and adrenal medullary transplant are unproven but hopeful. Thalamotomy, stereotactic pallidotomy, and deep brain stimulation have all shown varied efficacy.

Take Home Points

- The main pathologic event in PD is loss of dopaminergic neurons in the substantia nigra area of the brain.

- Classic manifestations are: bradykinesia, "cogwheel" rigidity, "pill rolling" tremor, and shuffling gait.
- Levodopa-carbadopa (Sinemet) is largely first line and serves to increase CNS dopamine levels.

Multiple Sclerosis

A neurologic disease with a commonly relapsing course caused by recurrent demyelination of neurons in brain and spinal cord white matter. Etiology remains unknown but both autoimmune and viral theories exist. Incidence is higher in women aged 20–40 years old and shows predilection for temperate climates and certain families.

Symptoms

Symptoms come and go in exacerbation/remission fashion. Usually in young women and often present with optic neuralgia and vision changes. Other symptoms are diplopia, gait disturbance, incontinence, vertigo, emotional lability, and scanning speech. Many symptoms are made worse by heat, infection, trauma, pregnancy and exercise.

Diagnosis

Diagnosis is clinical but must involve separation of attacks in "time and space" indicating multiple CNS lesions.

Physical exam: Internuclear ophthalmoplegia (impaired horizontal eye movement with weak adduction of the affected eye and abduction nystagmus of the contralateral eye), Lhermitte's sign (electric shock down spine on neck flexion), positive Babinski sign, clonus, hyperactive deep tendon reflexes, paresthesias, hyperesthesia, ataxia, and vertical nystagmus.

Labs: CSF reveals IgG/oligoclonal bands and myelin basic protein.

Imaging: MRI with and without contrast is diagnostic for demyelination plaques. CT and plain films are not helpful.

EMG shows characteristic slowing of conduction but must be correlated clinically.

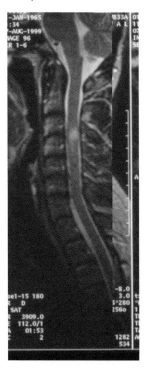

FIGURE 3.8 Multiple sclerosis of the cervical spinal cord. Note the lesion of acute demyelination at the C3 level of this sagittal T2-weighted image of the cervical spinal cord. Reprinted with permission from Warrell DA, Cox TM, et al. *Oxford Textbook of Medicine*, 4th edition. 2003, Oxford University Press.

Treatment

Steroids are the mainstay of medical therapy. Other meds may treat disease course, e.g. immunosuppressive agents such as azathioprine (Imuran), cyclophosphamide, interferon, methotrexate, mitoxantrone (Novantrone), and cyclosporine. Other medications are aimed at symptom relief, such as antispasmotics like baclofen (Kemstro). Remember to treat accompanying disorders such as psychosis, depression, infection, and seizures.

Take Home Points

- Symptoms are often made worse by heat, infection, trauma, pregnancy, and exercise.
- Diagnosis is clinical but must show attacks that are separated in "time and place."
- The McDonald criteria outline clinical guidelines for the diagnosis of MS and combine features including clinical attacks, MRI findings, and typical CSF findings.
- Treat with steroids and immunomodulators.

Amyotrophic Lateral Sclerosis (Lou Gehrig's Disease)

A neurodegenerative progressive, insidious disease characterized by symptoms of both upper and lower motor neuron degeneration which is almost universally fatal.

Symptoms

The most common initial presentation is asymmetric limb weakness followed by the next most common presentation of bulbar dysfunction seen as dysarthria and dysphagia. Other symptoms are many and variable and include fasciculations, personality changes, spasticity, and atrophy. Family history is positive in only 10% of patients.

Diagnosis

Physical exam: Proximal muscle weakness, hyperreflexia, spasticity, muscular atrophy and weakness. Extraocular muscles are sparred leading to the characteristic "locked in" syndrome. Eventual respiratory failure.
EMG: Widespread denervation in grouped atrophy fashion.

Treatment

Riluzole (Rilutek) produces modest improvement in morbidity and delay of mortality. Antispasmotics such as baclofen (Kemstro) may be helpful for spastic symptoms.

    Mechanical ventilator support needed later in disease.

    Recommend advanced directive.

Take Home Points

- ALS is a disease of both upper and lower motor neurons.
- EMG shows widespread denervation in a grouped atrophy fashion.
- Death is almost inevitable and occurs due to respiratory failure.

Huntington's Disease

An autosomal dominantly inherited neurodegenerative disorder involving progressive choreiform movements and dementia. The gene mutation for HD is located on chromosome 4 and results in an expanding trinucleotide repeat (C-A-G) sequence that in turn results in abnormal levels of neuronal protein buildup that eventually leads to cell death. Because of inheritance, offspring of HD patients have a 50% chance of being affected.

Symptoms

Age of onset is 30–50 years. Early signs develop insidiously and include chorea; and cognitive changes such as apathy, agitation, anhedonia, asocial behavior, irritability, bipolar symptoms, or schizophreniform disorder. Late manifestations include dysphagia, bladder and bowel incontinence, gait disturbance, hyperkinesias, dementia, tongue protrusion, facial grimacing, ataxia or dystonia.

Diagnosis

Clinical diagnosis based on typical symptoms and family history.
Imaging: CT or MRI scan of the brain may reveal marked atrophy of the neostriatum affecting the caudate nucleus more than the putamen.
Neuropsychologic testing may detect affected high risk individuals slightly earlier than clinically noted.

Treatment

There is no cure and treatment remains symptomatic.
> Antipsychotics such as haloperidol (Haldol) may help for psychotic symptoms.
> Chorea may respond to clonazepam (Klonopin) or reserpine.
> Muscle rigidity may respond to baclofen (Lioresal).
> Give SSRIs or TCAs for depressive symptoms.
> Genetic counseling (and possible testing for the gene mutation) is essential in offspring.

Take Home Points

- HD is autosomally dominant, which means offspring have a 50% chance of inheriting the disease.
- Choreiform movements and mental changes are two hallmarks of disease.
- No cure exists and treatment remains symptomatic.

Paraplegia/Quadriplegia

The paralysis of the lower limbs (paraplegia) or all four limbs (quadriplegia).

Symptoms

Often accompanying trauma, symptoms include complete or partial motor dysfunction of the skeletal musculature. Sensory impairment usually accompanies motor symptoms but not always. Autonomic dysfunction more commonly exists in quadriplegia and may involve temperature dysregulation, digestion, etc. Quadriplegia may also involve muscles of respiration, including the diaphragm which may require mechanical support.

Diagnosis

Evident on exam, which constitutes its diagnosis.
Imaging: MRI of the spine may show complete or partial transection in cases of trauma. Local edema of the cord and surrounding tissues is usual acutely.

CT/plain radiograph may be useful to show tumor or bony abnormality in subacute or progressive symptoms.

Brown-Sequard syndrome results from hemi-transection of the spinal cord which causes ipsilateral paralysis and loss of discriminatory and joint sensation with contralateral loss of pain and temperature sensation.

Treatment

Depends on the etiology. Trauma victims may benefit from immediate use of corticosteroids to reduce cord edema (although literature shows conflicting benefit vs. harm). Neurosurgery should be consulted for all cases including less acute presentation or demonstrable tumor.

After initial injury, physical therapy and rehabilitation play a vital role in reeducating the patient on limb movement and accessory muscle use. Some mobility of affected muscle may be seen with rehab but course is usually prolonged. Spinal cord transections usually never fully recover but partial recovery and learned use of accessory muscles often return some functional capacity.

Take Home Points

- Acquired paralysis may be due to trauma, cancerous growth, benign/space occupying growth, infection, autoimmune, toxic, metabolic, and idiopathic etiologies.

- In the trauma patient, consider steroids as soon as possible. Consult neurosurgery.

- Keep in mind quadriplegics may have accompanying autonomic dysfunction.

Seizure Disorder

A temporary and sudden electrically mediated change in cortical activity resulting in uncontrolled activation of motor or sensory neural pathways. This activation may be seen as a change in consciousness (generalized) or isolated to a certain body part without affecting consciousness (partial). Many different etiologies exist including febrile, epileptic, infectious, hypoxic, metabolic, diabetic, conversion, CVA, vascular malformations, and idiopathic.

Symptoms

TABLE 3.4 States of Seizure Disorder

Stage	Symptoms
Pre-ictal	Often associated with auditory, visual, or olfactory hallucinations (commonly familiar smell tips patient off to oncoming seizure)
Ictal	Seizure activity
Post-ictal	May range from sleepiness and lethargy to asymptomatic. Usually not cognitively impaired.

Types

Generalized tonic/clonic seizures are the classic "grand-mal" seizure that involves symmetric shaking of upper and lower extremities with transient disruption of consciousness.

Partial seizures involve one specific place of the cortex and thus affect isolated parts of the body. By definition, partial seizures occur with the preservation of consciousness. Classic presentation is of "Jacksonian March," which is seizure activity moving from one part of the body to another in a stepwise fashion as activity in the brain moves across the cortex. Partial seizures may be associated with Todd paralysis, which involves transient post-ictal paralysis of the affected limb. If a seizure starts out partial then progresses to involve a change in consciousness, it's termed "complex partial."

Febrile seizures—Commonly affect the pediatric population 3 months to 5 years of age and consist of generalized seizure activity associated with fever or hyperthermia.

Status epilepticus involves at least 30 minutes of uninterrupted tonic/clonic seizure activity or incomplete recovery between discrete seizures with an overall duration of at least 30 minutes.

Other seizure forms exist such as absence (usually seen in pediatric population involving rapid interruption in consciousness without post-ictal state), conversion (pseudoseizure), and drop seizures (often in children and involve generalized transient paralysis).

Diagnosis

Labs: Check screening BMP, CBC, glucose, drug screen, and TSH for possible derangements and etiology. CPK may be elevated due to significant muscle injury.

Imaging: CT/MRI can be useful if trauma, lesion, or tumors are suspected etiologies.

Shoulder X-ray may reveal posterior dislocation of the humoral head.

EEG: Considered standard for diagnosis but often falsely negative since done in inter-ictal period. Video monitored EEG with sleep deprivation may increase sensitivity of test.

Treatment

Many anticonvulsants exist and often require periodic medication levels to monitor effective ranges. Start with monotherapy and add more if needed. Almost all are contraindicated in pregnancy but weigh the risks/benefits.

Status epilepticus—ABCs then lorazepam (Ativan), thiamine, and glucose are classic. Add phenytoin (Dilantin) or fosphenytoin (Cerebyx) if seizure continues.

Generalized tonic/clonic—Phenytoin (Dilantin), carbamazepine (Tegretol), or valproate (Depakene).

Absence—Classically ethosuximide (Zarontin).

Partial—Clinically effective single or combinations of above medications.

Febrile—Treat increased temperature with acetaminophen, NSAIDs, or ice packs. Usually does not require anticonvulsants.

Conversion—Psychiatry referral.

Surgery: Stereotactic seizure focus ablation has showed effectiveness but is reserved for medically refractory cases.

Take Home Points

- Seizures may involve a pre-ictal prodrome and a post-ictal state.

- Genuine seizures do *not* involve hip thrusting (which can be used to distinguish from conversion/malingering).

- Status epilepticus involves 30 min of uninterrupted seizure or incomplete recovery between seizures lasting 30 min or more.

- Acute therapy involves lorazepam (Ativan), phenytoin (Dilantin), or fosphenytoin (Cerebyx).

Cerebral Palsy (CP)

A general disorder encompassing a group of patients with a permanent neurologic condition causing spasticity or postural abnormalities. Etiology may be due to neurologic insult acquired prenatally, perinatally, or in infancy. Types include spastic, athetotic (dyskinetic), mixed, and ataxic.

Symptoms

Early presentation of spastic movement disorders and paralysis predominate. Often, CP is associated with severe functional and cognitive impairment. Take a good history of maternal pregnancy and exposures to TORCH infections and toxins (including EtOH). Once thought to be caused by acute hypoxia at birth, this theory is being disproved by recent research.

Diagnosis

Labs: Genetic analysis and screening is indicated and applicable to possible future pregnancies.
Imaging: MRI is appropriate to look for possible structural causes but commonly shows normal findings. EEG is appropriate since seizure disorder is common with CP.

Treatment

Supportive and tailored to individual needs. Often surrogate caretakers are needed, sometimes on 24 hour basis.

Physical therapy is a mainstay to improve and maintain muscular ability. This can include specialized movement education programs that educate the patient on movement.

Nutritional support and special diets are indicated in severe cases.

Education is often in the special education category but CP patients may have average or better intelligence.

Anticonvulsant therapy is often indicated to control commonly accompanying seizure disorder.

Muscle relaxants such as baclofen (Lioresal) may be of some use. Botulinum toxin (Botox) IM injections have also been used to control spastic movement.

Take Home Points

- CP is the presence of permanent spastic movements or postural abnormalities present from early in life.
- Supportive care, maintenance nursing, and physical/occupational therapy are the mainstays of therapy.

Trigeminal Neuralgia

Sudden, usually unilateral, severe, brief, stabbing, recurrent episodes of pain in the distribution of one or more branches of the fifth cranial (trigeminal) nerve. Etiology is thought to be compression of the trigeminal nerve root at the point of entry into the pons causing localized demyelination, most commonly by an aberrant blood vessel.

Symptoms

Sharp, often stabbing paroxysmal facial pain that lasts seconds to minutes. Usually unilateral and occurs in the distribution of the trigeminal nerve ($V_{1,2,3}$). This pain occurs almost exclusively in mid-life to elderly patients (over 50 years) and may be exacerbated by trigger points.

Diagnosis

Physical exam: Exquisite tenderness to palpation of the affected areas of the face.
Imaging: MRI may be used to rule out neoplasm in cerebellopontine angle causing similar symptoms or mechanical compression. Occasionally, multiple sclerosis or similar disease is discovered to be the cause.

Treatment

Start with **carbamazepine (Tegretol)**, response is commonly considered diagnostic. May wane in efficacy over period of years and cause sedation as a side effect.

Gabapentin (Neurontin), baclofen (Lioresal), phenytoin (Dilantin), valproate (Depokene), pimozide (Orap), and clonazepam (Klonopin) alone or in combination can be tried. Some antiepileptic drugs such as lamotrigine (Lamictal) and topiramate (Topamax) have been reported to be useful. Oxcarbazepine (Trileptal), a derivative of carbamazepine, may also be effective.

Do not forget that some of these drugs need periodic blood level monitoring.

Surgery: Several surgeries exist and are effective for medically refractory cases: Microvascular decompression, radiofrequencey rhizotomy, glycerol rhizolysis, balloon decompression, Gamma knife radiosurgery, linear accelerator radiosurgery, peripheral nerve block, and peripheral neurectomy.

Take Home Points

- Sharp, stabbing, intermittent facial pain in the elderly is commonly trigeminal neuralgia.
- The medication of choice is carbamazepine (Tegretol).

Bell's Palsy

Partial or total paralysis of the muscles supplied by the facial nerve (CN VII) due to inflammation of the nerve as it passes through the facial canal on its way to muscular innervation. This commonly unilateral acute paralysis is most commonly idiopathic although HSV-1 has been implicated.

Symptoms

Unilateral facial nerve paralysis. History may reveal acute URI or head infection or history of herpes infection of the face.

Diagnosis

Commonly a clinical diagnosis.

Physical exam: Local swelling, ipsilateral numbness, paralysis, loss of taste, and loss of corneal reflex.

Imaging: MRI to image posterior fossa may be indicated to rule out tumor or central infarcts. Usually not needed.

EMG is very useful to confirm diagnosis although it usually does not influence management.

Treatment

Since patients often have difficulty blinking and wetting affected eye, patching is recommended. Monthly corneal inspections for abrasions are indicated throughout recovery course. Artificial tears may be useful as well.

Corticosteroids are commonly used if the patient presents within the first 4–6 days of onset. Commonly, they are combined with valacyclovir (Valtrex) or acyclovir (Zovirax) for suspected HSV involvement. These therapies remain controversial and unproven, however.

Surgery is only considered in very prolonged cases.

Vast majority are self limiting, but recovery is often over number of months.

Take Home Points

- Bell's palsy involves inflammation and entrapment of the facial nerve as it passes through the facial canal while exiting the brain.

- EMG testing confirms the diagnosis, especially early on.

- Recovery is usual and prognosis is better with partial paralysis.

Myasthenia Gravis

The autoimmune attack and resultant dysfunction of peripheral acetylcholine receptors, typically in the head and neck region. This disease does have a genetic component and occurs in females more than males.

Symptoms

Presentation often involves ptosis, difficulty chewing, and abnormal smile although the hallmark of disease is **muscular fatigability** (usually presenting after exercise). Extraocular muscles are often affected which produces diplopia. Dysarthria, dysphagia, and neck muscle pain are also seen. MG may eventually progress to respiratory compromise.

Diagnosis

Screening labs: Consider ANA, TSH, rheumatoid factor, and Vitamin B12 for screening of respective disorders.

Edrophonium (Tensilon or Enlon) test: Administration of edrophonium (an anticholinesterase inhibitor with short half-life) to the diseased patient produces acute, transient reversal of symptoms.

Chest CT may demonstrate a thymoma (approximately 15% of MG patients).

EMG produces characteristic stepwise results. Techniques include repetitive nerve stimulation testing and single-fiber electroyography.

Acetylcholine receptor antibodies (AChR-ab) can be detected in most affected patients, but their level does not correlate with clinical severity. MuSK antibodies are less common but may be present in AchR-ab negative patients.

Imaging: MRI/CT are useful to rule out the commonly associated **thymoma**.

Treatment

Pyridostigmine (Mestinon) is the classic treatment of choice. Dosing ranges from q4–6 hours to qd depending on disease severity. Side effects are GI upset/diarrhea, salivation and bronchial secretions (which are parasympathetic). Neostigmine (Prostigmine) can be used parenterally if in an emergency. Atropine is the antidote to this class.

Steroids also have a role, although dosage varies widely and duration of therapy is often prolonged. Side effects are many, so weigh the risks/benefits.

Azathioprine (Imuran) and cyclosporine may also be used for immunosuppressant therapy and may be useful to decrease the dose of steroids.

Plasmapheresis may be used in the severely ill hospitalized patient after other modalities fail.

Surgery: Thymectomy in patients with severe generalized form or thymoma is indicated.

Take Home Points

- MG is caused by autoimmune attack of peripheral acetylcholine receptors.
- Muscular fatigability is the hallmark of disease.
- Edrophonium may be used to diagnose, although also test plasma for AChR-ab antibodies.
- Treat with pyridostigmine (Mestinon), steroids, or immunosuppressants.

Guillain-Barré Syndrome

A heterogeneous disorder of acute, autoimmune mediated demyelination of peripheral nerves usually after intestinal viral or bacterial infection. Variants of disease include: acute inflammatory demyelinating polyneuropathy (AIDP), Miller-Fischer syndrome (involving ophthalmic and facial musculature), acute motor axonal neuropathy (AMAN), and acute motor and sensory axonal neuropathy (AMSAN).

Symptoms

An ascending and symmetric paralysis usually beginning with the lower extremities (see types above). History may reveal recent GI infection, cold/flu-like symptoms, surgery, or immunization. Acute, seemingly unrelated illness usually results and paralysis begins days to weeks later. Presenting complaints are often of weakness on walking, foot drop, and mildly decreased sensation. This progresses up the body, usually sparing the sphincters.

Diagnosis

Physical exam: Loss of deep tendon reflexes and complete paralysis of proximal muscles of affected limbs (although distal parts are commonly affected first). Sensation may also be impaired.
Lumbar puncture shows increased CSF protein and IgG later in course.
EMG shows slowed conduction velocities indicative of demyelination.

Treatment

Disease is usually self limited with maximal peak of symptoms in 2nd and 3rd weeks.

Plasmapheresis (plasma exchange) is the classic treatment but must be started early in disease course to be effective.

IVIG (intravenous immunoglobulin) infusion in hospitalized patients may be useful and is an equivalent alternative to plasmapheresis.

Steroids must be avoided due to worsening of disease.

This disease is indication for hospital admission and the patient must be closely monitored due to possible need for mechanical ventilation. Monitor for development of bed sores and/or DVT.

Take Home Points

- Guillain-Barré is commonly associated with GI infection; especially *Campylobacter* sp.
- Look for ascending paralysis weeks after infection, then lasting weeks to months.
- Plasmapheresis or IVIG infusion may be attempted for therapy. Avoid steroids.

Subarachnoid Hemorrhage (SAH)

Extravasation of blood into the subarachnoid space, basal cisterns, and CSF pathways. Cause is often due to rupture of saccular "berry" aneurysms, A-V malformations, or trauma. Polycystic kidney disease and coarctation of the aorta are associated with existence of berry aneurysms; hypertension leads to higher rates of aneurysm rupture.

Symptoms

Classically starts with a "thunder-clap" headache that is described as the **worst headache in the patient's life.** Further symptoms vary by the location of the bleed but anterior circulation bleeds produce focal neurologic deficit and hemiparesis. If in the posterior circulation, they produce alteration of consciousness, imbalance, nausea, vomiting, delirium, seizure, or coma.

Diagnosis

Physical exam: Conjugate eye deviation, ophthalmoplegia, irregular breathing, papilledema, retinal hemorrhage, or pinpoint pupil(s). Tachycardia, arrhythmia, and hypertension are commonly detected. Over the course of 24–48 hours, fever and nuchal rigidity may develop. Sequelae may occur in the less acute setting and go undetected, in which case symptoms often partially abate although some degree of neurologic impairment usually persists.

Imaging: CT is the best way to see hemorrhages in the brain; this is usually done with thin sections (3 mm) to detect possible small hemorrhages. CT should be done before lumbar puncture (LP) is attempted to avoid possible herniation. MRI is less useful to detect acute bleeds but may be used if CT is negative or to look for ischemic changes.

Lumbar puncture should be done if the CT is negative and if the clinical picture is still suggestive of SAH. LP should be uniformly bloody (as opposed to traumatic tap) and may be under increased pressure. Bilirubin and xanthochromia may be seen in the CSF but only after about 12 hours post-bleeding. Thus, general recommendations for highly suspected SAH in the setting of a negative CT scan include waiting at least 12 hours from the onset of symptoms and then obtaining CSF and analyzing it for bilirubin.

Cerebral angiography may be used to guide treatment and search for more extensive disease if bilirubin is found in the CSF.

ECG and continuous cardiac monitoring is indicated due to high rates of arrhythmias.

Treatment

Largely supportive. Place patient in quiet, dark room with head of bed elevated and cardiac monitoring. Give stool softeners to prevent straining and control headache with acetaminophen/codeine. Manage the airway with mechanical ventilation if needed. Give mannitol (Osmitrol) to decrease cerebral edema if present. Monitor fluid status.

Give seizure prophylaxis as needed.

Nimodipine (Nimotop) should be given to treat cerebral vasospasm.

Manage blood pressure to keep mean arterial pressure (MAP) < 125. Esmolol (Brevibloc) or enalapril (Vasotec) are good choices for this.

Surgery: May be an option for accessible bleeds and includes radiosurgery, endovascular obliteration, and AV malformation obliteration; all depending on neurosurgical evaluation of the case.

Take Home Points

- SAH often presents as "the worst headache of my life" reported by the patient.
- CT without contrast is the test of choice for evaluation of acute bleeding.

- If the CT is negative but clinical suspicion is still high, wait for 12 hours to pass since symptom onset and obtain CSF for bilirubin level.

- Management is supportive with control of hypertension (to avoid HTN emergency) and neurosurgical consultation.

Subdural and Epidural Hematomas

TABLE 3.5 Features of Subdural and Epidural Hematomas

	Subdural	Epidural
Etiology/associations	Rupture of bridging veins. May occur chronically.	Rupture of artery; middle meningeal. Look for "lucid interval" after the accident. Skull fracture often evident.
Prototypical age group	Elderly	Often young, after trauma
Evaluation	CT/MRI	CT/MRI
Treatment	Surgery can be lifesaving if large. Supportive care and monitoring if small-moderate.	Burr hole placement for decompression can be lifesaving.

Transient Ischemic Attack (TIA)

A transient episode of neurological dysfunction caused by focal brain, spinal cord, or retinal ischemia, without acute infarction. This has classically been defined as lasting < 24 hours. These symptoms occur due to transient blockage of small capillaries in the watershed areas of the brain causing transient ischemia. These symptoms mimic those of a larger stroke but are milder and are, by definition, temporary.

Symptoms

Depending on the anterior or posterior circulation, TIA may produce focal motor loss, slurred speech, blurred vision, diplopia, **amaurosis fugax** (ipsilateral unilateral visual loss characterized to resemble a shade being drawn over the eye), tinnitus, alteration of consciousness, headache, drop attacks, loss of sensation, or ataxia. History is often characteristic of symptoms and presence of risk factors for atherosclerosis, hypertension, cardiac arrhythmia, endocarditis, or embolic-producing disorder.

Diagnosis

Labs: Coagulation profile including INR, CBC, and chemistry panel should be examined routinely. Consider protein C/S, factor V Leiden, thrombin, lupus anticoagulant testing, antithrombin, or if coagulation profile is abnormal or patient is of younger age.

Imaging: Acutely, CT is the test of choice to evaluate for bleeding, however, it's not the test of choice for diagnosis. Diffusion weighted MRI is much more sensitive to find small infarcts if they're present. MRA (magnetic resonance angiogram) may be used if the posterior circulation is suspected to be the source.

Cardiac evaluation: ECG, Holter monitoring, and transthoracic echocardiogram (TTE) or transesophageal echocardiogram (TEE), are appropriate to evaluate for arrhythmias or possible sources of embolization.

Carotid evaluation: Carotid angiography is the gold standard for imaging the carotid arteries; however, it is invasive and fairly impractical. **Duplex ultrasonography** is practically the best test to evaluate the carotid arteries and will give an accurate percentage of stenosis.

Treatment

Admission to the hospital is reasonable in most cases.

The goal for obtaining neuroimaging in TIA patients is < 24 hours.

Depending on the results of the above investigation, if cardiac embolization, arrhythmia, or abnormality, treatment is aimed at the underlying disorder.

In many cases, rupture of atherosclerotic plaques in the carotids is the etiology and should be treated with attention to the degree of stenosis.

TABLE 3.6 Treatment Recommendations by Percent Carotid Artery Stenosis

Stenosis	Treatment
< 50%	Medical management
50–69%	Individual evaluation based on risk factors, ulceration of plaque, and symptoms
> 70%	Surgical candidate

Medical management may include anticoagulant therapy or antiplatelet therapy.

Anticoagulation should be started with heparin or low-molecular weight heparin (enoxaparin [Lovenox]), then warfarin (Coumadin).

Antiplatelet options include aspirin, clopidogrel (Plavix), or dipyridamole (Persantine). Combinations of these, including Aggrenox (dipyridamole/ASA), may be more effective than either agent alone. Ticlopidine (Tidlid) is an older drug once used but has fallen out of favor due to side effects (agranulocytosis).

Surgery: Carotid endarterectomy carries a risk based on the skill and experience of the surgeon as well as the degree of disease in the patient. Certain centers perform more per year than others and research has shown a clinically significant difference in effectiveness and morbidity/mortality to the patient. The extent of the patient's disease and the risk of the procedure must be taken into account.

Remember to control risk factors of disease. This may include tight glycemic control, dietary/medical control of hyperlipidemia, control of hypertension, and reduction of tobacco and alcohol use.

Take Home Points

- Amaurosis fugax and mild focal neurologic signs are classic symptoms for TIA.
- Evaluate the carotid circulation with duplex US; percentage of occlusion correlates with recommended treatment.
- The goal for obtaining neuroimaging in TIA patients is < 24 hours.
- Surgical management consists mainly of carotid endarterectomy (CEA).

Ischemic Stroke

Brain tissue ischemia from either cerebrovascular disease or cerebral embolism/thrombus blocking blood flow. Often occurring in distribution of the middle cerebral arteries (watershed areas). Risk factors include: age, hyperlipidemia, hypertension, coronary artery disease (CAD), smoking, diabetes, family history of CAD, atrial fibrillation, etc.

Symptoms

A variety of neurologic symptoms may be seen, including those in TIA. Classically, contralateral hemiplegia, hemianesthesia, and hemianopsia. Stroke may involve almost any neurologic presentation from very subtle stepwise deficit to evolving dementia to sudden coma or death.

Diagnosis

Physical exam: Increased temperature, change in mental status, focal neurologic changes such as paralysis, facial droop, "pronator drift," or focal anesthesia.

Labs: Coagulation profile including INR, CBC, electrolytes. Consider protein C/S, factor V Leiden, antithrombin, if coagulation profile is abnormal.

Imaging: Noncontrast CT is the standard first study to rule out bleeding. MRI remains the best test for diagnosis. MRA or arteriography may be useful in certain situations.

Carotid evaluation may be useful in the long term to find possible reversible cause but not useful in the acute setting. As in TIA, carotid duplex ultrasound is the standard.

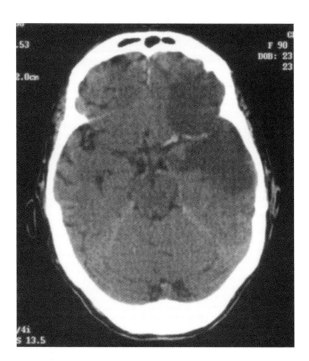

FIGURE 3.9 CT scan showing an acute middle cerebral territory infarction within a few hours of onset of neurological deficit. Note the increased density in the left middle cerebral artery representing a thrombus. The T2-weighted MRI scan of the same patient is shown in Figure 3.10. Reprinted with permission from Warrell DA, Cox TM, et al. *Oxford Textbook of Medicine*, 4th edition. 2003, Oxford University Press.

Treatment

Treatment of ischemic stroke should start with the ABCs, with particular attention to cardiac rhythm. Then be sure to give oxygen and fluids and obtain basic labs. Give antiplatelet medications as early as possible but only after intracranial hemorrhage is excluded with imaging.

Anticoagulation is controversial and under investigation. Giving heparin/warfarin must be done under strict guidelines and only after intercranial hemorrhage is definitively ruled out.

Antithrombotics such as tPA (Activase) or streptokinase are ultimately too complex for most test makers to ask about. Rules are extensive and these drugs should only be used on ideal, investigated candidates with symptom-onset-to-drug time ≤ 3 hours.

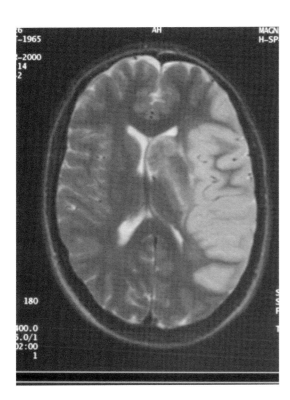

FIGURE 3.10 T2-weighted MRI scan of the same patient (Figure 3.9) showing the extensive high T2 signal affecting grey and white matter in the left middle cerebral artery territory. Reprinted with permission from Warrell DA, Cox TM, et al. *Oxford Textbook of Medicine*, 4th edition. 2003, Oxford University Press.

Blood pressure should only be controlled if very significantly elevated. Hypertension is a protective mechanism and should be allowed but monitored, even at hypertensive urgency levels.

After the stroke, control risk factors such as emboli source, hyperlipidemia, hypertension, smoking, diet, and exercise.

Rehabilitation is the main treatment of stroke. Significant function may be restored to affected areas by retraining with physical therapy and occupational therapy.

Take Home Points

- Ischemic strokes are commonly much less severe than hemorrhagic strokes.
- Localization of the affected area of the brain is the main diagnostic step. Most commonly, this may be done by symptom analysis rather than direct imaging.
- Rehabilitation is very important in stroke victim recovery.

Malignant Intracranial Neoplasm

Primary brain cancer is a result of undifferentiated cells in the brain. Different types include astrocytoma, medulloblastoma, oligodendroglioma, glioblastoma multiforme, glioma, schwannoma, ependymoma, meningioma, and craniopharyngioma. Secondary causes include metastasis commonly from breast, lung, kidney, and skin cancer.

Symptoms

In the broad sense, symptoms may be localizing or general and result from brain tissue effects localized to the lesion that may be peripheral, central, or specific. Mass effect may also develop, leading to generalized alteration of consciousness, seizure disorder, endocrine/electrolyte abnormalities, ocular problems, or herniation syndromes. Often, focal effects evolve slower than stroke or infection and may involve compensation mechanisms in the brain.

Diagnosis

Labs: Initial screening labs are important and should include electrolytes and renal function to evaluate for possible SIADH or other endocrine problems. CSF studies are rarely useful and should only be considered after a CT is performed to avoid herniation.

Imaging: CT to evaluate for mass effect, herniation, or acute bleeding. MRI is more accurate and may show lesions in better detail.

Biopsy by CT guided needle or examination after resection may indicate histology.

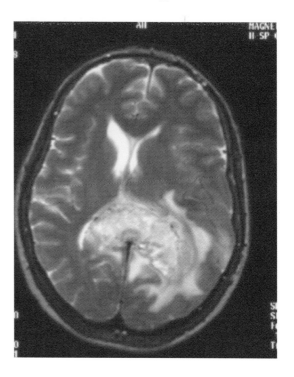

FIGURE 3.11 Axial T2-weighted image of a large glioblastoma involving the corpus callosum. Reprinted with permission from Warrell DA, Cox TM, et al. *Oxford Textbook of Medicine*, 4th edition. 2003, Oxford University Press.

Treatment

Treatment depends largely on the type of malignancy. Histology, stage, and progression determine therapeutic options in almost all cases.

Discrete lesions may be amenable to neurosurgery, radiation, or chemotherapy.

Consider palliative treatment as needed.

Discuss advanced directive choices with the patient and family.

Take Home Points

- The hallmark of intracranial tumor presentation is that of slow development of neurologic signs.

- Neurosurgical evaluation should be done with every intracranial lesion; however, due to the sensitivity of brain tissue and limited space available, palliation is commonly the only option.

Migraine

Etiology remains unclear, although undoubtedly involves intracranial vasculature. Types include: migraine with aura (classic migraine), without aura (common migraine), basilar, hemiplegic, ophthalmoplegic, menstrual, and chronic.

Symptoms

Classic type begins with aura that may consist of a smell or visual effect (commonly flashing lights or scotomata). Common type generally lacks this aura. Both are generally unilateral with severe pain, photophobia, phonophobia, nausea, vomiting, and may involve focal neurologic deficit. Migraine does not involve alteration of consciousness or seizure. The patient may state headaches are triggered by certain stimuli including bright lights, loud sounds, pungent odors, or other stimuli.

Diagnosis

Based mainly on typical history although exclusion with screening labs (CBC, BMP) and possibly brain imaging may be considered.

Imaging: May be clinically indicated in the non-typical patient, change in headache pattern, or onset of headaches at advanced age.

Treatment

Prophylaxis: Topoisomerase (Topamax) and β-blockers such as propanolol (Inderol) have been used with good success. Amytriptyline (Elavil) or other TCAs may also be useful. Valproate (Depokene) and verapamil have also been tried with mixed results.

Abortive: The triptan class has shown excellent results and includes sumatriptan (Imitrex), rizatriptan (Maxalt), naratriptan (Amerge), zolmatriptan (Zomig), and others. Ergots including dihydroergotamine (Migranal) and ergotamine/caffeine (Cafergot) may also be used but are absolutely contraindicated in pregnancy. Other combination drugs of the above with acetaminophen or NSAIDs exist.

Analgesics: Acetaminophen, ketorolac (Toradol), or NSAIDs may be very effective but may also not provide enough relief.

Patients with severe, acute symptoms may benefit from antiemetics (promethazine (Phenergan)) and, rarely, sedatives including non-hypnotics (zolpidem (Ambien)) or benzodiazapines.

Do not give opiates for migraine! Abuse potential is much too high!

Several natural remedies have also been tried but studies are lacking and conclusive evidence is scarce. These include such herbs as feverfew and butterbur.

Take Home Points

- Types include: migraine with aura (classic migraine), without aura (common migraine), basilar, hemiplegic, ophthalmoplegic, menstrual, and chronic.

- Imaging may be useful in new diagnosis or change in headache pattern to exclude other diagnoses, but should be normal in the migraine patient.

- Treatment should consist of the combination of prophylactic medications and as needed abortive medications. Further treatment should be symptom based.

Headache

TABLE 3.7 Common Headache Types

	Cluster	Tension	Caffeine Withdrawal
Symptoms	Usually unilateral, associated with periorbital and temporal areas. May involve tearing of the eye, nasal symptoms, facial sweating, ptosis, or miosis. Patients tend to be male and pace during acute attacks.	Bilateral and radiating from the posterior neck to frontal area. Often worse in the PM or after exhausting day.	Bilateral and stabbing. Occurs in patients with high caffeine intake or recent attempt at reducing/quitting.
Associations	More common in men. Characteristically waxes and wanes in frequency over period of months.	Associated with muscle spasm or tightness on exam.	Caffeine-related
Treatment	High flow oxygen with non-rebreather mask, verapamil for prophalaxis, systemic steroids, indomethacin (Indocin), or a triptan for abortive effect.	NSAIDs or acetaminophen. Massage can be effective.	Long absence of caffeine to break addiction. Some commercial analgesics contain caffeine (Excedrin) and thus are "very effective" at treating this headache.

Delirium

A temporary, reversible state of acute change in mental status, abnormal attention, or disorganized thinking. Reversible causes are most often seen in the advanced elderly and include infection, ischemia (cardiac or brain), metabolic insult, or psychiatric disturbance.

Symptoms

Very similar presentation to dementia. Differences include more rapid onset of global (as opposed to recent) memory loss. Sundowning that may include hallucinations, illusions, and delusions may coexist. Arousal level and attention span are impaired.

Diagnosis

Based on history and physical exam. There should be a demonstrable reason for the delirium and that, by definition, is reversible.

Labs: Vitamin B12/folate, thyroid function, electrolyte level, endocrine work up, VDRL, brain imaging, BUN/creatinine, and liver function should all be investigated as possible sources. Check CBC, UA/urine culture.

Imaging: Chest X-ray to investigate for infectious cause.

Consider "pseudodementia" and screen for depression.

Treatment

Treat the underlying cause! Reversal can be dramatic.

Take Home Points

- Distinguish between dementia and delirium by recognizing the causative agent of delirium.
- Exclude depression as a cause of pseudodementia.

Syncope

Syncope involves the transient loss of consciousness and may be associated with a fall. This disorder is often split into causes that affect the heart, such as arrhythmias or ischemia; or neurologic, such as seizure or anxiety. The most common benign cause is neurocardiogenic (vasovagal) syncope in which interplay between neurologic and vascular compensatory mechanisms for blood pressure preservation are not maintained, producing a transient lack of blood flow to the brain.

Symptoms

Associated symptoms may include aura if the cause is seizure, including: lightheadedness, vertigo, sweating, feeling of flushing/heat, tachycardia, fibrillations, chest pain, coughing, nausea, vomiting, micturition, or visual disturbance. History may indicate locking of the knees, sudden stress, rising quickly from seated/lying position, history of indicative cause, turning head abruptly, wearing tight collars (which suggest carotid sinus massage), or malingering.

Diagnosis

Largely based on history and physical. Assess volume status clinically and obtain postural blood pressures.
Labs: Glucose level, BUN/creatinine, electrolytes, and CBC. Consider cardiac ischemic enzymes in the high-risk patient.
Imaging: Generally not indicated unless trauma, mass effect, or intracranial tumor is suspected.
 ECG/Holter monitor may be helpful to investigate possible ischemia and arrhythmias.
 Echocardiology may be useful for structural abnormalities or steal syndrome.
 EEG to investigate possible seizures.
 Head-up tilt table (HUT) testing may be of use to elicit vasovagal response.
Carotid sinus massage: Can be dangerous and cause cardiac arrhythmias or asystole when used for diagnosis. For test purposes, do not use this as a screening test and only consider with cardiac monitoring and support personnel.

Treatment

Depends on the cause.
 Hydrate aggressively to eliminate possibility of dehydration etiology.
 Neurocardiogenic (vasovagal syncope) reaction: Behavioral modification and warning sign recognition. Breathing exercises have shown success in some people.
 Anticonvulsants for seizure disorder (see section on **Seizure Disorder**).
Referral and treatment of cardiac anomaly may be indicated.

Take Home Points

- Syncope should be classified as cardiac, neurologic, or other.
- Often, work up of both cardiac and neurologic systems needs to be complete before finding a definitive etiology.
- Diagnosis and treatment are especially important in older adults since falls may cause multiple serious injuries.

Tremor

TABLE 3.8 Tremor Types

Tremor Type	Symptoms	Associations/Diagnosis	Treatment
Resting	Fine tremor usually of the hands	Parkinson, Wilson	Physical measures such as weights or conscious control methods.
Intention	Oscillation intensifies on movement toward a target	Cerebellar outflow diseases such as multiple sclerosis	Treat underlying disease. Otherwise none effective.
Physiologic	Usually mild and may occur with rest or movement	Some degree is normal. Otherwise strongly associated with anxiety/stress.	Treat the cause or remove the stress. Infrequent benzodiazepines in low doses. Propranolol (Inderal) or primidone (Mysoline) may be effective for acute stressful states.
Essential (benign hereditary)	Noticed with skilled tasks. Affects hands, head, and voice.	Hereditary. Often seen in elderly.	Benzodiazepines in low doses. Propranolol (Inderal) or primidone (Mysoline) may be effective. Physical measures such as weights or conscious control methods.

Insomnia

The vast majority of individuals will experience insomnia at one time in their lives. However, pathologic insomnia refers to those who are unable to eventually achieve reliable sleep despite significant behavioral and lifestyle modification. In many cases, a thorough sleep history reveals lack of overall sleep time, excessive sleep time (inconsistent sleep hygiene), excessive stimulant intake (caffeine, etc), or occupational shift work.

Symptoms

Trouble falling asleep, staying asleep, or early morning awakening. History may reveal poor sleep habits, use of stimulants/caffeine in excessive amounts or frequency. Patients may report irregular sleep hours or travel and may have external arousals such as young children.

Diagnosis

A good sleep history and sleep diary are very useful. Evaluate specifically for caffeine, nicotine, alcohol, decongestant, prescription, or illicit drug use.
Labs: Obtain a TSH.
Screen for depression.
Sleep testing only in advanced, refractory cases.

Treatment

Behavioral modifications to include: regular sleep schedule, regular bedtime routine, sleep-conducive environment, relaxation techniques, regular exercise, avoidance of stimulants and diuretics.

Pharmacologic options include low addictive potential medications such as zolpidem (Ambien), zaleplon (Sonata), ramelteon (Rozerem), and eszopiclone (Lunesta). Other options include benzodiazepines including temazepam (Restoril), flurazepam (Dalmaine), triazolam (Halcion), estazolam

(Prosom), lorazepam (Ativan), and clonazepam (Klonopin). When prescribing these medications, keep in mind addiction potential is very high from both drug effect and psychological dependence.

Other medications include antihistamines such as: diphenhydramine (Benedryl), hydroxyzine (Vistaril), and TCAs such as amitriptyline (Elavil), mainly for their side effect of drowsiness. Trazodone (Desyrel) is also effective.

Valerian, melatonin, warm milk, and turkey are herbal and cultural alternatives but none, to date, have been conclusively shown with consistent research to benefit insomnia patients.

Take Home Points

- Insomnia is very common. History of sleep habits, stimulant or depressant ingestion, and accompanying symptoms usually reveals the etiology.

- Non-hypnotic sedatives have recently shown excellent advancement, leading to a significant increase in pharmacologic options. However, monitor for psychological dependence.

Coma

The abnormal state of inarousability and decreased consciousness. Etiologies are many including metabolic disturbance, traumatic brain injury, stroke (ischemic or hemorrhagic), global anoxia, as well as many others.

Symptoms

Profound inability to arouse consciousness through any means including painful stimuli. Primitive neurologic reflexes may be present upon stimuli and include decorticate/decerebrate posturing. Often, history is unknown, but if witnesses are present may reveal underlying disorder. Breathing may be irregular if metabolic derangement is present, e.g. Cheyne-Stokes respiration.

Diagnosis

Physical exam: Evaluate Glasgow coma score, breathing pattern, and breath odor. Evaluate pupil reactivity and appearance.

TABLE 3.9 Glasgow Coma Scale

Eye	Verbal	Motor
Non spontaneous	No verbal	No motor response
Response to pain	Unintelligible sounds	Extension to pain
Response to verbal	Inappropriate speech	Flexion to pain
Spontaneous	Confused	Withdrawal from pain
	Oriented	Localizing to pain
		Obeys commands
4	5	6

Scored 3–15
≥ 13 Mild brain injury
9–12 Moderate brain injury
≤ 8 "Intubate"

Labs: Glucose level, ABG, drug screen (including EtOH), ammonia level, CBC, basic metabolic panel, coagulation panel, liver function and transaminases (AST/ALT), blood cultures, d-dimer, and calcium. Consider gastric lavage if poisoning is on the differential.

Imaging: Acutely obtain CT and evaluate for possible bleed/herniation. MRI may also be useful but is much slower. Don't forget to get a chest X-ray.

Lumbar puncture is indicated if CT/retinal exam is not indicative of increased ICP.

EEG may be performed if all other tests are negative and may give clue to nonconvulsive status epilepticus.

Treatment

Treat the underlying cause.

Minimal treatment usually includes ABCs, thiamine (before glucose), oxygen, temperature control, and fluids (with dextrose depending on glucose level).

Don't give reversal drugs such as naloxone (Narcan) or flumazenil (Romazicon) unless you are confident of the cause.

Control shock if present.

Take Home Points

- Causes: AEIOU TIPPS: Alcohol, Epilepsy/Electrolytes, Insulin, Opiates, Uremia, Trauma, Infection, Poison, Psych, Stroke.

- Obtain CT scan of the brain and toxicology screen on anyone presenting with coma if the cause is not otherwise obvious.

Brain Death

This condition may be equated to death itself although organs and tissues other than the brain may continue to live. This is an important condition since many states/countries classify brain death as legal demise.

Diagnosis

Exclude etiologies that may mimic condition such as neuromuscular blockade, toxins, metabolic derangement, hypothermia, and hypotension. Remember "nobody's dead until they're warm and dead," i.e. warm all patients to exclude possibility of hypothermia.

Inform or make reasonable attempt to contact next of kin.

Tests of Brain Death

Oculocephalic/oculovestibular reflex: When turning head rapidly from side to side patient does not exhibit "doll's eyes" as a normal person would.

Reactivity of pupils to light is negative.

Gag reflex is negative.

Caloric response reflex: Flushing the ears with cold water does not produce nystagmus.

Apnea test: Stopping mechanical ventilation for at least 8 minutes and monitoring respiratory movement. $PaCO_2$ must increase >20 mmHg from pretest baseline or rise above 55 mmHg for adequate test.

EEG shows electrical silence.

Four vessel cerebral angiography shows no blood flow.

The special tests above should be done at least twice, 2 hours apart, if both batteries are negative, the person is brain dead.

Take Home Points

- Brain death is considered legal demise in many states/countries.

- Tests for evaluation include: oculocephalic/oculovestibular reflex, pupil reactivity, gag reflex, caloric response reflex, apnea test, EEG, and four vessel cerebral angiography.

- Check with legal counsel for specific definitions in individual cases.

4   Special Senses

Ophthalmology

Diabetic Retinopathy

Primarily, diabetic retinopathy is related to the relative hyperglycemic state of diabetes mellitus (DM) patients although the exact pathogenesis remains unknown. Death of retinal pericytes and microvascular endothelial cells leads to thickening of the retinal basement membrane and formation of microaneurysms which exude lipids and proteinacious material, causing ischemia and the release of vasoproliferative compounds. After some time, these changes cause occlusion of the retinal microvasculature leading to rupture and more ischemia, causing this harmful cycle to repeat.

Symptoms

May present as gradual visual loss, difficulty reading, blurred vision, halos around lights, or dark spots in visual field. Neovascularization can be a leading cause of vision loss; evidence is seen on exam.

Diagnosis

Retinal exam may show "dot and blot" or "flame-shaped" hemorrhages which are caused by retinal vessel occlusion and leakage or "cotton wool" spots that occur from microinfarcts, resulting in decreased retinal perfusion. Retinal edema may also be seen and if long standing can lead to visible leakage from microaneurysms termed "hard exudates."

Imaging: Fluorescein angiography may be used to further evaluate disease.

Stages of development of diabetic retinopathy

Background diabetic retinopathy

Preproliferative diabetic retinopathy

Proliferative diabetic retinopathy

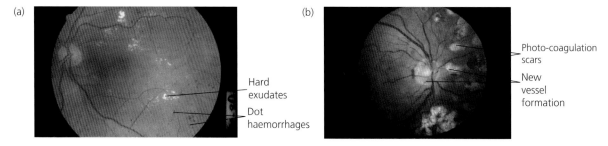

FIGURE 4.1 Diabetic retinopathy. (a) Background retinopathy, (b) proliferative retinopathy. Reprinted with permission from Cox NLT, Roper TA. *Clinical Skills*. 2005, Oxford University Press.

Treatment

Diabetics should be referred for ophthalmology exam annually.

Otherwise good control of glucose levels and blood pressure are very effective.

Panretinal laser photocoagulation may be helpful in proliferative retinopathy with neovascularization.

Treatment of nonproliferative retinopathy consists of laser photocoagulation only to the affected area.

For retinal hemorrhage, vitrectomy may be indicated.

Take Home Points

- This is the most common cause of blindness in diabetics.
- Diabetic retinopathy results from hyperglycemia-related damage and neovascularization of the retina.
- Treatment consists of referral to ophthalmology and use of laser photocoagulation.

Age-Related Macular Degeneration

Age-related central vision loss which is classified into two types:

Dry type (atrophic/non-exudative)—Due to macular focal/geographic chorioretinal thinning, subretinal drusen deposits, and pigment epithelial changes. Course is often slowly progressive.

Wet type (neovascular/exudative)—Growth of abnormal vessels in the choroidal circulation which are characterized by leaking and collections of subretinal fluid, and localized exudative retinal detachment and/or bleeding. The course is more acute than dry type, taking weeks to months to affect vision.

Symptoms

Painless visual loss often accompanied by visual distortion when looking at straight lines. Loss of vision affects the central visual field, not peripheral.

Risk factors include:

- Age
- Caucasian race
- Smoking
- Hypertension
- Vascular disease
- Fatty diet
- UV light exposure

Diagnosis

Retinal exam shows pigmentary or hemorrhagic disturbance in the macular region accompanied by drusen deposits.

Amsler chart of gridlines is often used to diagnose. Patient will see distorted lines. Fluorescein angiography also shows a neovascular membrane beneath the retina.

Treatment

Prevention with antioxidant use (vitamins A, C, E, zinc, and beta carotene) may prevent some degree of disease.

Dry type—Laser photocoagulation may be useful, although neovascularization is a significant complication. For others, assistive visual aides are the only treatment.

Wet type—Treatment may benefit some patients and includes: intravitreous injection of a vascular endothelial growth factor (VEGF) inhibitor (ranibizumab (Lucentis), bevacizumab (Avastin)), thermal laser photocoagulation, photodynamic therapy, and macular translocation surgery.

Both types benefit from risk factor control as a means of prevention.

Take Home Points

- Macular degeneration is one of the most common causes of visual loss.
- ARMD is caused by two types: the gradual dry type or brisk wet type.
- Treatment depends on type but prevention benefits either.

Retinal Detachments, Defects, and Disorders

TABLE 4.1 Retinal Detachments, Defects, and Disorders

Disorder	Description	Associations/Diagnosis	Treatment
Central retinal artery occlusion	Blockage of the central retinal artery, producing unilateral blindness.	Sudden, painless onset. Caused commonly by atherosclerosis, emboli (TIA), or **temporal arteritis**. Exam shows "cherry red" spot on retina.	Treatment must be immediate and consists of acetazolamide, ophthalmologic beta blocker, **manual massage** to closed eyelid, or anterior chamber paracentesis. Also important to protect other eye by treating temporal arteritis (if present) with systemic steroids.
Central retinal vein occlusion	Blockage of the central retinal vein producing gradual blindness/vision defects.	Gradual, painless vision loss. Commonly in elderly with glaucoma, DM, HTN. Exam often shows retinal hemorrhages in single quadrant of retina. Neovascularization is apparent. Fluorescein angiography can diagnose.	No good treatment available.
Retinal detachment	Separation of neural retina from underlying retinal pigment epithelium.	Associated with trauma but is painless vision loss. Floaters and flashes or curtain falling is classic. Direct visualization is key.	Immediate referral to ophthalmologist is key. Retinal reattachment or laser surgery may correct vision loss.

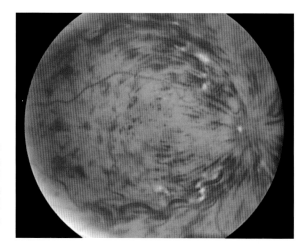

FIGURE 4.2 Central retinal vein occlusion. Note the "bloodstorm" appearance with profuse flame hemorrhages forming between the nerve fibers in all quadrants. Cotton wool spots representing microinfarcts are also present. Reprinted with permission from Warrell DA, Cox TM, et al. *Oxford Textbook of Medicine*, 4th edition. 2003, Oxford University Press.

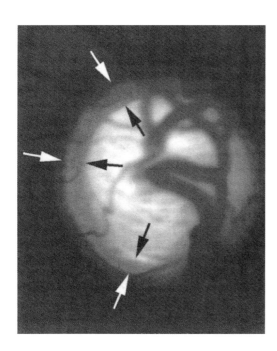

FIGURE 4.3 Retinal exam in open angle glaucoma. Note increased cup size (black arrows) as compared to optic disc (white arrows). Reprinted with permission from Silberstein SD, Lipton RB, Dalessio DJ. *Wolff's Headache and Other Head Pain*, 8th edition. 2007, Oxford University Press.

Glaucoma

A progressive ocular neuropathy with characteristic optic nerve changes and loss of peripheral visual fields. The causative factor is thought to be increased intraocular pressure (above 21–22 mmHg) which occurs due to several factors depending on the subtype of disease, although outflow tract obstruction to draining aqueous humor is the common theme.

Symptoms

This disorder affects peripheral visual fields.

Open angle glaucoma: This type represents 90% of glaucoma cases. Pressure ranges are commonly 20–30 mmHg. **Painless bilateral** visual loss is gradual over the course of years. Risk factors include black race, age > 60 years, DM, HTN, myopia, and family history.

Closed angle glaucoma: Rare type that is often tested but almost never seen. Sudden, **painful unilateral** vision changes. Halos around lights, red eye, nausea/vomiting, and vision loss are common.

Screening: The U.S. Preventative Services Task Force (USPSTF) found no evidence supporting a screening schedule for normal adults. The American Academy of Ophthalmology recommends yearly screening after age 20 at varying intervals. Since the test is quick and easy, at least screening of high risk groups is a reasonable approach.

Diagnosis

Screen by tonometry to assess intraocular pressure (IOP). Visual field testing and gonioscopy are also useful. Further imaging may include optical coherence tomography (OCT) to measure neurofiber layer thickness.

Open angle glaucoma: Exam reveals optic nerve changes with increased cup-to-disc ratio.

Closed angle glaucoma: Exam reveals fixed, dilated pupil with intraocular pressure > 30 mmHg. Palpation of globus with closed eyelid reveals noticeably hard eye. Retina reveals **cupping of the optic disc**.

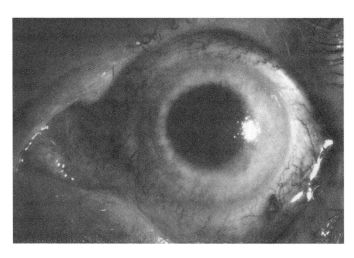

FIGURE 4.4 Acute angle-closure glaucoma. Note typical characteristics of the eye including edematous cornea, "steamy" dull appearance of light reflex, mid-dilated, somewhat irregularly shaped pupil, and injected conjunctiva. Reprinted with permission from Silberstein SD, Lipton RB, Dalessio DJ. *Wolff's Headache and Other Head Pain*, 8th edition. 2007, Oxford University Press.

Treatment

Open angle glaucoma: Start with medical treatment and progress to surgery after concurrent use of 3 agents fails. Classes of medications include: Miotics (pilocarpine, physostigmine, neostimine), carbonic anhydrase inhibitors (acetazolamide), α_2-selective adrenergic agonist (apraclonidine), β-blockers (Timolol), prostaglandins (Latanoprost), and osmotic diuretics (Mannitol, Glycerin).

Surgery includes argon laser trabeculoplasty, trabeculectomy (filtering surgery), shunt placement, or ciliary body ablation.

Closed angle glaucoma: Immediate referral to ophthalmology. Treat on the way with **pilocarpine, acetazolamide, timolol, and mannitol or glycerin**. Surgery may be warranted and includes peripheral iridectomy, argon laser iridotomy, or argon laser gonioplasty.

Take Home Points

- Glaucoma is commonly open angle, although acute painful glaucoma signals a closed angle.
- Screening is reasonable although beginning age and interval is not agreed upon.
- Treat with intraocular pressure lowering medications or surgery.

Cataracts

Opacification of the lens which occurs in a localized or generalized pattern. This is the leading cause of worldwide blindness and is associated with several types, including: age related (senile), congenital, toxic/nutritional (steroid use), systemic disease associated (myotonic dystrophy, atopic dermatitis), metabolic (diabetes, hypocalcemia, Wilson disease), complicated (uveitis associated with juvenile rheumatoid arthritis (JRA), sarcoid, etc.), or trauma (thermal burn, etc.).

Visual Field Defects

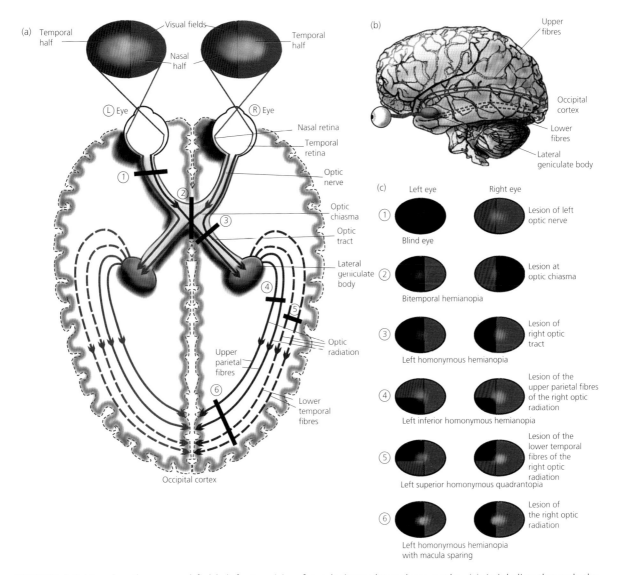

FIGURE 4.5 Visual pathways and field defects arising from lesions along these paths. (a) Axial slice through the brain at the level of the eyes, (b) lateral view of the brain, (c) visual defects associated with lesions indicated. Nerve impulses travel down the optic nerves (nasal fibers crossing at the optic chiasm) before traveling along the optic tracts to relay in the lateral geniculate bodies. The impulses then travel along the optic radiation to terminate in the occipital cortex. Ultimately the right occipital cortex is responsible for the left half of the visual fields and the left occipital cortex is responsible for the right. The brain is able to synthesize the visual stimuli and correct the inversion of the images to produce meaningful vision. Reprinted with permission from Cox NLT, Roper TA. *Clinical Skills*. 2005, Oxford University Press.

Symptoms

Painless, progressive loss of vision usually presenting at older age but may be congenital. Risk factors include old age, female gender, estrogen exposure, sunlight exposure, alcohol consumption, chronic or frequent steroid use, DM, and trauma (lightning strikes).

Diagnosis

Physical exam: Loss or absence of red reflex or grossly opacified lens on exam. Slit lamp exam indicated for diagnosis.

Treatment

Surgery is the mainstay and is one of the most commonly performed surgeries in the U.S. Replacement of the opacified lens with artificial implants dramatically corrects the problem. Surgery may, however, be postponed until significant disturbance in lifestyle is reported.

Take Home Points

- The majority of the geriatric population at some point will develop cataracts.
- The surgery is easy and very common; therefore a low threshold for surgery should be applied to this type of visual loss.

Visual Disturbances

TABLE 4.2 Types of Visual Disturbances

Term	Definition
Myopia	Nearsightedness. Focal point of incoming light is before it reaches the retina.
Hyperopia	Farsightedness. Focal point of incoming light is behind the retina.
Presbyopia	Age-related loss of ability to accommodate.
Astigmatism	When the cornea is steeper in one meridian than the other or the globe is irregularly shaped. Thus, light is not properly focused on the retina.
Diplopia	Double vision, i.e. seeing two images of a particular object. When diplopia exists after covering one eye, it's either malingering or corneal related. When it resolves when one eye is covered, it's likely neurological.

Treatment

Corrective devices such as glasses or contacts are usually very effective. New surgeries such as laser in situ keratomileusis (LASIK) or photorefractive keratectomy (PRK) are gaining popularity and are becoming very safe. Others include radial keratotomy (RK) and astigmatic keratotomy (AK) for mild myopia and astigmatism, respectively.

Conjunctivitis

Conjunctivitis is the inflammation of the conjunctiva which is the mucus membrane that lines the inside surface of the lids and covers the surface of the globe up to the limbus (the junction of the sclera and the cornea). Common etiologies include viruses, bacteria, allergic reaction, or mechanical irritation.

Symptoms

Redness, pain, irritation, tearing, and watering of the affected conjunctiva. Prominent features are almost always irritation and watering. Patients report waking up with "crusted over" eye. If viral, history of similar symptoms in casual contact and/or spread from contralateral eye is common. If bacterial, suspect *N. gonorrhoeae/Chlamydia trachomatis* in a neonate or sexually active adult. Allergic conjunctivitis is usually bilateral and involves trigger mechanisms leading to inflammation of the conjunctiva; history may reveal other concurrent symptoms. Mechanical conjunctivitis may be produced by foreign body, wind, snow reflection, dust, or smoke.

Diagnosis

Physical exam: Hyperemia and lacrimation of the affected eye. Vision and cornea are normal (unless foreign body is present). Slit lamp and glaucoma testing may be needed if history suggests foreign body or risk factors for glaucoma. If disease presents in the neonate after silver nitrate eye drops are placed (as in many newborn protocols; < 24 hours of life) source of irritation is most likely chemical.

Culture and gram stain may be taken of the discharge to evaluate for bacterial cause (Gram stain especially for *N. gonorrhoeae*); however, treat before results return if clinical suspicion is high.

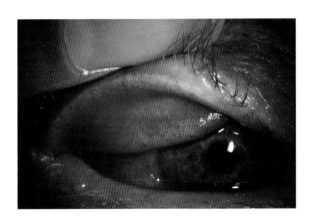

FIGURE 4.6 Severe conjunctivitis. Note the involvement of the upper eyelid's opposing conjunctival lining. Reprinted with permission from Cox NLT, Roper TA. *Clinical Skills.* 2005, Oxford University Press.

Treatment

Neonate:
   N. gonorrhoeae/Chlamydia (always treat the mother and treat for both organisms)→Ceftriaxone (Rocephin) and erythromycin.
Suppurative non-gonococcal, non-chlamydial:
   Bacitracin-polymixin B ophthalmic ointment/drops or erythromycin opth ointment.
Bacterial contact lens wearers (*Pseudomonas*):
   Tobramycin (Tobrex) or gentamicin (Genoptic) *plus* pipercillan or ticarcillan eye drops q15–60 minutes around the clock × 1–3 days.
Viral:
   Herpes simplex I or II—Trifluridine (Viroptic) eye drops.

Unknown viral:

Supportive care with cool artificial tear drops may help. Vasoconstrictors such as naphazoline (Nafcon) may help symptomatically.

Allergic:

Artificial tear drops, vasoconstrictors, and antihistamines such as azelastine (Optivar) and epinastine (Elestat). Other anti-allergy systemic medications may be used as indicated.

Take Home Points

- Conjunctivitis is most commonly caused by viruses, but other etiologies include bacterial, allergies, and mechanical irritation.

- Judgment should be made as to the presence of bacterial infection, thus, the need for antibiotics.

Disorders of the Eyelid and Lacrimal System

TABLE 4.3 Disorders of the Eyelid and Lacrimal System

Disorder	Associations/Diagnosis	Treatment
Dacryostenosis (nasolacrimal duct obstruction)	Common in the newborn period. Can be congenital or acquired. Exam shows overflow tearing and mild erythema of lacrimal opening.	Gentle fingertip **massage** BID is usually enough treatment but should resolve by 6 months. If not, dilation and probe may be needed.
Blepharitis	Presents with lid edema, pain, loss of eyelashes, and conjunctival irritation. May occur with seborrheic dermatitis. Usually *Staph Aureus*.	Bacitracin-polymixin B ointment and warm compresses. Monitor for common resistance.
Hordeolum (stye)	Usually *Staph* infection on single eyelid gland or eyelash follicle. Often seen after blepharitis.	**Warm compresses**. Will quickly form a small abscess that can then be squeezed or incised. If internal, PO nafcillin/oxacillin. Topical antibiotics usually ineffective.

Orbital Cellulitis

Cellulitis involving the tissues proximal to the orbital septum may be considered orbital and a true ophthalmic emergency. Distinguishing between orbital and pre-septal (periorbital) cellulitis is key to the urgency of treatment and prognosis of recovery. True orbital cellulitis may lead to permanent visual damage or even death from extension of infection from the optic nerve to the brain.

Symptoms

Orbital cellulitis involves severe pain around the eye, swelling, proptosis, impaired mobility of the eye, conjunctival hyperemia and edema, fever, and malaise. History of sinusitis, dental infection or procedure, or trauma may reveal inciting event.

The key point of exam is to determine if the condition is preseptal or orbital cellulitis. Orbital cellulitis has features including: proptosis, painful or impaired ocular motility, decreased visual acuity, or decreased color vision. Preseptal cellulitis does not.

Diagnosis

Exam: Increased temperature, eyelid swelling, erythema, painful or impaired ocular motility, decreased visual acuity, decreased color vision and proptosis.

Imaging: Stat CT scan. Features of orbital cellulitis include diffuse orbital infiltrate, proptosis with or without sinus opacity, and orbital abscess.

MRI is superior to CT scan but is less commonly used due to impracticality, greater availability of CT, and higher level of difficulty with pediatric patients.

Orbital ultrasound is useful in following orbital abscess resolution but less commonly available and is operator dependant.

Labs: Make sure to take local conjunctival cultures as well as blood and nasal discharge cultures.

Treatment

IV antibiotics to include cefuroxime (Ceftin), cefoxitin (Mefoxin), and cefotetan (Cefotan). Add nafcillin or vancomycin for better control of MSSA or methicillin-resistant *Staphylococcus aureus* (MRSA) coverage, respectively.

Consider surgical drainage if not resolved or improved in 36 hours.

Monitor closely for signs of spread to CNS and optic neuritis.

Ophthalmology consult is indicated in most cases.

Take Home Points

- Distinguish between orbital and preseptal cellulitis both clinically and with CT scan.

- Treatment is with admission and administration of IV antibiotics.

Pediatric Strabismus

Misalignment of one eye in relation to the other. The key complication of early strabismus in children is the development of amblyopia; a permanent defect of central visual processing leading to reduced visual field acuity (in the absence of structural abnormality).

Symptoms

Often observed in otherwise normal newborns in which the misalignment shows no specific favorite direction.

Esotropia: Strabismus in which the visual axes converge.

Exotropia: Strabismus in which the visual axes diverge.

Diagnosis

Physical exam: Disconjugate gaze.

Treatment

Treatment is generally only needed if strabismus persists beyond **4 months of age**.

Referral to ophthalmology is in order but therapy is likely to consist of corrective lenses, orthoptic training, and possibly surgery.

At the point of amblyopia, patching of the normal eye may be used to suppress the two unmatched images and thus force the affected eye into normal sight.

Take Home Points

- Newborn strabismus often corrects spontaneously.

- Correction should be made if strabismus persists beyond 4 months of age.

- Classic treatment for amblyopia remains patching of the good eye although corrective lenses or surgery may be used at the discretion of the ophthalmologist.

Nystagmus

A physical exam finding that shows rhythmic movements of the eyes, usually in unison.

Possible causes include: alcohol intoxication, illegal drug use, vestibular apparatus disease, vertigo, Meniere disease, water or fluid in outer or middle ear, or primary neurological disorder such as multiple sclerosis, stroke, or tumor.

Diagnosis

The vestibular system of each ear may be tested by installation of water in varying temperatures into the external ear canals. The direction of the resultant horizontal nystagmus (in the normal functioning patient) will be the same as in the pneumonic **COWS**→ **C**old **O**pposite, **W**arm **S**ame. Keep in mind "direction" indicates the direction of the short beat.

Imaging: MRI may be of value to find neurologic cause.

 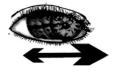

FIGURE 4.7 Nystagmus of the left eye on looking to the left. Reprinted with permission from Cox NLT, Roper TA. *Clinical Skills.* 2005, Oxford University Press.

Treatment

Treat the underlying cause. In vertigo (see Chapter 3: Diseases of the Nervous System), scopolamine (Scopace) or meclizine (Antevert) may be useful.

Take Home Points

- Nystagmus indicates derangement in the bodies or natural vestibular system, either peripherally or centrally.
- The most common cause of nystagmus is EtOH intoxication.
- Vertical nystagmus points toward multiple sclerosis or other central brain disease.

Uveitis

Uveitis is a term used to describe inflammation of the uveal tract including the iris, ciliary body, and choroid, and often includes adjacent structures such as the vitreous, retina, and optic nerve. Acute anterior uveitis accounts for about 90% of disease and involves the inflammation of the iris (iritis) and ciliary body (iridocyclitis) and may be associated with idiopathic disease, HLA-B27 carriers, infection (viral, bacterial, spirochetal, protozoan, netomatode, and fungal), systemic disease states (such as diabetes, sarcoidosis, etc.), vascular disease, renal disorders (such as IgA nephropathy), or other causes (Kawasaki disease, Schwartz syndrome, Posner-Schlossman syndrome, etc.).

Symptoms

Anterior uveitis commonly involves decreased visual acuity, deep eye pain, photophobia, conjunctival vessel dilation, or small pupillary size. Intermediate or posterior uveitis may present with decreased visual acuity, bilateral symptoms, floaters, and minimal pain or redness.

Diagnosis

Physical exam: Anterior uveitis: conjunctival vessel dilation, perilimbal dilation of vessels (ciliary flush), and fever, fatigue, etc if associated with systemic disease. Intermediate or posterior uveitis: visible inflammation of the chorioretinal structures on retinal exam and detection of leukocytes in the vitreous humor.

Slit lamp exam may be of particular use in anterior uveitis and show leukocytes and a haze termed "flare," representing protein accumulation in the aqueous humor.

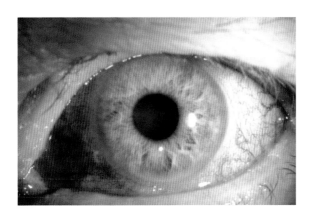

FIGURE 4.8 Anterior uveitis. Reprinted with permission from Cox NLT, Roper TA. *Clinical Skills*. 2005, Oxford University Press.

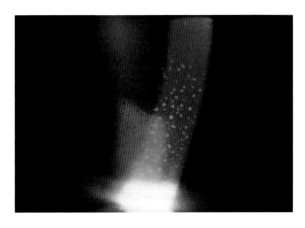

FIGURE 4.9 Slit lamp view of anterior uveitis associated with ankylosing spondylitis. Note cells in the anterior chamber which have sedimented on the interior surface of the cornea as white keratic precipitates. Reprinted with permission from Warrell DA, Cox TM, et al. *Oxford Textbook of Medicine*, 4th edition. 2003, Oxford University Press.

Treatment

Uveitis due to infection should be treated promptly with the appropriate anti-microbial therapy such as antiviral or antibacterial agents.

Anterior uveitis not due to infection can be given topical glucocorticoids and cycloplegics for pain control such as scopolamine (Isopto Hyoscine), homatropine (Isopto Homatropine), or cyclopentolate (Cyclogyl). Referral to ophthalmology is important.

Intermediate or posterior uveitis not due to infection usually does not respond to topical steroids and may benefit from systemic, periocular injection, intraocular injection or implant placement of glucocorticoids.

Systemic NSAID therapy may help for pain control.

Take Home Points

- Uveitis is the inflammation of the internal structures of the eye.
- Most commonly, uveitis occurs in the anterior structures.
- The cornerstone of treatment is glucocorticoid therapy and ophthalmologic referral.

Pterygium

A triangular elevated mass arising from the conjunctiva that invades the cornea. This may impede vision if invasion is extensive enough to involve the pupil. It may be related to sunlight, wind, previous chemical insult, or heat exposure. Usually this disease is not painful but may be unsightly and uncomfortable.

Treatment

Consists of referral to ophthalmologist and likely surgery. Medical treatment is ineffective.

Take Home Points

- Pterygium may impede vision if it extends to the pupil.
- Refer to ophthalmology for surgical treatment.

Corneal Abrasion

Corneal abrasion involves superficial corneal wounds and commonly occurs due to minor trauma to the eye but may also accompany foreign body injury. Thus, in evaluation of corneal abrasion, always examine carefully for foreign bodies.

Symptoms

Exquisite and extreme unilateral eye pain. Often the feeling of foreign body is present even if none actually exists in the eye. Other signs are excessive tearing, hyperemia, and photophobia.

Diagnosis

Fluorescein staining and Wood's lamp (blacklight) exam are very useful in making diagnosis. If positive, do a slit lamp exam to show defect in better detail. Make sure to examine closely with lid eversion for foreign bodies.

Treatment

Topical anesthetic is certainly warranted. Consider irrigation of the eyes for at least 15 minutes if history suggests chemical splash or metal foreign body.

Give erythromycin, tobramycin (Tobrex), or bacitracin-polymyxin B eye drops for antibacterial coverage.

Systemic opioids for pain relief.

Avoid contact lens use.

The cornea is one of the fastest healing tissues of the body. Symptoms should significantly improve in 48 hours.

Take Home Points

- Corneal abrasion and foreign body often present together.
- Pain is usually exquisite so pain control will be a priority to the patient.

Mastoiditis

Inflammation and purulent discharge within the mastoid air cells, most commonly from extension of otitis media.

Symptoms

Ear pain, postauricular or supra auricular swelling, erythema, pain, hearing loss, fever, and headache are most common.

Diagnosis

Physical exam: Erythematous, bulging, and possibly suppurative tympanic membrane. Palpable mass, swelling, and tender area either above or behind the ear.

Labs: CBC may show leukocytosis.

Imaging: Plain mastoid films may reveal clouding of the air cells. CT shows air cells in better detail and may show loss of septation between them.

Myringotomy may yield fluid for culture and gram stain for organism identification and sensitivities.

Treatment

Treat acute otitis media (AOM) before complications can develop. Empiric antibiotic choice is same as for AOM.

Myringotomy with placement of pressure equalization (PE) tube with culture of the fluid. Tailor antibiotic regimen to cultures.

Complications include subperiosteal abscess or extension of infection into the neighboring meninges and brain. Monitor for these complications.

Mastoidectomy is reserved for refractory or complicated cases (CNS involvement).

Take Home Points

- Mastoiditis commonly occurs in conjunction with otitis media.
- Monitor for CNS complications.

Otitis Media

A disease of mostly children, otitis media is thought of as an inflammatory state of the middle ear. A joint committee of the American Academy of Pediatrics (AAP) and the American Academy of Family Physicians (AAFP) determined the need for three clinical criteria for the diagnosis of acute otitis media. These include: history of acute presentation with typical symptoms, signs/symptoms of acute middle ear inflammation, and presence of middle ear effusion. Classic organisms are *S pneumoniae*, *H influenza*, and *M catarrhalis*, although many infections are idiopathic or of mixed flora.

Symptoms

Ear pain, otorrhea, fever, ear fullness, decreased or loss of hearing. Often after upper respiratory infection or rhinitis. Non-modifiable risk factors include low socio-economic factors, young age, Native American or Eskimo ethnicity, or family history. Modifiable risk factors include exposure to tobacco smoke, pacifier use, "bottle propping" when bottle feeding, and sleep position.

Diagnosis

Physical exam: Erythematous, inflamed tympanic membrane (TM). TM may be bulging, retracted, show air fluid level (indicating middle ear effusion), resistant to pneumatic movement, or show rupture. Pus may be present in external canal. Fever is often present in the young.

Treatment

Remember, monitoring without antibiotics is an option! Especially in the older child or adult when diagnosis is not clear.

Control pain with NSAIDs, Tylenol, or topical analgesics like benzocaine (Auralgan).

Treat with antibiotics in young child if diagnosis is certain or in children < 6 months old even if not. Recommendations are for amoxicillin or amoxicillin/clavulonate (Augmentin) for 7–10 days. Use ceftriaxone (Rocephin) for three days as an alternative.

Control modifiable risk factors.

Consider tympanostomy in:

- Children who have structural damage to the tympanic membrane or middle ear.

- Children who have otitis media of 4 months duration with persistent hearing loss or other signs/symptoms.

- Children with recurrent or persistent otitis media who are at risk of speech, language, or learning problems, regardless of hearing status.

- Close follow up in 48–72 hours is strongly recommended.

Take Home Points

- Otitis media is diagnosed by the presentation of acute onset of symptoms, signs/symptoms of middle ear inflammation, and middle ear effusion.

- Distinguish otitis media from non-inflammatory middle ear effusion (MEE).

- Treat with watchful waiting, antibiotics, or tympanostomy if certain criteria are met.

Cholesteatoma

A tumor-like growth of desquamated, stratified, squamous epithelium within the middle ear space. As keratin desquamates from the epithelial lining of the middle ear canal, it gradually enlarges, causing eventual erosion of the ossicles, mastoid air cells, and external auditory structures. Formation of a cholesteatoma typically occurs after a retraction pocket has formed in the posterior/superior quadrant and may be linked to recurrent otitis media, tympanic membrane trauma, or inflammatory/iatrogenic perforation.

Symptoms

Sensineural or conductive hearing loss, vertigo, disequilibrium, facial paralysis (from pressure on the facial nerve), and if left untreated may progress to meningitis, brain abscess, or sepsis.

Diagnosis

Physical exam: Otoscopy may reveal a tumor-like structure in the posterior/superior quadrant of the visible TM or perforation of the TM. External ear canal may contain mucopurulent or granulation tissue. Magnification otoscopy gives a more accurate exam.

Imaging: CT scan may be helpful but MRI with visualization of the middle ear is best.

Audiology assessment should be done as part of the standard work up.

Treatment

Surgical excision is the standard and may consist of tympanomastoidectomy.

Take Home Points

- Cholesteotomas are significant sources of hearing loss in adults and children.
- Imaging consists of MRI and treatment is surgical.

Vertiginous Disorders

Disorders that cause vertigo or dizziness are varied and include medications (benzodiazepines, opiates, diuretics), infection (labyrinthitis, otitis media/interna, HIV), metabolic derangement (hyponatremia, diabetes), oncologic (Schwannoma, primary brain cancer), primary CNS disorders (MS, temporal lobe epilepsy), and idiopathic causes (benign paroxysmal positional vertigo, Meniere disease). Vertigo tends to occur with greater frequency in the elderly.

Symptoms

Vertigo, dizziness, lightheadedness. These may be accompanied by ear pain, blurry vision, tinnitus, or nausea/vomiting. Many etiologies exist but a strong history of when symptoms are worse and when they started is key. Focus history on trauma, recent viral infection, alcohol use, drug/medication use, or vasculitis.

Diagnosis

Physical exam: Nystagmus is common. Neurologic signs such as focal deficits, agnosia, or ataxia may be present. Ear exam may show hemotympanum, or ear inflammation. Perform Rhomberg test for balance and Weber and Rinne tests (to distinguish sensorineural from conductive hearing loss).

Tests include caloric stimulation test and Dix-Hallpike maneuver.

Imaging: MRI is best for imaging brain and cerebellum, thin cut CT useful in evaluation of acute stroke in cerebellum.

Treatment

Depends on disease and etiology.

Various maneuvers (Epley, Brandt-Daroff, etc.) exist for therapy of benign paroxysmal positional vertigo.

Medications include the standard; meclizine (Antivert), scopolamine (Scopace), dimenhydrinate (Dramamine), or diphenhydramine (Benedryl). However, all have side effect of drowsiness and care must be taken in the elderly. Prochlorperazine (Compazine), promethazine (Phenergan), metoclopramide (Reglan), and ondansetron (Zofran) are very effective for nausea and vomiting. Benzodiazepines may also be used for sedation.

Take Home Points

- Vertigo may be due to a myriad of causes and is more common in the elderly.
- Treatment may consist of anticholinergics or antihistamines.

Tinnitus

Perceived sound that is not associated with an external source. Types include continuous, intermittent, or pulsatile. Categories of etiology are vascular, neurogenic, eustachian tube dysfunction, or others.

Ototoxic drugs may be found in the history and are often aminoglycosides, ACE-inhibitors, or anti-malarials, just to name a few. Approximately 50 million people in the U.S. have this disorder, with a majority reporting a significant impact on their daily life.

Symptoms

Patient may experience buzzing, ringing, whistling, roaring, or hissing. Obtain detailed history of tone, timing, characteristic, and quality to determine possible areas of dysfunction.

Diagnosis

Physical exam: Otoscopy is important; also look for neurologic symptoms, nystagmus, possible vascular disease, etc. No one physical exam trait reveals diagnosis.

Imaging: Head imaging with MRI, CT, or angiography may be reasonable based on history, looking for vascular or tumor origin.

Audiometry is a must.

Treatment

Treat the underlying cause if identified.

Tinnitus retraining therapy, masking devices, biofeedback techniques, and cognitive behavioral therapy are also proven options.

Take Home Points

- Tinnitus may occur due to dysfunction anywhere along the hearing axis.

- There is no cure for tinnitus but therapy may lessen symptoms.

Hearing Loss

Obvious hearing loss or deafness may follow a sudden or gradual course and be associated with acute or chronic loud noises, systemic disease, metabolic derangements, localized ear disease, drugs (aminoglycosides, etc.), or ear trauma.

Symptoms

Sudden, acute hearing loss may be associated with sound trauma such as an explosion or percussion event. Presbycusis, or age-related hearing loss, starts with loss of high frequency sound that progresses. Other causes have unique presentations but all are unified by decrease in hearing sense.

Diagnosis

Physical exam: Otoscopy important to evaluate for infection, tympanosclerosis, cerumen impaction, middle ear effusion (MEE), or TM perforation.

Weber test: Apply tuning fork to midline vertex of the head, if sound is loudest in the deaf ear, conductive hearing loss is present; if loudest in normal ear, sensorineural hearing loss is present.

Rinne test: Apply tuning fork to mastoid process of each ear, then next to ear without touching the head. Time in seconds until the sound is not heard is recorded. Normally, air conduction hearing is 2 times longer than bone conduction. If bone conduction longer than air, conductive hearing loss is present. If air conduction is less than twice as long as bone, sensorineural hearing loss is present.

Audiometry is a must.

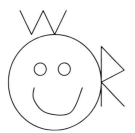

FIGURE 4.10 Simple figure to show placement positions of tuning fork for Weber and Rinne tests.

Imaging: Consider MRI, CT scan to evaluate for CNS lesion or cholesteatoma.

Treatment

Treat etiology if simple and identified.

Most conditions warrant referral to an otorhinolaryngologist who will evaluate for treatment. Some conditions require surgery or targeted therapy. Don't miss the treatable causes such as acoustic tumor, cholesteatomas, acute rupture, otosclerosis, etc. Treatment also includes hearing aids or cochlear implants.

In acute sound trauma hearing loss, consider a course of oral steroids to prevent localized inflammation. Steroid use is not definitively proven effective but is practiced by many experts.

Refer to ENT as needed.

Take Home Points

- Presbycusis (age-related hearing loss) results in the loss of high frequency sounds.
- Treat the underlying cause, if possible.

Peritonsillar Abscess (Quinsy)

Infection and abscess formation in the retropharyngeal space between the anterior and posterior tonsillar pillars and the superior pharyngeal constrictor muscle. This space is especially vulnerable to abscess formation from extension of acute tonsillitis or pharyngitis.

Symptoms

Extreme sore throat, odynophagia, dysphagia, trismus, fever, "hot potato voice," or drooling or pooling of saliva in the mouth.

Diagnosis

Physical exam: Erythematous posterior pharynx, unilaterally swollen tonsil, contralaterally displaced uvula, and cervical lymphadenopathy.
Labs: CBC reveals leukocytosis; culture any aspirated fluid.
Imaging: Ultrasound often shows fluid-filled cavity. CT scan also shows abscess pocket well.

Treatment

Incision and drainage under operative conditions or needle aspiration have shown equal efficacy. Culture the fluid in either case. When performing the procedure, have capabilities for intubation ready if needed. Recurrence after drainage and antibiotic use is uncommon.

If recurrence occurs, consider tonsillectomy.

Classic antibiotic is penicillin. Start with IV or IM dosing then switch to PO. Add metronidazole (Flagyl) if gram negative coverage needed. Alternatives include cephalosporins. Tailor regimen to cultures if possible.

Take Home Points

- Peritonsillar abscess often occurs in conjunction or after acute pharyngitis or tonsillitis.
- Abscess formation or complications of it may cause airway obstruction.
- Needle aspiration or I/D (incision and drainage) procedure are indicated with concomitant antibiotic administration.

Allergic Rhinitis

A rhinitis syndrome characterized by the allergen-mediated hypersensitivity reaction involving IgE antibody controlled mast cell degranulation and release of several inflammatory mediators such as histamine and prostaglandins. This release results in local infiltration of eosinophils, neutrophils, basophils, and mononuclear cells.

Symptoms

Congestion, nasal stuffiness, rhinorrhea (usually clear), sneezing, watery/ reddened eyes, and itching of the eyes, nose, and palate. Often allergic rhinitis is seasonal but it may be triggered by known allergens such as pet dander or dust.

Diagnosis

Physical exam: Red, runny, and possibly swollen turbinates. Blood may be present from local irritation. Look for associated nasal polyps.
Labs: Often unnecessary, but nasal washings show many eosinophils.
Patch skin testing or RAST (radioallergosorbent test) may be useful in finding the specific allergy. Often does not add anything to treatment.
Imaging: Radiographs may show opacity of nasal areas, CT for sinus evaluation is often unnecessary.

Treatment

Avoid the allergen if known.
Intranasal, oral, or ophthalmic medications as listed.

TABLE 4.4 Treatment of Allergic Rhinitis

Class	Examples
Antihistamines (H1 blockers)	Diphenhydramine (Benedryl) Hydroxyzine (Atarax)
Antihistamines (second generation)	Loratadine (Claritin) Fexofenadine (Allegra) Cetirizine (Zyrtec)
Decongestants	Pseudoephedrine Phenylephrine nasal spray
Mast cell stabilizers	Cromolyn (Nasalcrom, Gastrocrom) Olopatadine (Patonol) eye drops

(continued)

TABLE 4.4 Continued

Class	Examples
Leukotriene antagonist	Montelukast (Singular)
Intranasal steroids	Fluticasone (Flonase) Mometasone (Nasonex) Budesonide (Rhinocort) Flunisolide (Nasalide, Nasarel)
Intranasal anticholinergic	Ipratropium (Atrovent nasal)
Direct vasoconstrictor	Oxymetazoline (Afrin) Warning: do not use > 5 days
Saline nasal spray	Saline water

Allergy shot desensitization is useful in some but requires referral to allergist.

Take Home Points

- Eliminate infectious causes of rhinitis before assuming allergies are present.
- Intranasal steroids or antihistamines (2nd generation) are commonly used as first line therapy.
- Restrict or avoid use of direct vasoconstrictor medications such as oxymetazoline (Afrin) due to the side effect of reactive congestion upon d/c.

Nasal Malformations

TABLE 4.5 Nasal Malformations

Disorder	Associations	Treatment
Nasal polyps	Asthma, nose picking, aspirin sensitivity	Surgery
Deviated nasal septum	Snoring, breathing problems	Surgery

Epistaxis

Bleeding from the anterior or posterior nasal mucosa. Occurrence is extremely common in children but recurrent and uncontrollable bleeds should prompt investigation of blood dyscrasia or intranasal abnormality.

Symptoms

Blood loss from the nares signifies an anterior source such as Kiesselbach's plexus.

Blood loss from posterior nasal opening causing post nasal drip, hemoptysis, hematemesis, anemia, or melena is most often a posterior nasal source.

History may reveal cause including trauma, sensitivity to low humidity, coagulopathy, foreign body, or intranasal drug use.

Diagnosis

Physical exam: Standard otoscopy may reveal source. Pharyngeal exam may show blood but this is not solely indicative of posterior bleeding.

Labs: CBC for hematocrit. Consider toxicology screen if drug use suspected. PT/aPTT/INR to evaluate for bleeding dyscrasias.

Imaging: Often unnecessary unless fracture or tumor is suspected. Plain radiographs or CT may be helpful for these.

Nasal endoscopy if the source can't be identified and bleeding is not controlled (which also makes the procedure difficult).

Treatment

Apply direct pressure to the anterior nares (with or without packing) for 15–20 minutes. This stops the majority of bleeds.

Anterior bleeds: Phenylephrine nasal spray or oxymetazoline (Afrin) may vasoconstrict adequately. Anterior nares packing is also effective. Tampons are very useful for this and may be expanded by adding water after insertion.

Posterior bleeds: Often otorhinolaryngologist is consulted. Placement of specialized inflatable packing balloons (rhino-rocket) is ideal. A Foley catheter balloon will suffice if packing balloon not available. Insert through anterior nares and inflate for tamponade effect.

Packing or balloon tamponade usually left in place for 1–3 days.

Surgical cauterization with laser or electrocautery may be needed if bleeding uncontrolled and perfuse.

Take Home Points

- Anterior epistaxis accounts for the vast majority of nasal mucosal bleeding.
- Direct pressure or nasal packing is commonly effective.

Sinusitis

Inflammation in the paranasal sinuses leads to sinus outflow tract blockage and retained secretions which then become susceptible to secondary bacterial infection and worsening local inflammation.

Acute: Disease < 4 weeks duration.

Chronic: Disease > 8–12 weeks duration.

Symptoms

Unilateral facial pain above or below the eyes, increased pain on leaning forward, maxillary toothache, purulent rhinorrhea, headache, or fever. History importantly may reveal **"second sickening,"** meaning symptoms initially improved then worsen. Patient may also report history of sinusitis.

Diagnosis

Physical exam: Swollen, erythematous turbinates with purulent discharge. Unilateral frontal or maxillary sinus tenderness. Maxillary tooth tenderness, facial erythema or swelling, visual changes, or change in mental status are particularly concerning.

Imaging: Acute sinusitis often does not need imaging. Plain x-ray (either 4-view standard or **Waters' view**) in a chronic setting may reveal air-fluid levels, mucosal thickening, or opacification of sinuses although these are low specificity. Plain x-ray is limited, depending on which sinus is suspected of disease. Limited sinus CT scan may be helpful to determine possible anatomic etiology (tumor, polyp, abscess, etc.) in the chronic setting. MRI shows better detail but is often unneeded.

Nasal endoscopy may be performed by a specialist and cultures may be taken; this is the gold standard.

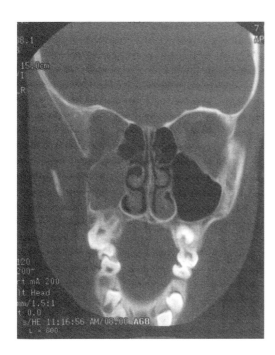

FIGURE 4.11 Coronal CT scan of the sinuses demonstrating normal left sided anatomy and right maxillary sinus opacification. Reprinted with permission from Silberstein SD, Lipton RB, Dalessio DJ. *Wolff's Headache and Other Head Pain*, 8th edition. 2007, Oxford University Press.

Treatment

Determine if viral or bacterial etiology by clinical presentation. If mild disease, antibiotics will likely not be effective. If moderate to severe, antibiotics are reasonable.

High dose **amoxicillin** is commonly first line if no prior antibiotic use is reported, or amoxicillin-clavulonate (Augmentin) if there has been. Alternatives include co-trimoxazole (TMP/SMX) (Bactrim, Septra), cefdinar (Omnicef), azithromycin, or ceftriaxon (Rocephin). Duration is 10–14 days or up to 21 days with chronic presentation.

Nasal decongestants are often helpful. Nasal steroids are controversial.

Systemic decongestants such as pseudoephedrine (Sudafed) or mucolytics are anecdotally effective.

Saline nasal spray often improves symptoms.

Endoscopic sinus surgery if chronic, recurrent, refractory, or complicated disease is present.

Take Home Points

- Sinusitis is commonly viral but may become secondarily infected, leading to worsened symptoms.

- Amoxicillin or amoxicillin-clavulonate (Augmentin) is often effective for 10–14 day course.

- Reserve antibiotics for bacterial disease only.

Dental Caries

Infection of the tooth due to bacteria commonly from supragingival plaque origin. *Strep mutans S sobrinus,* and *lactobacillus* are the main bacteria causing caries and which use fermentation of simple sugars to produce acid that causes localized decay. Two main types exist: coronal caries occur on the superior surface of the tooth and root caries which occur between or on the sides of the tooth itself.

Symptoms

Dental pain is the most common symptom. May be seen by parent or caregiver as a black dot on the tooth area. History often reveals young age, excess sugar consumption, no exposure to supplemental fluoride, or previous caries.

Diagnosis

Physical exam: Characteristic black or discolored area of tooth. Often tender to manipulation and rubbery in texture. Look for surrounding gum inflammation, swelling, erythema, or drainage that may indicate abscess or gingivitis.

Treatment

Prevention with tooth brushing after every meal, use of fluorinated water or toothpaste, and low sugar diet.

Monitor for complications such as pulpitis or periodontal abscess. Treatment of an abscess involves incision and drainage.

Refer to dentist.

Filling with various amalgams and filling material is common and effective.

Take Home Points

- Dental caries are tooth infections which should be treated by a dentist.
- Filling of the infected area before invasion of the inner tooth structures is the treatment of choice.
- Prevent caries with tooth brushing and fluoride use.

Temporomandibular Joint Syndrome

Temporomandibular joint (TMJ) syndrome is the presence of symptoms of pain and discomfort centered around the TM joint and masticatory muscles. TMJ syndrome is thought to arise due to stress, jaw malocclusion, jaw clenching, bruxism, other musculoskeletal problems (such as degenerative joint disease, internal joint derangements, etc.), and rarely from trauma. This disorder occurs more often in women in the 3rd and 4th decades of life.

Symptoms

Pain, clicking, popping, locking, or catching with jaw movement. May progress to headache, facial, neck, or ear pain. History may reveal comorbid conditions such as anxiety, fibromyalgia, rheumatoid arthritis, osteoarthritis, gout, or other arthropathy.

Diagnosis

Physical exam: Tenderness or audible symptoms on jaw range of motion. Erythema, swelling, ecchymosis, or deformity may reveal fracture.

Imaging: Single-contrast videoarthrography helpful in demonstrating joint dynamics and disc movement. Consider plain radiographs for bone structure but are otherwise rarely useful. MRI is most helpful for visualization of structures.

Treatment

Dependent on etiology and dysfunction.

General measures include jaw rest, analgesics, NSAIDs, local heat application, and soft diet.

Stress reduction and therapy may help some with psychosomatic cause.

Orthodontic guidance appliance may be indicated. Teeth guard at night may help to reduce nocturnal tooth grinding problems. Tricyclic antidepressants taken at night are often helpful, with amitriptyline (Elavil) being most efficacious. Oral muscle relaxants such as cyclobenzaprine (Flexeril) may be helpful.

Steroid injections to TMJ are efficacious acutely. Use mix of methylprednisolone and lidocaine for best effect.

Botulinum toxin (Botox) injection has recently shown benefit.

Long term treatment of comorbid psychiatric disorders will likely improve this syndrome.

Surgical referral indicated for refractory cases or those with significant displacement or damage to disc.

Take Home Points

- Screen for structural abnormalities for a reason of TMJ pain before this syndrome is diagnosed.

- The presence of TMJ syndrome may eventually be classified as a chronic pain disorder in a particular patient but only after elimination of correctable causes.

- Treatment consists of a combination of oral pain medications, heat application, soft diet, use of orthodontic devices including teeth guard, stress reduction, antidepressant use, and steroid or botulinum toxin injection.

Laryngeal Carcinoma

The second most common head and neck cancer, laryngeal carcinoma is overwhelmingly squamous cell in origin. Three areas divide the disease according to anatomic location, including: supraglottic, glottic, and subglottic regions.

Symptoms

Persistent hoarseness is the most common presentation, which is often accompanied by stridor, dysphagia, hemoptysis, weight loss, neck mass, or neck pain. History often reveals age > 40 and smoking/drinking.

Diagnosis

Physical exam: Palpable mass in the neck, fullness of throat region, or regional lymphadenopathy.
Labs: Chem 7 for electrolyte abnormalities, hepatic function panel for possible metastatic liver disease.
Imaging: Laryngoscopy with biopsy is the gold standard. Biopsy reveals histology and may help in staging. CT or MRI for better visualization. These may be used on other areas to rule out metastasis. Order a bone scan and CXR to rule out likely areas of metastasis.

Treatment

Early disease may be treated with local excision, laser vocal cordectomy, and/or radiation. Every effort is made to attempt vocal cord sparing treatment, especially in early stages.

More advanced cases require laryngectomy with follow up radiation.

Metastatic disease often responds to chemotherapy.

Stop smoking/drinking to prevent this cancer.

Take Home Points

- Hoarseness is often the presenting symptom of laryngeal carcinoma.

- Treatment is based on stage with high priority on voice-sparing treatment.

Cancer of the Lip, Oral Cavity, and Pharynx

Cancers of the lip, oral cavity, and pharynx are overwhelmingly squamous cell in origin and many are directly linked to the use of tobacco products, including dip/chew, smoking, or heavy alcohol use.

Symptoms

Symptoms depend on site.

Lip cancer presents with ulceration or exophytic lesion with pain and bleeding. Local involvement of the mental nerve may lead to numbness or pain of chin area.

Oral cavity cancer presents with nonhealing mouth ulcers, loosening of teeth, ill-fitting dentures, dysphagia, odynophagia, weight loss, bleeding, or referred otalgia.

Pharyngeal cancer presents much later in the course with pain, bleeding, or a neck mass. Look for history of smoking and alcohol abuse.

Diagnosis

Physical exam: Palpable mass in the neck, lymphadenopathy, ulceration, or tumor in the oral cavity or pharynx.

Labs: Chem 7 for electrolyte abnormalities, hepatic function panel for possible metastatic liver disease, alkaline phosphatase for bone involvement. Fine needle aspiration of either the tumor in question or locally enlarged nodes is helpful to determine histology. Direct biopsy is best if possible.

Imaging: CT scan and MRI are used widely for staging and evaluation of local disease as well as evaluation of distant organ/tissue metastasis. Obtain a bone scan for screening for metastasis. PET or integrated PET-CT scanning is also useful and has high sensitivity and specificity.

Treatment

Surgically excise early disease.

Radiotherapy is often added to reduce chances of recurrence.

Chemotherapy, although effective at controlling local disease, is controversial without metastatic spread.

Consult oncology for treatment recommendations.

Plastic surgery may be needed for disfiguring surgical excisions due to this cancer.

Stop smoking/drinking.

Take Home Points

- Tobacco and alcohol use are major risk factors for this disease.

- Direct biopsy is often the best strategy for analysis of a suspected oral lesion.

- Surgery may be disfiguring but is often necessary.

5   Cardiovascular Disease

Hypertension

Primary (essential, benign, idiopathic) hypertension accounts for > 90% of all hypertension cases and has no true known etiology, although the multifactorial influence of cardiac output, muscular arterial wall tension, and renal factors all contribute.

Secondary hypertension refers to that hypertensive state which is caused by a specific organic source. Secondary reversible causes should be eliminated before diagnosis of primary hypertension is made.

Symptoms

Typically, hypertension is asymptomatic with the possible exclusion of headache. Symptoms from associated conditions such as retinal disease, cerebrovascular disease, or congestive heart failure may be present.

Diagnosis

The Joint National Committee on Detection, Evaluation, and Treatment of High Blood Pressure (JNC) reported the following guidelines and treatments for hypertension.

TABLE 5.1 JNC Classification of Hypertension

Classification	BP Range
Prehypertension	120–139/80–89
Stage I	140–159/90–99
Stage II	$\geq 160/\geq 100$

Two separate blood pressures must be taken on separate days to constitute hypertension.

Exam may reveal signs of left ventricular hypertrophy (LVH), including displaced PMI (point of maximal impulse) or S4. Fundoscopic retinal exam may show AV nicking or "copper-wire" appearance of vessels.

A workup should be done to exclude secondary causes of hypertension (see section on Secondary Hypertension). This should include an electrocardiogram and urinalysis; basic chemistry including blood glucose, serum potassium, creatinine, calcium; CBC for hematocrit; and a lipid profile.

Treatment

The goal of treatment is to reduce blood pressures to < 140/90, or < 130/80 in diabetics and renal insufficiency patients.

Consider that some medications increase blood pressure, such as oral contraceptives and NSAIDs.

If the patient is less than 20/10 mmHg from goal, lifestyle modifications can be tried first. These include: weight reduction, eating the Dietary Approaches to Stop Hypertension (DASH) diet, dietary sodium reduction, physical activity, and moderation of alcohol consumption. These lifestyle changes should also be implemented when the patient is started on medication.

Medications: Best first line is a **thiazide diuretic**. Add additional meds from other classes as needed to obtain the desired effect (calcium channel blockers, beta blockers, ARBs [angiotensin receptor blockers], α-blockers, ACE-Is, β-blockers). Manage comorbidities as needed and control other diseases (e.g., diabetics should receive an ACE-I or ARB). Consider individual risk factors to tailor the patient's regimen.

TABLE 5.2 Hypertension Medications

Medication	Special Considerations	Side Effects
Thiazide diuretics	First line; indicated especially in African Americans; contraindicated in gout and nephrolithiasis patients	Increased urination upon starting, gouty flares, calcium based kidney stones
β-blockers	Protective in ischemic heart disease; contraindicated in asthmatics	Bradycardia, alopecia, erectile dysfunction
ACE-I	Indicated especially in diabetics	Cough, angioedema, hyperkalemia
ARB	Indicated as next alternative for patients intolerant of ACE-I	Hyperkalemia
Calcium channel blockers		Lower extremity edema

Take Home Points

- Hypertension starts at 140/90, or 130/80 in diabetics and renal insufficiency patients.
- Patients don't die of hypertension; they die of the *consequences* of hypertension, i.e., stroke, MI, etc.
- Consider starting the DASH diet and other lifestyle changes in conjunction with or before using medications.
- Start with a thiazide diuretic, and then tailor the regimen to the individual patient risk factors.

Hypertensive Urgency/Emergency

Hypertensive Urgency—The generally accepted definition includes blood pressure > 180/120, although there still is some debate about the absolute numbers. Hypertensive urgency is also commonly thought of as extremely high blood pressure without evidence of direct, acute organ damage.

Hypertensive Emergency—Extremely high blood pressure (generally > 180/120) with the presence of direct, acute end-organ damage.

Symptoms

Hypertensive urgency is, by definition, asymptomatic or only mildly symptomatic (headache, minor chest pain, etc.). Hypertensive emergency may present with mental status change, vision change, palpitations, presyncope, syncope, hematuria, or seizure/coma (constituting hypertensive encephalopathy). The greatest risk factors for either of these conditions are failing to comply with a prescribed anti-hypertensive medication regimen and new, previously undiagnosed hypertension.

Diagnosis

Physical exam: Retinal exam may reveal papilledema, retinal hemorrhages, or exudates. Lung exam may reveal rales indicating pulmonary edema. Heart exam may show murmur. Abdominal exam may show renal artery bruit or mass.

Labs: Obtain complete chemistry to include renal function, electrolytes, liver transaminases, bicarbonate, and glucose. Also order urinalysis for protein and microscopic analysis. Direct further testing toward specific suspect causes, e.g., pheochromocytoma, acute MI, etc.

Imaging: Obtain CT scan of the head for acute bleeding or evidence of herniation. Consider CT scan of the abdomen for possible endocrinologic source. Obtain chest x-ray and consider pulmonary edema/effusion or aortic dissection.

Consider ECG and V/Q lung scan or CT scan of chest for pulmonary embolism (PE) if suspected.

Treatment

Hypertensive urgency—Generally can be treated with oral medications to reduce blood pressure. However, do not reduce it too fast as further complications (such as cerebral hypoperfusion) may develop. A rule of thumb is 25% in the first 24 hours or to ≤ 160/100. To accomplish this, adjust the patient's current medication regimen to maximize each before adding another. If the patient is a candidate for additional medications or is a new hypertensive, give oral β-blockers (atenolol, metoprolol), calcium channel blockers (nifedipine), ACE-Is (captopril, enalapril, lisinopril), or a small dose of clonidine. There is little evidence of benefit of one medication over another.

Hypertensive emergency—Admit the patient to the hospital. Generally, parenteral administration of anti-hypertensive medications is best. Drip infusions are most common and include nitroprusside, hydralazine, nicardapine, labetalol, nitroglycerine, or esmolol. Final choice depends on the patient's comorbid conditions and end-organ damage in question. Stabilize; give therapy for end-organ damage, then switch to oral medication.

A word of warning: In head injury or intracranial bleeding, systemic blood pressure may be elevated to preserve intracranial pressure and thus perfusion; therefore, eliminate brain injury as a cause of hypertension before lowering the blood pressure!

Take Home Points

- The difference between urgency and emergency is the presence of direct, acute end-organ damage.

- Hypertensive urgency may be managed as an outpatient; admit hypertensive emergency.

- Make sure there is no intracranial pathology before lowering the BP with parenteral medications.

End-Organ Hypertensive Effects

Three commonly affected organ systems include cardiac, neurologic, and renal. These are all affected in separate ways, but the common theme is damage to the arterial walls and coexistence of atherosclerotic disease.

Symptoms

Symptoms of left ventricular hypertrophy (LVH), including those of congestive heart failure or ischemic phenomenon, may eventually affect the patient. These symptoms include shortness of breath, dyspnea on exertion, cough, paroxysmal nocturnal dyspnea (PND), peripheral edema, or ascites. For the neurologic system, ruptured brain aneurysm may produce acute focal neurologic deficits, dementia, mental status change, or sudden death. Symptoms of renal disease are often lacking until significant failure exists; however, general decrease in energy and possible mental status change are sometimes presenting symptoms.

Diagnosis

If uncontrolled hypertension has existed for a significant amount of time, obtain EKG for likely LVH or arrhythmias, basic chemistry for electrolytes and BUN/creatinine → calculate creatinine clearance to estimate the glomerular filtration rate (GFR), order a TSH, and obtain U/A for protein and urine microalbumin.

Imaging: Obtain chest x-ray for cardiomegaly or pulmonary edema (seen by Kerley B lines, diffuse opacities, increased vascular markings, and cephalization) indicating heart failure.

Echocardiography for LVH, ejection fraction, and any possible wall motion abnormalities.

Treatment

Control blood pressure to prevent these disorders.

Use β-blockers and ACE-Is to control blood pressure preferentially after damage has occurred. In congestive heart failure (CHF), spironolactone and other diuretics also show benefit. ACE-Is are especially important in controlling renal disease (although their use in renal failure is contraindicated).

Avoid NSAIDs.

Take Home Points

- Commonly affected systems are neurologic, cardiac, and renal.
- Investigate individual systems by targeted labs and imaging.
- Control the BP early since these effects tend to develop after long term HTN has existed.

Secondary Hypertension

Extensive differential diagnosis may include:

- Sleep apnea
- Drug-induced
- Chronic kidney disease
- Pregnancy (preeclampsia/eclampsia)
- Primary aldosteronism
- Renovascular disease such as renal artery stenosis
- Chronic steroid therapy
- Cushing syndrome
- Pheochromocytoma
- Coarctation of the aorta
- Thyroid or parathyroid disease
- OTC dietary supplements (e.g. ephedra, ma haung, bitter orange)
- Cocaine, amphetamines, other illicit drugs
- Nonsteroidal anti-inflammatory drugs
- Cyclooxygenase 2 (COX-2) inhibitors

Symptoms

Symptoms are varied since the etiology of disease is varied. Isolated hypertension may, however, be associated with headache or other diffuse complaints.

Diagnosis

The JNC 7 recommends ECG and laboratory evaluation per the following: electrocardiogram; urinalysis for protein; basic chemistry including blood glucose, serum potassium, creatinine, and calcium; CBC for hematocrit; fasting lipid profile; and optional microalbumin measurement.
If history/physical dictates, add the following:

- TSH
- Chest x-ray
- Provocative renal nuclear scans
- Selective arteriography
- Plasma/urine catecholamines
- Plasma renin
- Aortogram
- Renal biopsy
- CT scan of abdomen
- 24-hour urine cortisol

Treatment

As appropriate for each condition after identification.

Cardiology or nephrology consultation may be appropriate if diagnosis is not found. Don't be afraid to ask for help!

Take Home Points

- Patients < 30 years old or with a paucity of risk factors for HTN should have a secondary hypertension workup before starting treatment.
- Repeat the secondary hypertension workup in a patient whose hypertension is unusually hard to control.

Acute Myocardial Infarction

Myocardial infarction (MI) is one of the leading causes of death in the U.S. The pathophysiology includes coronary atherosclerotic build up and plaque rupture leading to occlusion of the artery and ischemia/infarction of the territory downstream. MI may be divided into Q-wave or non-Q-wave types. Q-wave MI occurs due to complete occlusion of the vessel and transmural infarction, while non-Q-wave MI results from non-transmural infarction and only severe, acute narrowing of the artery. Because of acute clot formation, many therapies are aimed at reducing clotting mechanisms in the blood while others are aimed at reducing myocardial oxygen demand, and still others dilate the blood vessel to increase blood flow around the clot.

Symptoms

Classically, symptoms include left-sided crushing chest pain that radiates down the left arm or up to the jaw, especially with **exertion**. Diaphoresis, shortness of breath, nausea, or lightheadedness may be present. In the elderly or diabetics, these symptoms may or may not be present (silent MI). History may reveal risk factors such as angina, coronary artery disease equivalents (e.g., diabetes), male gender, African descent, smoking, significant EtOH use, hyperlipidemia (especially LDL), obesity, sedentary lifestyle, "type A" personality, or age ≥ 40 years.

Diagnosis

Exam may show signs of acute heart failure, including pulmonary rales, increased jugular venous pulsation, S3, S4, or arrhythmia.

Obtain stat ECG: Look for Q-waves, T-wave inversion, ST segment depression (ischemia) or elevation (infarction), new left bundle branch block, new heart block, shifted axis, or arrhythmia (especially V-tach). Order old records and ECGs for comparison. Changes occur in contiguous leads.

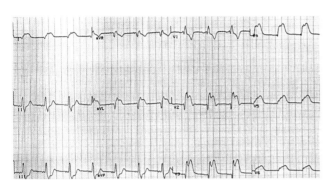

FIGURE 5.1 Acute anterior/lateral myocardial infarction. Reprinted with permission from Cox NLT, Roper TA. *Clinical Skills*. 2005, Oxford University Press.

Laboratory: On admission, obtain CBC, BMP, TSH, coagulation profile. Importantly, get cardiac enzymes which include CK, CK-MB, and troponins. Cardiac enzymes should be taken every 6–8 hours x 3.

TABLE 5.3 Ischemic Injury Localization by Leads of the 12 Lead ECG

I Lateral (LCA)	aVR	V_1 Septal (LCA, LAD)	V_4 Anterior (LCA, LAD)
II Inferior (RCA)	aVL Lateral (LCA)	V_2 Septal (LCA, LAD)	V_5 Lateral (LCA)
III Inferior (RCA)	aVF Inferior (RCA)	V_3 Anterior (LCA, LAD)	V_6 Lateral (LCA)

Acronyms in parentheses indicate vessel affected. LCA = left circumflex artery, RCA = right circumflex artery, LAD = left anterior descending.

Nitroglycerin is sometimes used in diagnosis, in that if chest pain is relieved→ cardiac cause. This is low sensitivity since most chest pain of any origin is relieved by nitro.

Imaging: Chest x-ray for pneumonia or dissection.

If work up is negative for acute injury, obtain fasting lipid profile and cardiac stress test (via exercise or chemical stress) and consider thallium nuclear medicine imaging. This will help risk stratification.

Treatment

Stabilize the patient if unstable. Consider ACLS protocols.

Start IV fluids.

Remember **MONA**: **m**orphine, **o**xygen, **n**itroglycerin, **a**spirin as first line when patient presents.

Make the patient NPO.

After above are done and while labs, imaging, and ECG are pending, obtain history and physical. If clinical suspicion is high for cardiac origin of symptoms, place patient on oxygen, have them chew an aspirin for antiplatelet action, give MSO_4 (morphine sulfate) for vasodilation/pain control, and nitroglycerine (IV, sublingual, transdermal) for pain control and vasodilation. Then consider IV β-blocker for cardioprotection, ACE-I for post MI benefits, and heparin or low molecular weight heparin (Lovenox) for anticoagulation.

If ischemia is proved ongoing (either by dynamic ECG changes or cardiac enzyme abnormalities), order cardiac catheterization with balloon angioplasty, ASAP. The cardiologist will evaluate for coronary artery bypass graft (CABG).

Thrombolytics (tPA, streptokinase) must be given within 6 hours of symptom onset, and have many contraindications. Review the patient's inclusion and exclusion criteria to find out if they are a candidate for thrombolytics.

If found to be having NSTEMI (non ST segment elevation MI), consider glycoprotein IIb/IIIa inhibitors (Integrilin, abciximab).

After event (and if found *not* to have had an acute ischemic origin to symptoms), risk stratify and place on aspirin (or clopidogrel (Plavix)). Lower risk factors such as obesity, smoking, hypertension, and control diabetes.

Look for post-MI complications including depression.

Take Home Points

- MI commonly presents with chest pain; however, beware the diabetic or elderly with neuropathy!
- Diagnosis is key, common practice is the "rule out MI" in which the patient is held in the hospital for serial ECGs and 3 sets of cardiac enzymes. If MI is ruled out, they are often discharged in just under 24 hours.
- Remember: "MONA greets all patients with chest pain."
- Remember: "Time is myocardium."

Angina Pectoris

Chest-related symptoms (commonly chest pain/pressure) caused by myocardial ischemia which does not progress to infarction.

Stable angina: Chronic or recurrent condition of angina with exertion.

Variant (Prinzemetal) angina: Spasm of coronary vessels with temporary or partial occlusion resulting in angina. May be associated with cocaine use.

Unstable angina: Recent onset of angina at rest or worsening of existing symptoms with regard to character or frequency.

Symptoms

Substernal pain, pressure, tightness, heaviness, or sharp pain of relatively short duration. Diaphoresis, nausea, dyspnea, or radiation of pain or numbness down left arm or up to jaw may be present. This feeling is not pleuritic and classically may be relieved by rest or nitroglycerin.

Diagnosis

Physical exam: S_4, new murmur, rhythm, rate, or signs of heart failure should be noted.

Resting ECG often is negative but may show signs of ischemia if ongoing angina is present.

Labs: Obtain CBC for hematocrit, TSH, lipid profile, Basic chemistry for electrolytes and glucose; in acute setting obtain 3 sets of cardiac enzymes (CK, CK-MB, troponin) to evaluate for MI.

Imaging: Chest x-ray. Consider CT of the chest if aortic dissection thought possible.

Special testing:

Echocardiography for valvular or structural abnormality.

Exercise stress testing to evaluate for ECG changes during cardiac stress (exercise or chemical).

Stress echocardiography to visualize wall motion abnormalities.

Radionuclide testing (thallium, persantine thallium, etc.) to visualize myocardial blood flow.

Coronary angiography to visualize and quantify degree of coronary blood vessel occlusion.

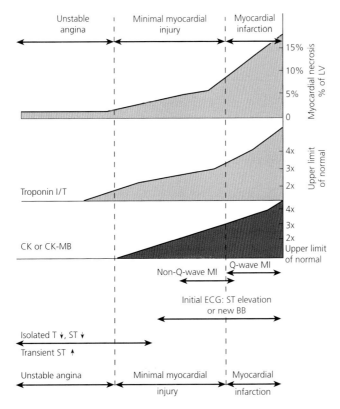

FIGURE 5.2 Schematic of the spectrum of acute coronary syndromes. The relationship between the extent of myocardial necrosis and the release of cardiac enzymes (troponin I or T, or CK or CK-MB) and ECG changes. The schematic illustrates that unstable angina is associated with myocardial ischemia without the release of CK or CK-MB but with the release of troponin in approximately one-third of cases. With minimal myocardial injury, more extensive myocardial necrosis is associated with the release of cardiac enzymes and ECG changes (non-ST elevation MI). With Q-wave MI the most extensive myocardial necrosis and release of cardiac enzymes occurs in association with the ECG changes. Reprinted with permission from Warrell DA, Cox TM, et al. *Oxford Textbook of Medicine*, 4th edition. 2003, Oxford University Press.

Treatment

Aggressive management of contributing diseases such as diabetes and hypertension are essential. Control of risk factors such as obesity, smoking, hyperlipidemia, etc.

TABLE 5.4 Angina Medications

Agent	Effect
Intermittent short-acting (nitroglycerin) or long-acting nitrates (isosorbid di/mono nitrate)	Reduce preload stress
β-blockers	Reduce cardiac output and cardiac exercise response as well as provide cardioprotection against ischemic injury
Calcium channel blockers	Reduce myocardial contraction demands and cause vasodilation; very effective especially in spasm-associated angina
Aspirin or clopidogrel (Plavix)	Exert antiplatelet effects and inhibition of prostaglandins

Surgery: Cardiac catheterization with balloon angioplasty or stent placement. Coronary artery bypass grafting (CABG) is also a possibility.

Take Home Points

- Angina is a symptom of ischemia of the myocardium. Take this as a warning sign of MI.
- Risk stratification should be done on new patients with angina to assess for risk of future MI. This includes exercise stress testing as well as investigation of risk factors.
- The progression of angina may be mediated by medications, although angina usually signifies the progressive disease of atherosclerosis.

Pericarditis

Inflammation of the pericardial sac. The most common etiologies are viral illness and idiopathic causes. Others include TB, systemic lupus erythematosus (SLE), medications, rheumatoid arthritis, bacterial infection, and neoplasm. Effusion is often seen with pericarditis and may lead to tamponade.

Symptoms

Subacute onset of retrosternal chest pain. May be pleuritic and radiate to neck or jaw. Classically it's relieved with leaning forward. Fever, myalgias, anorexia, or pleuritic component to chest pain may be seen. History may reveal recent URI or other minor infection.

Diagnosis

Physical exam: Classic pericardial friction rub. Distant heart sounds may be heard if effusion is present. Look for signs of tamponade including increased facial plethora and jugular venous distension.
Lab: CBC may show increased WBCs, ESR or CRP will likely be increased. Investigate other causes with ANA, rheumatoid factor, etc.
Imaging: Chest x-ray may show pericardial effusion with "boot shape" appearance of heart. Chest CT may reveal effusion or constrictive thickened pericardial sac.

ECG: Pan-elevation of ST segment. This is classic difference from MI. If significant effusion is present, electrical alternans may be seen (which is alteration of axis of QRS between beats (rare)). Look for altered axis if effusion is seen.

Echocardiography: May show effusion or constriction. Effusion may be new or worsening.

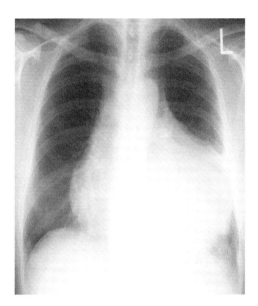

FIGURE 5.3 Chest x-ray showing typical "boot" shape of the heart with a large pericardial effusion. Reprinted with permission from Thomas J, Monaghan T. *Oxford Handbook of Clinical Examination and Practical Skills.* 2007, Oxford University Press.

Treatment

Give NSAIDs, classically aspirin.

Oral or IV steroids if NSAIDs ineffective.

Surgery: Pericardiectomy/pericardiotomy if hemodynamic compromise. Pericardiocentesis with needle aspiration may be needed if effusion present.

Take Home Points

- Classically, leaning forward relieves chest pain caused by pericarditis.
- Look for pan-elevation of the ST segment.
- Chest x-ray may reveal "water bottle" shaped heart, indicating effusion.
- Give NSAIDs.

Cardiomyopathy

Types of cardiac muscle disease include: dilated, arrhythmogenic, restrictive, hypertrophic, and unclassified. Actual etiologies for each type are many; these represent the interference of the heart muscle to provide adequate pumping power for the heart.

Symptoms

Symptoms parallel heart failure. Dyspnea, syncope, presyncope, angina, fatigue, or palpitations for left heart dysfunction. Edema, ascites, and hypervolemic states for right heart dysfunction.

Diagnosis

Labs: Screening labs such as CBC, Basic chemistry for electrolytes and renal function. Consider b-type natriuretic peptide (BNP), ESR.

Imaging: Chest x-ray for cardiac dilation or signs of pulmonary edema/congestion. Consider CT scan of chest.

ECG for increased QRS voltage indicating dilation, arrhythmia, signs of ischemia, or altered axis. Previous MI may be elicited.

Echocardiography for visualization, wall motion abnormalities, chamber dilation, or restriction.

Stress testing for reversible ischemia.

Multiple-gated acquisition scan (MUGA) may help in determining the ejection fraction.

Treatment

Treat for heart failure (see section on Congestive Heart Failure).

Consider dual chamber pacemaker to improve contractility.

Heart transplant in severe cases is definitive although low long-term survival.

Take Home Points

- Types of cardiomyopathy vary and include dilated, arrhythmogenic, restrictive, hypertrophic, and unclassified.

- Signs often parallel heart failure as does treatment.

Hypertrophic Cardiomyopathy

Synonyms: Idiopathic hypertrophic subaortic stenosis (IHSS), hypertrophic obstructive cardiomyopathy (HOCM), or cardiomyopathy with asymmetrical involvement of the interventricular septum.

A form of cardiomyopathy, this disease is caused by a thickened septum impinging on the anterior mitral valve leaflet during systole, causing outflow obstruction and thus increasing ventricular filling pressures leading to further diastolic dysfunction. This is an autosomal dominant disease with high penetrance; therefore screening of first degree relatives is indicated.

Symptoms

Note that symptoms result from both systolic and diastolic dysfunction. Dyspnea, syncope, presyncope, angina, fatigue, paroxysmal nocturnal dyspnea (PND), or palpitations. Symptoms of limited cardiac output response to exercise, exertional syncope, or LV hypertrophy may be the clinical presentation. Sudden cardiac death is the worst sudden discovery of disease. History may reveal relatively young athlete with no prior knowledge or symptoms of heart disease.

Diagnosis

Physical exam: Harsh crescendo/decrescendo systolic murmur that lengthens with valsalva, S_4, laterally displaced PMI.

Labs: Screening labs such as CBC, CMP, coagulation profile are indicated but none are diagnostic.

ECG: Increased QRS voltage suggesting LVH, nonspecific ST changes, T waves inversions, Q waves in anterior and lateral leads mimicking MI, P wave abnormalities indicating left atrial enlargement (LAE), or short PR interval. A fib is a late and concerning finding.

Imaging:

Chest x-ray: May show normal or increased cardiac size. Pulmonary congestion and edema may present due to diastolic dysfunction.

Echocardiography is the best initial procedure. This shows asymmetric septal hypertrophy, LVH, left atrial enlargement, small ventricular chamber size, and mitral or aortic valve irregularities.

Cardiac catheterization: Reveals often patent vessels, obstruction to ventricular outflow, and abnormal diastolic ventricular filling.

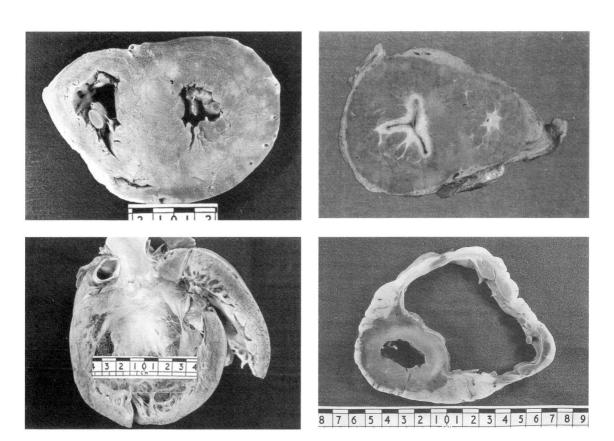

FIGURE 5.4 Transverse short axis section through the ventricles from a patient with ventricular hypertrophy from hypertrophic cardiomyopathy. Reproduced with permission from Davies MJ, Colour Atlas of Cardiovascular Pathology. 1998 Oxford University Press.

Treatment

Avoid strenuous exercise or situations.

Medications are aimed at reducing contractility to allow for increased ventricular filling. Thus, avoid digoxin or afterload reducers such as nitrates or diuretics.

Therapy includes β-blockers (metoprolol, propanolol) and calcium channel blockers (primarily verapamil).

Pacemaker placement is the standard.

Surgery: Left ventricular myomectomy is recommended for severe cases and has a generally good outcome.

Take Home Points

- Most patients with hypertrophic cardiomyopathy die from sudden cardiac death, leading to several well known examples in the sports arenas.

- Diagnosis, ideally, is with echocardiogram and shows the classic hypertrophied septum.

- Restrict strenuous exercise in young athletes if this is suspected.

Congestive Heart Failure

Congestive heart failure (CHF) is the clinical state in which cardiac output does not meet the demands needed to properly profuse bodily tissue. Etiologies include: idiopathic, myocarditis, ischemia/infarction, hypertension, Chagas disease, HIV infection, and drug toxicity (e.g., doxorubicin). Remember, the most common cause of right heart failure is left heart failure.

TABLE 5.5 New York Heart Association Classification of CHF

Class I	No limitation of activities; they suffer no symptoms from ordinary activities.
Class II	Slight, mild limitation of activity; they are comfortable with rest or with mild exertion.
Class III	Marked limitation of activity; they are comfortable only at rest.
Class IV	Patients who should be at complete rest, confined to bed or chair; any physical activity brings on discomfort and symptoms occur at rest.

Source: American Heart Association, Inc.

Symptoms

Shortness of breath, dependent edema, ascites, fatigue, weakness, right upper quadrant pain, anorexia, dyspnea on exertion, or paroxysmal nocturnal dyspnea (PND). If in acute exacerbation, look for coughing up **frothy sputum.**

Diagnosis

Physical exam: Basilar rales, pitting edema, increased PMI, jugular venous distention, hepatomegaly, hepatojugular reflex, cool extremities, ascites (abdominal distention, fluid wave, etc.), and S_3 or S_4 gallop. In severe cases, cyanosis, pulsus alternans, anasarca, and Cheyne-Stokes respirations may be seen.

Labs: Screening CBC for WBCs and possible anemia, Basic chemistry for electrolytes (hyponatremia) and renal function, LFTs for bilirubin, TSH, and HIV. Obtain **BNP (B-type natriuretic peptide)** if the patient is suspected of having heart failure-caused symptoms in the acute setting. Consider cardiac enzymes for possible ischemia. Consider an ABG if lung function is considerably impaired. Directed laboratory investigations such as iron studies for hemochromatosis or ANA for autoimmune causes as warranted.

Imaging: Chest x-ray may show cardiomegaly, cephalization (prominent upper lobe vasculature), and signs of pulmonary edema (Kerley B lines in periphery and general "bat wing" distribution), or effusions.

ECG may show increased QRS voltage indicating LVH or RVH, signs of ischemia, or arrhythmia.

Echocardiography: Best test which may show structural abnormalities including LVH, wall motion abnormalities, and decreased **ejection fraction**.

Radionucleotide imaging may also be used to evaluate systolic cardiac function and ejection fraction.

Cardiac catheterization to evaluate for possible narrowing of coronary vessels.

TABLE 5.6 Framingham Criteria for Heart Failure

Major	Paroxysmal nocturnal dyspnea
	Increased central venous pressure (> 16 cm H_2O at right atrium)
	Distended neck veins
	Pulmonary rales
	Hepatojugular reflex
	S3 gallop
	Cardiomegaly on chest x-ray

(continued)

TABLE 5.6 Continued

	Pulmonary edema on chest x-ray
	Weight loss > 4.5 kg in five days in response to treatment of presumed heart failure
Minor	Bilateral leg edema
	Nocturnal cough
	Dyspnea on ordinary exertion
	Hepatomegaly
	Pleural effusion
	Tachycardia (heart rate 120 beats/min)
	Decrease in vital capacity by one-third from maximum recorded

This scale represents one set of criteria used to diagnosis heart failure. Diagnosis of CHF consists of the existence of two major or one major criteria combined with two minor criteria that aren't attributable to another disease process. Adapted from McKee PA, et al. The natural history of congestive heart failure: the Framingham study. *N Engl J Med.* 1971; 285(26): 1441–6.

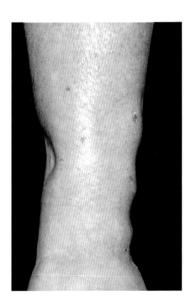

FIGURE 5.5 Pitting leg edema as seen in congestive heart failure. Reprinted with permission from Cox NLT, Roper TA. *Clinical Skills.* 2005, Oxford University Press.

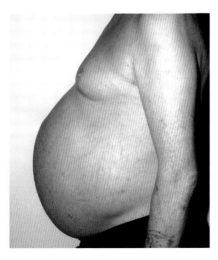

FIGURE 5.6 Ascites seen in CHF patient. Reprinted with permission from Cox NLT, Roper TA. *Clinical Skills.* 2005, Oxford University Press.

Treatment

Properly control hemodynamically unstable patients.

Place on O_2 therapy and low sodium diet.

Acutely, reduce extravascular fluid volume by giving diuretics (furosemide). Consider addition of metolazone (Zaroxolyn) for synergy and/or spironolactone for hypokalemia. This will often reduce respiratory problems (but has not shown decrease in mortality).

Morphine can reduce respiratory drive, anxiety, and decreases preload.

Vasodilators such as IV nitroglycerin may show short term benefit by reducing preload, afterload, and systemic resistance.

Digoxin is the classic drug to improve contractility (inotrope) but make sure there is no MI, hypertrophic cardiomyopathy, or aortic stenosis present.

ACE-Is, ARBs, and β-blockers show good effectiveness in decreasing mortality and are considered first line.

Use dopamine or dobutamine for short-term improvement in admitted, severe cases.

As outpatient, control risk factors such as hypertension and smoking. Low sodium diet is critical.

Surgery may be indicated for valve replacement, biventricular pacing, or even heart transplant in severe cases.

Take Home Points

- Congestive heart failure may be classified as systolic or diastolic or right or left sided. These are mainly characterized by the related sets of symptoms associated with the HF.

- Diagnosis is clinical, although several tests are routinely relied upon including echocardiography and BNP.

- Diuretics are the mainstay of therapy to reduce extravascular fluid accumulation. Other antihypertensives also reduce mortality. Consider the addition of an inotrope (digoxin) if not contraindicated.

Cor Pulmonale

Cor Pulmonale (CP) is pathophysiologic right heart failure caused by pulmonary hypertension (increased right ventricular afterload). Pulmonary hypertension is most commonly caused by lung dysfunction including primary pulmonary disease (COPD, asthma, pneumonitis), pulmonary vasculature disease (CREST, sickle cell disease, PE, HIV) or thoracic diseases contributing to pulmonary dysfunction (obesity, sleep apnea, kyphoscoliosis).

Symptoms

Acutely, symptoms may consist of severe dyspnea, anxiety, chest pain, air hunger, or cyanosis. Chronically, symptoms mimic that of right-sided heart failure and include orthopnea, tachypnea, voice hoarseness (from compression of left recurrent laryngeal nerve by expanding vasculature), fatigue, lethargy, dyspnea on exertion, cough, chest pain, ascites, or edema.

Diagnosis

Physical exam: Pallor, tachypnea, diaphoresis, jugular venous distention with inspiration (Kussmaul sign), murmur, split S_2, S_3 gallop, peripheral edema, hepatomegaly, hepatojugular reflex, or cyanosis.
Lab: CBC, Basic chemistry, TSH. Consider ABG for hypoxemia or A-a gradient supporting PE.

Imaging: Chest x-ray may show prominent pulmonary trunk and hilar vessels. Look for possible primary lung disorders such as sarcoidosis, etc.

ECG may be helpful and show rightward axis deviation, right bundle branch block, and/or increased P wave in leads II, III, and aVF.

Echocardiography remains the best single test to evaluate right ventricular hypertrophy and large vessel dimensions.

Thallium myocardial scintigraphy, MRI, or CT angiography may also be helpful but generally only ordered by cardiologist.

Consider pulmonary function testing to assess lung function.

Treatment

Oxygen therapy has shown good benefit by reducing pulmonary arterial resistance.

Treat the underlying cause. Commonly this includes pulmonary therapy consisting of bronchodilators such as albuterol, metaproterenol, ipratropium, terbutaline, and theophylline. Sildenafil (Viagra) has also recently been proven effective at selective pulmonary vasodilatation without increasing pulmonary hypertension.

Diuretics such as furosemide and spironolactone are helpful for fluid excess symptoms.

Vasodilators have previously been used as the next step and include hydralazine, nifedipine, diltiazem, and prazosin and may help with moderately-advanced disease. However, primary administration during right heart catheterization to record benefit of therapy is recommended to prove effect in a particular patient, obviously the job of a cardiologist.

For advanced disease, bosentan (Tracleer) may be used but requires advanced monitoring and should be followed by an experienced cardiologist.

Take Home Points

- Cor Pulmonale is caused by pulmonary hypertension most commonly secondary to pulmonary disease.

- If suspected, obtain echocardiography for right ventricular hypertrophy (RVH).

- Look for right axis deviation on ECG indicating RVH.

- Treat pulmonary disease to reduce afterload on the right ventricle.

Myocarditis

Inflammation of the myocardium. Etiologies are most commonly made up of infections including viral (coxsackie B virus, HIV, echo, etc), bacterial (diphtheria, TB), mycotic, rickettesial, protozoal, and helminthic. Toxins such as alcohol and cocaine or systemic diseases such as sarcoidosis and systemic lupus erythematosis may also be involved.

Symptoms

Symptoms can be variable but include chest pain, unexplained fatigue or sinus tachycardia, palpitations, symptoms of CHF, or symptoms of pericarditis. History may reveal recent URI or enteritis illness.

Diagnosis

Physical exam: Fever, sinus tachycardia (out of proportion to fever), S_3 or S_4, irregular rhythm indicating arrhythmia, murmur, or friction rub.

Lab: CBC and Basic chemistry tend to show nonspecific findings. Cardiac enzyme (troponin, CK-MB, CK) findings may mimic myocardial infarction.

ECG: Often mimics pericarditis or MI with ST changes or T wave flattening/inversions. May also show arrhythmia or heart block.

Chest x-ray: Possible cardiomegaly, increased pulmonary vasculature or pulmonary edema as in CHF.

Echocardiography: Clinically, most valuable test. May show dilated cardiomyopathy, wall motion abnormalities, characteristic appearance of myocardial tissue, valvular dysfunction, or thrombi.

Cardiac MRI: May be helpful to show local cardiac muscle damage or edema.

Endocardial biopsy is the gold standard although is rarely used because of inherent risk. Criteria to evaluate the biopsy are called the **Dallas criteria** and basically outline degrees of inflammation.

Treatment

Nonspecific and supportive care is the standard.

Restrict exercise to prevent undue stress on inflamed myocardium.

IVIG (IV immunoglobulin) has recently shown evidence of benefit.

Treat specific causes if known.

Otherwise, provide O_2 as needed, treat CHF symptoms, and monitor course.

In advanced cases, cardiac transplant may be considered.

Take Home Points

- Myocarditis is the inflammation of heart tissue; most commonly caused by a virus.

- Give supportive care and restrict exercise.

- Clinical distinction from MI may be difficult due to ECG and cardiac enzyme similarities.

Arrhythmias

Heart Block

TABLE 5.7 First Degree Heart Block

Degree	Characteristic on ECG	Treatment
First	Prolonged PR interval (> 0.2 s)	Generally none Avoid β-blockers or Ca channel blockers

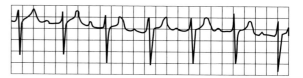

FIGURE 5.7 First degree heart block. Reprinted with permission from Brown J. Oxford American Handbook of Emergency Medicine. 2008 Oxford University Press.

TABLE 5.8 Mobitz Type IAV Block

SecondDegree	Characteristic on ECG	Treatment
Mobitz I (Wenckebach)	Elongating PR interval until dropped QRS	Atropine and transcutaneous pacing if symptomatic acutely. Consider permanent pacemaker if symptomatic chronically.
Mobitz II	Consistent, predictably dropped QRS with normal PR intervals	Pacemaker placement

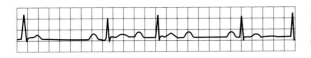

FIGURE 5.8 Mobitz type I AV block. Reprinted with permission from Brown J. *Oxford American Handbook of Emergency Medicine.* 2008, Oxford University Press.

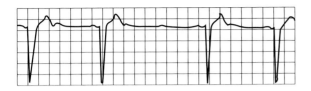

FIGURE 5.9 Mobitz type II AV block. Reprinted with permission from Brown J. *Oxford American Handbook of Emergency Medicine.* 2008, Oxford University Press.

TABLE 5.9 Third Degree Heart Block

Degree	Characteristic on ECG	Treatment
Third	Total atrial/ventricular disassociation. P waves and QRS unrelated.	Pacemaker placement

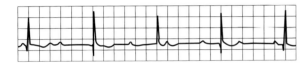

FIGURE 5.10 Third degree heart block. Reprinted with permission from Brown J. *Oxford American Handbook of Emergency Medicine.* 2008, Oxford University Press.

Atrial Fibrillation

A chronic or paroxysmal atrial arrhythmia characterized by chaotic multifocal electrical discharges. Because of multiple electrical signals from the atria, ventricular response is irregular and often tachycardic (rapid ventricular response). History may reveal alcohol abuse (holiday heart), known heart failure, hyperthyroidism, hypertension, or prior MI.

Symptoms

Often asymptomatic but may present with palpitations, lightheadedness/presyncope, tiring easily, dyspnea on exertion, symptoms of heart failure (dependent edema, pulmonary congestion, etc.), or unexplained fatigue. Be aware of possible thrombotic events that may lead to symptoms of TIA (transient ischemic attack)/stroke.

Diagnosis

Physical exam: Irregularly irregular rhythm.

Lab: Obtain screening Basic chemistry, hepatic function panel, CBC. Obtain cardiac enzymes to evaluate for MI. Order TSH.

ECG: P waves are absent. "F" waves appear like P waves but are usually smaller and unassociated with QRS segments. QRSs are **irregularly irregular** and ventricular rate is anywhere between 90 and 170 bpm.

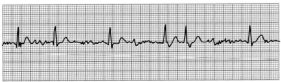

Rhythm strip 1—atrial fibrillation.

FIGURE 5.11 Atrial fibrillation. Reprinted with permission from Thomas J, Monaghan T. *Oxford Handbook of Clinical Examination and Practical Skills.* 2007, Oxford University Press.

Echocardiogram:

Transthoracic for structural abnormalities and evaluation of heart function.

Transesophageal for possible left atrial thrombi if duration of atrial fibrillation is unknown or > 48 hours.

Chest x-ray for lung or cardiac abnormalities.

Consider Holter monitoring for paroxysmal atrial fibrillation.

Treatment

If unstable, remember ACLS (advanced cardiac life support) guidelines and perform external cardioversion.

If stable, "Control the rate or convert the rhythm." This can be done by various antiarrhythmic drugs such as β-blockers, non-dihyrdropyridine Ca channel blockers (verapamil, diltiazem), digoxin, or amiodarone. Consensus for best agent is controversial. Diltiazem (Cardizem) is a popular choice for outpatient therapy. Electrocardioversion is also an option but clinically rarely used.

Anticoagulation and cardioversion:

Guidelines from the Seventh American College of Chest Physicians (ACCP) Consensus Conference on Antithrombotic Therapy and the ACC (American College of Cardiology) recommend that outpatients who have been in A fib for more than 48 hours should receive three to four weeks of warfarin (Coumadin) prior to *and* after cardioversion. An alternative strategy supported by the AAFP (American Academy of Family Practice) and ACP (American College of Physicians) states that transesophageal echocardiography is sufficient to rule out atrial thrombi. If negative, cardioversion without pre-anticoagulation is safe.

After cardioversion, anticoagulation with warfarin (Coumadin) should be maintained for 3–4 weeks. Keep the INR between 2 and 3.

Chronic A fib patients should be maintained on warfarin (Coumadin) or aspirin long term.

Routine use of antiarrhythmic drugs for maintenance of sinus rhythm was not shown beneficial in the large, multicenter AFFIRM trial.

Surgery: Electrical ablation procedures exist but are rarely indicated or used.

Take Home Points

- Atrial fibrillation is a perfusing rhythm with an irregularly irregular rhythm.
- If suspected, obtain an ECG which is diagnostic.
- Control the rate or convert the rhythm.
- Place the patient on warfarin (Coumadin) for a variable amount of time.
- Keep the INR between 2 and 3.

Ventricular Tachycardia

Tachycardia from impulses originating inferiorly to the A-V node, causing a wide QRS complex. May be polymorphic or monomorphic in nature. Both involve etiologies that are commonly idiopathic, structural, ischemia based, or more complex (Brugada syndrome, arrhythmogenic right ventricular dysplasia (ARVD), or catecholaminergic polymorphic VT).

Diagnosis

ECG:

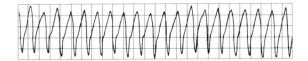

FIGURE 5.12 VT with a rate of 235 beats/min. Reprinted with permission from Flynn JA. *Oxford American Handbook of Clinical Medicine.* 2007, Oxford University Press.

Three or more consecutive, wide QRS (ventricular origin) beats at a rate of 100–200 bpm. AV dissociation is the hallmark since the ventricles are beating independently of the atria.

Monomorphic—one general shape.

Polymorphic—more than one shape. When associated with prolonged Q-T and appears to revolve around a stable baseline it is termed Torsades de pointes.

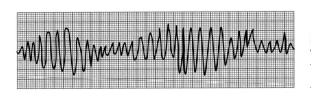

FIGURE 5.13 Torsades de pointes, a form of polymorphic VT. Reprinted with permission from Thomas J, Monaghan T. *Oxford Handbook of Clinical Examination and Practical Skills.* 2007, Oxford University Press.

Treatment

If unstable, immediate synchronized cardioversion is indicated. Use standard protocol of 200 J, 200–300 J, 360 J for monophasic defibrillator or equivalent if biphasic. Between shocks, give either amiodarone 150 mg IV over 10 min or lidocaine 0.5 to 0.75 mg/kg IV push.

If stable, (or while preparing for cardioversion) consider treatment with antiarrhythmics such as procainamide, lidocaine, β-blockers, magnesium, or amiodarone.

Take Home Points

- A "run" of V tach constitutes ≥ 3 consecutive wide QRS beats at a rate of 100–200 bpm.
- V tach commonly occurs due to idiopathic, ischemia based, or complex etiologies.
- May be seen as monomorphic or polymorphic on ECG.
- Convert this rhythm, ASAP.

Ventricular Fibrillation

Chaotic multifocal electrical discharges originating from the ventricles. This is a rhythm commonly associated with structural heart disease and coronary heart disease (CHD) including unstable angina/MI.

Symptoms

Since this is an unstable rhythm, patient drops to the ground and is inherently cardiovascularly unstable. **Associated with myocardial infarction**.

Diagnosis

ECG: Rapid wide complex ventricular beats with no recognizable rhythm. Inherently a non-perfusing rhythm.

(a)

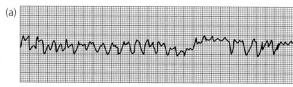

Rhythm strip 2—ventricular fibrillation (VF).

(b)

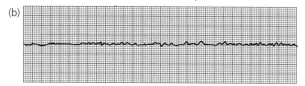

Rhythm strip 3—"fine" ventricular fibrillation.

FIGURE 5.14 (a) Ventricular fibrillation (b) "fine" ventricular fibrillation, which can easily be mistaken for asystole. Reprinted with permission from Thomas J, Monaghan T. *Oxford Handbook of Clinical Examination and Practical Skills.* 2007, Oxford University Press.

Treatment

DC cardioversion (unsynchronized) is the most effective action. Use the standard protocol of 200 J, 200–300 J, 360 J if monophasic defibrillator or equivalent if biphasic.

Between shocks, give epinephrine 1 mg IV push or vasopressin 40 mg IV push. If unsuccessful, reattempt DC cardioversion and consider further antiarrhythmics such as amiodarone, lidocaine, magnesium, etc.

In the rare patient with recurrent VF, an implantable cardiac defibrillator (ICD) may improve survival.

Take Home Points

- Ventricular fibrillation is inherently unstable and often associated with sudden cardiac death.
- ECG is characteristically irregular and erratic.
- Unsynchronized electrical cardioversion should not be delayed.

Asystole/Pulseless Electrical Activity (PEA)

No or minimal electrical activity occurring anywhere in the heart. By definition, no pulse can be elicited anywhere in the body.

For PEA, consider the Hs and Ts.

TABLE 5.10 Causes of PEA

Hs	Ts
Hypovolemia	Toxins
Hypoxia	Tamponade, cardiac
Hydrogen ion (acidosis)	Tension pneumothorax
Hypo/Hyper-kalemia	Thrombosis (coronary or pulmonary)
Hypoglycemia	Trauma
Hypothermia	

Diagnosis

ECG shows:

In asystole, the absence of electrical activity. Make sure fine V fib is not present (the difference being VF is shockable, asystole/PEA is not).

In PEA, diagnosis is made by presence of uncoordinated electrical activity without result of pulse.

Treatment

Make sure ECG reading is accurate and patient is unresponsive.

Start CPR and obtain IV/IO access.

Asystole/PEA are *NOT* shockable rhythms.

Give epinephrine 1 mg IV/IO and repeat every 3–5 min.

Or give vasopressin 40 U IV/IO to replace 1st, 2nd doses of epinephrine.

Consider atropine 1 mg IV/IO and repeat every 3–5 min.

Correct the cause of the arrhythmia, ASAP (Hs and Ts).

Take Home Points

- Asystole/PEA are NOT considered shockable rhythms.
- Find and correct the Hs and Ts, ASAP.

Wolff-Parkinson-White (WPW) Syndrome

WPW results from impulse conduction through an accessory pathway which bypasses the AV node leading to unregulated excitation of the ventricles. There are several types of WPW resulting in rhythms such as reentrant SVT, antidromic tachycardia (anterograde conduction through the accessory pathway and retrograde conduction through the AV node), and atrial flutter or fibrillation. The manner of sudden cardiac death from WPW is atrial fibrillation that progresses to conduct rapidly through the accessory pathway leading to ventricular fibrillation.

Symptoms

Clinically, may range from mild palpitations to syncope. Severe palpitations may also be a presenting sign. Uncommonly, further arrhythmias such as ventricular fibrillation may develop and lead to death acutely.

Diagnosis

ECG: Characteristic short P-R interval with a **delta wave**.

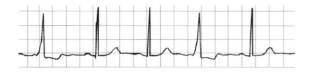

FIGURE 5.15 WPW syndrome with delta waves apparent in 1st and 4th beats. Notice how the delta wave both broadens the ventricular complex and shortens the PR interval. Reprinted with permission from Flynn JA. *Oxford American Handbook of Clinical Medicine.* 2007, Oxford University Press.

Provocation or dysrrhythmia and risk stratification can be done with electrophysiologic testing but this is generally done by a cardiologist.

Treatment

Immediate cardiology referral is indicated.

Restrict vigorous physical activity and sports participation until seen by a cardiologist.

Avoid digoxin, adenosine, β-blockers and Ca channel blockers which can slow conduction through the AV node and isolate conduction through the accessory pathway!

Radiofrequency ablation of the accessory pathway is the standard!

In the unstable patient, consider IV procainamide acutely.

Drugs that may be used in the intermittently symptomatic patient are: quinidine, disopyramide (Norpace), procainamide (Pronestyl), and propafenone (Rythmol).

In asymptomatic patients without concern for further progression after workup, no therapy may be indicated.

Take Home Points

- WPW is associated with delta waves and shortened PR interval on ECG.

- Three types of WPW exist depending on the anatomy of the accessory pathway.

- Refer to cardiology, which may result in radiofrequency ablation of the accessory pathway.

Valvular Disease

TABLE 5.11 Common Valvular Diseases

Lesion		Associations/Exam	Treatment
Mitral	Stenosis	May be caused by Rheumatic heart disease. Atrial fib is an uncommon complication. **Diastolic** blowing murmur with/without opening snap.	Rate control with digoxin or β-blocker as needed. Anticoagulate if atrial fib is present. Antibiotic prophylaxis for dental procedures. Treat with balloon valvuloplasty or valve replacement.
	Regurgitation	Holo**systolic** murmur made louder with valsalva.	Valvular repair or replacement if symptomatic or ejection fraction < 60%.
Mitral valve prolapsed (MVP)		Chest pain, anxiety, palpitations, dyspnea, and possibly panic attacks. **Mid systolic click**, late **systolic** murmur.	Reassurance that MVP rarely leads to cardiac problems.
Aortic	Stenosis	Syncope, CHF, angina, sudden death. After symptoms develop, short term mortality is high. May be associated with rheumatic heart disease if mitral valve is also affected. Harsh, **systolic** crescendo/decrescendo murmur. Made softer with valsalva.	Antibiotic prophylaxis for dental procedures. Valvular replacement is the standard (unless severely elderly).
	Regurgitation	Associated with endocarditis, rheumatic heart disease, collagen vascular disease, aortic dissection, bicuspid aortic valve, and syphilis. Look for widened pulse pressure. High pitched, **diastolic**, decrescendo murmur.	Afterload reduction with Nifedipine or ACE-Is. Valvular replacement is definitive and often best treatment.

Infectious Endocarditis

Inflammation of the cardiac valvular or mural endocardium. Septic vegetation formation within the cardiac chambers or attached to a valve presents a common source of embolization to the systemic circulation. Major risk factors are IV drug use (more commonly causing a right heart endocarditis) or valvular disease.

Symptoms

Fever, chest pain, rigors, malaise, back pain, anorexia, weight loss, conjunctival hemorrhage, painful hand or toe lesions (**Osler's nodes**), CHF symptoms, or symptoms of systemic embolization including TIA or stroke.

Diagnosis

Physical exam: New murmur with increased intensity upon deep inspiration, cardiac friction rub, Osler's nodes (painful, deep, lesions on fingers and toes), **Janeway lesions** (small skin infarctions), nail bed splinter hemorrhages, and Roth spots (retinal exudates) may occur especially with advanced cases.

Blood cultures: Take three different cultures from 2 different sites. *Strep viridans* is the most common bacterial cause. Others include the classic HACEK organisms (*Haemophilus aphrophilus, H parainfluenzae, Actinobacillus actinomycetemcomitans, Cardiobacterium hominis, Eikenella corrodens, Kingella kingae*) although isolation by culture may be difficult.

Labs: CBC for WBC and Hct, ESR, CMP for screening, UA for hematuria, rheumatoid factor.

Echocardiography: Transthoracic echo should be done first but if negative obtain a transesophageal echo to look for vegetations.

Clinical tool: Duke criteria are the classic clinical tool for diagnosing infective endocarditis.

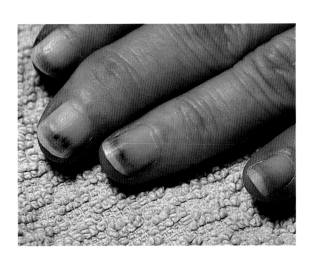

FIGURE 5.16 Splinter hemorrhages in a case of infective endocarditis. Reprinted with permission from Warrell DA, Cox TM, et al. *Oxford Textbook of Medicine*, 4th edition. 2003, Oxford University Press.

TABLE 5.12 Duke Criteria for Diagnosis of Endocarditis

Criteria	Description
Major	Positive blood cultures for infective endocarditis
	Positive echocardiogram
	New valvular regurgitation

(continued)

TABLE 5.12 Continued

Criteria	Description
Minor	Predisposition i.e., preexisting valvular condition or IV drug use
	Fever (temp > 100.4 F)
	Vascular phenomena, e.g., arterial emboli, mycotic aneurysm, Janeway lesions, conjunctival hemorrhages
	Immunologic phenomena, e.g., glomerulonephritis, Osler's nodes, Roth spots, RF positive
	Microbiologic evidence: positive blood culture but not meeting a major criterion or serologic evidence of active infection with organism consistent with endocarditis

Definite infective endocarditis: Two major criteria *or* one major criteria and 3 minor criteria *or* five minor criteria.

Treatment

Prevent with antibiotic prophylaxis in selected heart disease patients; obviously, avoid IV drug use.

Give oxygen.

Start antibiotics empirically. If likely to be skin organisms, start antistaphylococcal penicillin such as oxacillin or nafcillin *plus* penicillin G or, alternatively, ampicillin *plus* gentamicin. If MRSA (methicillin-resistant *S. aureus*) is possible, replace penicillin with vancomycin. Cultures should then guide treatment. Treatment should continue for 4–6 weeks. Don't forget to check gentamicin and vancomycin peaks and troughs.

Surgery: Valvular replacement may be indicated depending on severity of case and presence or absence of emboli.

Take Home Points

- Two major risk factors for endocarditis are valvular abnormalities and IV drug use.
- Use the Duke criteria for diagnosis.
- Assess risk factors for skin bacteria and start empiric antibiotics. Adjust the regimen based on culture results (multiple cultures needed).

Congenital Heart Disease

TABLE 5.13 Congenital Heart Disease

Defect	Associations	Exam	Treatment
Ventricular Septal Defect	If lesion is large, sx of CHF, frequent respiratory infections, or FTT. Often close on their own. Most common congenital heart defect. Eisenmenger syndrome: pulm HTN → RVH → conversion to R to L shunt causing cyanosis.	Pansystolic vibratory murmur	Follow small lesions annually for closure. Surgery for large lesions as soon as possible.

(continued)

TABLE 5.13 Continued

Defect	Associations	Exam	Treatment
Atrial Septal Defect	Often asymptomatic until adulthood. Sx of CHF are late finding of large defects. Eisenmenger syndrome is possible late.	Fixed split S2, systolic ejection murmur.	Small, asymptomatic defects do not need closure. Large defects may be surgically repaired. Antibiotics prior to dental procedures.
Patent Ductus Arteriosus (PDA)	Not diagnosed due to physiologic PDA in first few days of life. Produces L to R shunt. Associated with prematurity, high altitude, 1st trimester rubella.	Machinery murmur, wide pulse pressure, bounding peripheral pulses.	Eliminate possibility of other heart defects before treating. Child may depend on PDA for life! Keep open with prostaglandin E$_1$ if indicated. Close with indomethacin (Indocin) or other NSAID.
Coarctation of the Aorta	Turner syndrome, male sex, bicuspid aortic valve. Rib notching on chest X-ray.	Higher blood pressure in upper than lower extremities. Diminished lower extremity pulses. Systolic murmur.	Surgical correction is the standard. Balloon angioplasty is possibility depending on defect.
Tetralogy of Fallot	Features 1. Pulmonary stenosis 2. RVH 3. Overriding aorta 4. VSD "Tet spells"-child stops running/exercising to stop and squat. Chest X-ray shows boot-shaped heart.	Systolic ejection murmur, single S2. Cyanosis.	If cyanotic at birth, give PGE. Surgery is the standard of care and requires several different procedures. Treat tet spells with O$_2$, knee/chest position, morphine, and β-blockers.
Transposition of the Great Vessels	Congenital condition of pulmonary and systemic circulations existing in parallel. Life depends on PDA or VSD for oxygenated blood mixing, otherwise incompatible with life.	Cyanosis, tachycardia, and respiratory failure at birth. CHF signs may be present.	Prostaglandin E$_1$ (alprostadil) to keep PDA open. Surgery includes balloon septostomy to delay surgery if needed. Then staged surgical redirection early.

Abdominal Aortic Aneurysm (AAA)

A focal dilatation of the aortic segment within the abdomen having at least a 50% larger diameter than expected in that segment. Greater than 90% occur below the renal artery anastomoses and the most common risk factor is atherosclerosis although others include hypertension, tobacco use, male gender, age, and family history.

Symptoms

Commonly this disorder is asymptomatic. The patient may present with a pulsatile or vague epigastric mass or pain, urethral obstruction (and symptoms), or back pain from vertebral body erosion. The triad of **shock, abdominal pain, and pulsatile mass** suggests rupture. Obtain family history for Marfan syndrome or Ehlers-Danlos syndrome. Check blood pressure and obtain smoking and coronary artery disease (CAD) risk factors. These relate directly to diagnosis and treatment options.

Diagnosis

Physical exam: Palpable, pulsatile mass in the abdomen.
Imaging: Ultrasound (US) is the initial standard. May use US to measure unruptured aneurysm but need to obtain CT if rupture suspected. CT is also the best preoperative test.

MRI is a good choice if the patient is unable to tolerate CT contrast, can wait somewhat longer for the test, and is hemodynamically stable.

Treatment

Control risk factors such as smoking and hypertension.

β-blockers are the agent of choice for HTN in conjunction with AAA.

Surgical correction is the best option but size does matter. Indications are size greater than **5.5 cm or growth greater than 0.5 cm per 6 months**.

For medium-sized aneurysms (3.5–5.5 cm), watchful waiting and control of risk factors is best. Serial ultrasounds are indicated **every 6 months** to track expansion.

Aortic stents have recently been used but are of uncertain benefit thus far.

Take Home Points

- The triad of shock, abdominal pain, and pulsatile mass suggests AAA rupture.
- Obtain US to diagnosis and monitor the AAA.
- Refer to surgery AAAs that are ≥ 5.5 cm in size or grow ≥ 0.5 cm/6 months.

Aortic Dissection

The primary event in aortic dissection is a tear in the aortic intima, forming a secondary "false" lumen within the aortic wall. The most common risk factor remains hypertension, although others include preexisting aortic aneurysm, collagen vascular diseases (Marfan/Ehlers-Danlos), vasculitities, or conditions of genetic predisposition such as Turner syndrome, coarctation of the aorta, or bicuspid aortic valve.

Stanford classification:
Type A: Dissection involving the ascending aorta and aortic arch.
Type B: Dissection involving the descending aorta.

Symptoms

The most common complaint is a "tearing" or "ripping" sensation in the chest. This is commonly reported as sharp and well-localized pain. This sensation may radiate to the back, between scapulae, or shoulder region. Depending on severity (or survivability of the primary event), symptoms may also include syncope, limb ischemia, abdominal pain, angina, Horner syndrome, fever, or newly raspy voice. Remember, aortic dissection is "the other life-threatening chest pain" besides MI.

Diagnosis

Physical exam: Distant heart sounds, systolic murmur, hypotension, pallor, or diaphoresis.

Imaging: Chest x-ray may show widened mediastinum, enlargement of the aortic knob, double density of the descending aorta, or pleural effusion.

CT scan is used most often in the hemodynamically stable patient although spiral CT has shown significant improvement over conventional CT.

MRI is also useful if available in the stable patient.

Transthoracic echocardiography (TTE) is less useful due to inability to visualize the descending aorta.

Transesophageal echocardiography (TEE) is commonly used in the hemodynamically unstable patient with high sensitivity/specificity. However, its success is highly dependent on the operator's level of experience.

Aortography has largely been replaced with noninvasive accurate methods.

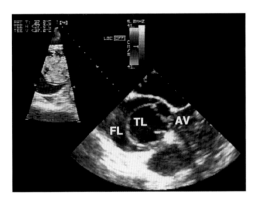

FIGURE 5.17 Transesphageal transverse two-dimensional and color Doppler echo images of the ascending aorta showing a dissection membrane partitioning the true (TL) and false (FL) lumens. Upper left panel shows systolic flow in the true lumen (but none in the false lumen). Reprinted with permission from Warrell DA, Cox TM, et al. *Oxford Textbook of Medicine*, 4th edition. 2003, Oxford University Press.

Treatment

Manage hemodynamically unstable patients aggressively.

Acute instability with confirmed or highly suspected aortic dissection necessitates prompt surgery.

Type A dissections (ascending aorta/aortic arch) are most commonly treated with surgery or stent placement. Lower the blood pressure acutely if needed. Start with IV β-blockers (propanolol, esmolol, labetalol) then switch to nitroprusside.

Type B dissections (descending) are most commonly treated with medical therapy and tight hypertension control. If the patient continues to be symptomatic, stent placement or surgery is considered.

Refer the patient for definitive treatment.

Take Home Points

- Aortic dissection is the "other life-threatening chest pain."
- Patients often feel a tearing or ripping sensation.
- CT scan is often the first confirmatory test used in practicality.
- In both types, lowering the blood pressure is an effective first step.
- Definitive treatment often depends on type; however, referral is almost always indicated.

Peripheral Vascular Disease

Atherosclerotic narrowing with eventual slowing or complete occlusion of blood flow to peripheral arteries, most commonly affecting the lower extremities. Risk factors parallel those for coronary artery disease such as hyperlipidemia, hypertension, obesity, sedentary lifestyle, age, smoking, etc.

Symptoms

Intermittent claudication is the most common symptom and is pathognomonic. This pain commonly occurs in the lower extremities but may present in the back and buttocks. Impotence may be seen in men.

Diagnosis

Physical exam: Lower extremity appearance is often cold, pale, shiny, and hairless.
Ankle-brachial index (ABI)—ratio of ankle and brachial blood pressures is often abnormal. Normal range is between 0.90 and 1.3.

> Exercise treadmill testing with pre and post ABI is often used.
> Segmental limb pressures may be helpful in further evaluation.
> Doppler ultrasound can be used to establish degree of flow.

Angiography and MRA are useful but are used before surgery, not for diagnosis.

Treatment

Control of risk factors such as smoking, hyperlipidemia, diabetes, hypertension, etc. is critically important.

> **Graded exercise training** is the single most effective treatment.
> Antiplatelet agents such as aspirin, dipyridamole (Persantine), and clopidegril (Plavix) have all been shown to have some benefit. Other antiplatelet agents such as cilostazol (Pletal) and pentoxifylline (Trental) have also been used with success.
> Surgery is reserved for severe cases of larger vessels.

Take Home Points

- Ankle-brachial index is a key measurement for PVD.

- Graded exercise training can significantly improve this condition. Consider addition of antiplatelet medications as well.

Arterial Embolism/Thrombosis

The acute occlusion of an artery or arteriole by an embolic event or locally formed thrombus. The primary event is then propagated by stagnant blood flow in the vessel causing acute ischemia or infarction to the distal territory. The most commonly affected age group is the geriatric population, although this disease may also be seen in the IV drug user.

Symptoms

Rapid onset extremity pain or numbness.

Diagnosis

Physical exam: Loss of pulse, loss of capillary refill, redness, and swelling may be seen. Signs of complications such as compartment syndrome must be considered.

Arterial Doppler ultrasound to establish flow.

Ankle-brachial index may be measured and is often profound.

Angiography is not useful in diagnosis but may play a role in preoperative imaging.

Labs: D-dimer (if positive, further testing needs to be done before test is useful), coagulation panel. Chest pain or symptoms may warrant cardiac enzymes.

EKG as indicated.

Treatment

Oxygen

Pain medications as needed.

Aspirin

Anticoagulation with heparin or LMW heparin (Lovenox).

Consider thrombolytics but make sure they are not contraindicated in the patient. These include tPA and streptokinase.

If in early stages, surgery such as balloon embolectomy may be considered.

If in late stages with evidence of infarction/gangrene, amputation of distal portion should be considered.

Take Home Points

- Look for signs of compartment syndrome occurring in the affected limb.

- The "golden" period is 4–6 hours after onset and represents the time before infarction takes place and the maximal time to affect outcome.

Raynaud Disease/Phenomenon

Raynaud disease—idiopathic vasospasm of distal extremity vessels causing symptoms. This commonly bilateral and symmetric disease is associated with the following risk factors: female sex, age 15–45 years old, and family history.

Raynaud phenomenon—due to underlying syndrome or cause (other than primary Raynaud disease). Often unilateral or localized to individual digits. Overall, morbidity is worse than primary Raynaud disease.

Symptoms

Symptoms most often occur with exposure to cold, alcohol, emotional distress, or smoking. First distal extremity or digits loose sensation, turn white or show notably increased pallor. Upon warming, pain and parasthesias, swelling, and erythema set in which can be debilitating. In severe cases, symptoms may progress to atrophy of fat pads and eventual autoamputation.

Diagnosis

Physical exam: White or pale appearance to distal digit with well demarcated transition line in finger, loss of sensation or tenderness to distal digit. Swelling or erythema may be present after event.

Cold challenge (with immersion in cold water) may be diagnostic.

Nailfold capillary exam is suggestive of secondary causes if capillary loops appear enlarged or distorted.

Test for secondary causes and obtain ANA, TSH, ESR, CBC, coagulation profile.

Treatment

Treat secondary causes of disease (e.g., Lupus, scleroderma, etc.).

Avoid cold exposure via gloves or insulated foot wear. Behavioral modification after symptom recognition to abort attacks with warm water, windmill arm motion, etc. may be useful.

Medications:

Avoiding cold weather, long-acting, calcium channel blockers (nifedipine, amlodipine, etc) have been shown effective. Aspirin or topical nitroglycerin may be added as the next step.

In severe cases, IV prostaglandin/prostaglandin analogues or chemical sympathectomy with lidocaine or bupivicaine may be indicated.

Take Home Points

- Raynaud disease is often bilateral and symmetric while the phenomenon is unilateral or asymmetric and associated with an underlying disease state.

- Treat any identifiable causes of underlying disease. Behavioral modification with glove wearing and cold/smoking avoidance often helps.

Superficial Thrombophlebitis

An inflammatory disorder of the superficial veins leading to/or caused by local thrombosis. This disorder may be septic or aseptic in nature. Risk factors include hypercoagulable states such as postpartum status, pregnancy, use of oral contraceptive pills, smoking, or genetic disposition. The leading risk factor for septic disease remains the presence of indwelling venous catheters.

Symptoms

Pain, tenderness, erythema, and local swelling along the affected superficial vein. If septic, may be associated with fever and signs of infection.

Diagnosis

Physical exam: Classically reveals a tender, **palpable "cord"** commonly with surrounding erythema.
Labs: Obtain CBC for WBCs to evaluate for possible septic thrombus or cellulitis, β-hCG, coagulation profile, platelet studies, protein C & S levels, antithrombin III level, ANA, factor V level, and other blood clotting disease as indicated.
Imaging: Ultrasound may be used to both confirm the presence of a superficial venous thrombosis and exclude deep venous thrombi.

Treatment

Warm compresses, NSAIDs, and elevation are the standard treatments.

Remove any possibly thrombosed catheters.

Anticoagulate only if associated with DVT. Otherwise, it is not needed.

Treat coagulation disorder.

Measures against embolism are not indicated as are in DVT.

Antibiotics and surgical exploration may be indicated if thrombus is septic.

Take Home Points

- Superficial thrombosis patients often have an underlying hypercoagulable state present.

- Septic thrombosis is more common in hospitalized patients with indwelling catheters.

Deep Venous Thrombosis (DVT)

Thrombosis located in the "deep" veins, most commonly of the pelvic or lower extremity region. Lower extremity thrombi are commonly split into two categories: proximal (thigh), referring to those occurring proximal to the popliteal trifurcation; and distal (calf), referring to those occurring distal to this. Proximal DVTs are more likely to embolize, distal DVTs often cause local symptoms.

Symptoms

Pain, swelling, erythema in the lower extremities. History often reveals hypercoagulable state, prolonged sitting or stasis, or injury (Virchow's triad-stasis, hypercoagulable state, endothelial damage). This may include OCP use, pregnancy, hormone replacement therapy, long plane flight, smoking, recent injury, factor V Leiden mutation, or blood clotting disorder such as protein C/S deficiency.

Diagnosis

Physical exam: May reveal positive Homans' sign (pain in calf on dorsiflexion of ankle), erythema, swelling, warmth, and tenderness of affected limb.

Labs: D-dimer is classic, but if positive simply indicates further testing needs to be done. If negative, is fairly reliable. Combination of the D-dimer and use of the **Wells score** has recently been shown very accurate in predicting DVT presence. CBC for platelet count and Hct, coagulation profile, fibrinogen, complete metabolic panel, and urinalysis. Further testing is indicated if cause remains idiopathic and may include protein C/S levels, factor V Leiden, factor VIII level, ANA, and PSA in men over 50 years.

Imaging: Doppler compression ultrasound is most widely used and considered most accurate but beware that this is only reliable for clots in femoral and popliteal areas.

Contrast venography is the gold standard but involves contrast and is not the first line test.

MRI may be a good alternative to contrast venography but is second line to Doppler U/S.

Impedance plethysmography may also be used, where available, but is much less common.

Clinically consider pulmonary embolism. If suspected, do a chest CT or V/Q scan.

TABLE 5.14 Wells Score for Probability of DVT Presence

Clinical Element	Point
Active cancer	1
Paralysis, paresis, recent plaster immobilization of lower limb	1
Recently bedridden for > 3 days or major surgery in past 4 weeks	1
Localized tenderness along distribution of deep venous system	1
Entire leg swollen	1
Calf swelling > 3 cm when compared to asymptomatic leg below the tibial tuberosity	1
Pitting edema	1
Collateral superficial veins (nonvaricose)	1
Alternative diagnosis as likely or more likely than that of DVT	–2

Probability
High   ≥ 3 points
Intermediate   1–2 points
Low   ≤ 0 points

Treatment

Low molecular weight heparin, enoxaparin (Lovenox) (1 mg/kg SC bid) or heparin IV or SC should be started immediately. Enoxaparin is most convenient and avoids excess monitoring needed with heparin. However, is most appropriate for uncomplicated disease.

Start warfarin (Coumadin) at the same time as enoxaparin/heparin and overlap these by several days to allow the INR (international normalized ratio) to achieve a level between 2–3. Then enoxaparin or heparin may be discontinued.

Duration of warfarin (Coumadin) use varies with level of complication of DVT. If uncomplicated and likely due to temporary coagulation defect, three months is adequate. If complicated with hereditary or acquired (malignancy) hypercoagulable state, surgery, need for prolonged inactivity, or pulmonary embolism, longer therapy may be required and last from 6–12 months to indefinite.

IVC (inferior vena cava) filters may be an option for those who are not candidates for anticoagulation but do have increased risk of recurrent DVT.

Thrombolytics are still being researched and are not currently recommended for treatment of DVT.

Remember to place all hospitalized patients on DVT prophylaxis of some sort (commonly enoxaparin (Lovenox) 40 mg SC qd for the non hip/knee replacement patient).

Take Home Points

- Virchow's triad—stasis, hypercoagulable state, and endothelial damage.
- Doppler US is the first line test for lower extremity DVT.
- Overlap the use of heparin or LMWH with starting warfarin (Coumadin) to avoid a theoretic transient hypercoagulable state.
- Keep the INR between 2 and 3 when on warfarin therapy.

Varicose Veins

Tortuous and dilated superficial veins with incompetent valves. They are most commonly found in the legs but may occur in almost any other area. Risk factors include pregnancy, occupations which require prolonged standing, older age, female sex, and obesity.

Symptoms

Often noticed by the patient to be unsightly, purple, tortuous veins on lower extremities. Usually non-tender (although large lesions may be painful), but patient may fixate on them. Only rarely are they inflamed or erythematous unless there is an overlying skin infection. Skin breaks and subsequent bleeding is rare. These may be accompanied by telangectasial lesions in the same areas.

Diagnosis

Physical exam: Tortuous enlarged veins and telangectasias usually of the lower extremities.

Treatment

Prevention with support stockings and frequent breaks for those with jobs requiring long standing or foot work.

Injection sclerotherapy with hypertonic saline or sodium tetradecyl sulfate, electrocauterization, or laser treatment are effective for telangectasial lesions.

Surgery: Vein ligation and stripping, removal with subsequent skin grafting, or stab avulsion phlebectomy are effective in management but careful consideration of extent of disease should be done before referral.

Take Home Points

- Varicose veins occur more often in older females.
- Treatment should be attempted with injected sclerosing agents, laser, or electrocautery before attempting surgery.

Atherosclerosis

The disease course of lipoid plaque formation within the intima and inner media of arteries and arterioles. Plaque make-up consists of cholesterol deposits, lipoid material, and lipophages. This process begins as early as childhood as "fatty streaks" on vessel walls. In the acute setting, plaque rupture leads to activation of the clotting cascade, leading to thrombus formation and occlusion of the vessel, which in turn can lead to ischemia and infarction downstream.

Symptoms

The disease itself is asymptomatic but complications include peripheral vascular disease, angina, myocardial infarction, stroke, etc. Look for symptoms of each. History is important and may reveal risk factors such as diabetes, smoking, obesity, hyperlipidemia, alcoholism, or hypertension.

Diagnosis

Atherosclerosis is not directly diagnosed or necessarily tested for. Testing for risk factors includes lipid levels, blood pressure measurement, markers of global inflammation, and direct end organ damage (renal function, suspected AAA, etc.).

Direct measurement of narrowing of vessels is tested for by carotid artery ultrasound and coronary artery catheterization when indicated.

Treatment

Lifestyle modification to slow progression of developing atherosclerosis is very effective. Increase activity, stop smoking, lose weight, and control diabetes.

Medications: Aspirin may be used for antiplatelet effects for prophylaxis or if an atherosclerotic plaque ruptures.

Statins (Lovastatin, Simvastatin, etc.) have been shown to reduce cholesterol levels and increase HDL, thus slowing progression of the disease. See section on Hyperlipidemia for further discussion.

Research has shown that with significant control of risk factors, atherosclerosis can be reversed.

Take Home Points

- Atherosclerotic risk factors include diabetes, smoking, obesity, hyperlipidemia, alcoholism, and hypertension.
- Coronary artery catheterization and carotid artery ultrasound are isolated examples of direct measurement of atherosclerosis.
- Treat and prevent disease with the use of lifestyle modification and statin medication.

Hyperlipidemia

The disease state of elevated blood lipid levels including total cholesterol, LDL cholesterol, and triglycerides. Other markers may be used for hyperlipidemia and essentially contribute to the diagnosis; these include Lp(a), VLDL, ultrasensitive CRP, etc.

Symptoms

Commonly asymptomatic, although consequences of atherosclerosis may be evident.

The Third Report of the National Cholesterol Education Program (NCEP) Expert Panel on Detection, Evaluation, and Treatment of High Blood Cholesterol in Adults (Adult Treatment Panel III), or ATP III, has set forth the following definitions.

Major Risk Factors (Exclusive of LDL Cholesterol) That Modify LDL Goals:

- Cigarette smoking

- Hypertension (BP ≥ 140/90 mmHg or on antihypertensive medication)

- Low HDL cholesterol (< 40 mg/dl)*

- Family history of premature CHD (CHD in male first degree relative <55 years; CHD in female first degree relative < 65 years)

- Age (men ≥ 45 years; women ≥ 55 years)

* HDL cholesterol ≥ 60 mg/dL counts as a "negative" risk factor; its presence removes one risk factor from the total count.

Coronary Heart Disease (CHD) risk equivalents:
Diabetes mellitus
Clinical CHD
Peripheral vascular disease
Symptomatic carotid artery disease
Abdominal aortic aneurysm

Diagnosis

Labs: Obtain blood lipid levels after 9–12 hour fast.

Tables 5.15–20 are from the Third Report of the Expert Panel on Detection, Evaluation, and Treatment of High Blood Cholesterol in Adults (Adult Treatment Panel III).

TABLE 5.15 LDL Cholesterol Levels

LDL-Cholesterol Levels	
< 100 mg/dL	Optimal
100–129 mg/dL	Near optimal/above optimal
130–159 mg/dL	Borderline high
160–189 mg/dL	High
≥ 190 mg/dL	Very high

TABLE 5.16 Total Cholesterol Levels

Total Cholesterol Levels	
< 200 mg/dL	Optimal
200–239 mg/dL	Borderline high
≥ 240 mg/dL	High

TABLE 5.17 HDL Cholesterol Levels

HDL-Cholesterol Levels	
< 40 mg/dL	A major risk factor for heart disease
40–59 mg/dL	The higher the HDL, the better
≥ 60 mg/dL	An HDL of 60 mg/dL and above is considered protective against heart disease

TABLE 5.18 Triglyceride Levels

Triglyceride Levels	
< 150 m g/dL	Normal
150–199 mg/dL	Borderline-high
200–499 mg/dL	High
≥ 500 mg/dL	Very High

TABLE 5.19 LDL Goals and Intervention Levels

Risk Category	LDL Goal	LDL Level at Which to Initiate Therapeutic Lifestyle Changes (TLC)	LDL Level at Which to Consider Drug Therapy
CHD or CHD Risk Equivalents	< 100 mg/dL	≥ 100 mg/dL	≥ 130 mg/dL (100–129 mg/dL: drug optional)
2+ Risk Factors	< 130 mg/dL	≥ 130 mg/dL	≥ 130 mg/dL ≥ 160 mg/dL
0–1 Risk Factor	< 160 mg/dL	≥ 160 mg/dL	≥ 190 mg/dL (160–189 mg/dL: LDL-lowering drug optional)

Consider the patient's individual risk factors and CHD status.

Treatment

For those with CHD or equivalents, start with therapeutic lifestyle changes (TLC) in conjunction with lipid-lowering agents immediately upon diagnosis.

For those without CHD or equivalents, start with therapeutic lifestyle changes (TLC) for three months followed by retesting and evaluation.

TLC changes:
TLC diet:

Saturated fat < 7% of daily calories, cholesterol intake < 200 mg/day
Consider increasing soluble fiber (10–25 g/day) and plant sterols (2 g/day)

Weight management
Increased physical activity

TABLE 5.20 Medications by Class for Hyperlipidemia

Drug Class	Agents and Daily Doses	Side Effects	Contraindications
HMG CoA reductase inhibitors (statins)	Lovastatin Pravastatin Simvastatin Fluvastatin Atorvastatin Cerivastatin	Myopathy Increased liver enzymes	Absolute: • Active or chronic liver disease Relative: • Concomitant use of certain drugs
Bile acid sequestrants	Cholestyramine Colestipol Colesevelam	Gastrointestinal distress Constipation Decreased absorption of other drugs	Absolute: • Dysbeta-lipoproteinemia • TG > 400 mg/dL Relative: • TG > 200 mg/dL
Nicotinic acid	Immediate release (crystalline) nicotinic acid, extended release nicotinic acid (Niaspan), sustained release nicotinic acid	Flushing Hyperglycemia Hyperuricemia (or gout) Upper GI distress Hepatotoxicity	Absolute: • Chronic liver disease • Severe gout Relative: • Diabetes • Hyperuricemia • Peptic ulcer disease
Fibric acids	Gemfibrozil Fenofibrate Clofibrate	Dyspepsia Gallstones Myopathy	Absolute: • Severe renal disease • Severe hepatic disease
Intestinal cholesterol absorption inhibitors	Ezetimibe	Few; possibly myopathy and elevation of liver enzymes	Relative: Liver dysfunction
Omega 3 acid ethyl esters	Lovaza	Foul (fishy) smelling breath Nausea GI bloating Flatulence	None specifically

Take Home Points

- Hyperlipidemia is a risk factor for the development of atherosclerosis and related diseases.
- Consider the patient's CHD status and risk factors to formulate a treatment plan.
- For average risk patient (1–2 risk factors), approximate levels should be: total cholesterol < 200 mg/dL, LDL < 130 mg/dL, HDL > 40 mg/dL, triglycerides < 130 mg/dL.
- Treat with both TLC and medications!

6   Respiratory Medicine

Acute Bronchitis

Inflammation of the trachea, bronchi, and/or bronchioles, resulting most commonly from viral infection, although bacterial causes should be considered. Infectious agents involve adenovirus, influenza A and B, parainfluenza, *Bordetella pertussis*, RSV, *H influenzae*, and *S pneumoniae*.

Symptoms

Usually seen in combination with other URI type symptoms. Symptoms consist of malaise, chills, mild to moderate fever, chest congestion, chest fullness, and cough. The most persistent of these is cough, which may be present for weeks after successful treatment.

Diagnosis

Generally, clinical assessment is all that is necessary.

Physical exam: Mild scattered rhonchi throughout bilateral lung fields, mild anterior cervical lymph-adenopathy, low grade fever.

Labs: If significantly ill with increased temperature, prolonged illness despite treatment, or concomitant underlying disease such as COPD, sputum culture and Gram stain may be indicated. If done, base treatment with antibiotics on sensitivities achieved.

Chest X-ray: May be used to exclude other common respiratory infections such as pneumonia but will be negative with genuine bronchitis.

Treatment

Supportive care is most effective since the vast majority of cases are caused by viruses.

Increasing hydration or oral guaifenesin (Robitussin) may be useful as mucolytics.

Steam inhalation may help for a short time.

If cough is productive avoid suppressing it with medication.

Antibiotics are useful if high suspicion of a bacterial cause or if underlying respiratory illness exists. Use amoxicillin or azithromycin PO.

Take Home Points

- The diagnosis of bronchitis should not necessitate antibiotics. Commonly, this disease is caused by a virus.

- Don't suppress a productive cough.

- If bronchitis is prolonged, consider investigation for pneumonia.

Acute Bronchiolitis

Most commonly caused by a virus, bronchiolitis is thought of as a wheezing, respiratory illness in patients **under the age of 2 years**. This may or may not include respiratory distress. The most common virus is respiratory syncytial virus (RSV), although others do exist. This diagnosis may be given if others such as pneumonia, foreign body, or atopy are excluded.

Symptoms

Fast, labored breathing is common. Since this is mostly observed by caregivers, wheezing or signs of respiratory distress may also be reported.

Diagnosis

Physical exam: Tachypnea, intercostal and subcostal retractions, and audible wheezing. The chest may appear hyperexpanded. Findings on auscultation include any combination of wheezing, prolonged expiration, crackles, or fine rales. In severe illness, signs of respiratory distress may be present, including increased work of breathing and cyanosis.

Labs: Oxygen saturation may be lower than clinically suspected. CBC may show an increase in WBCs (adjust for age of patient) and often shows lymphocytic predominance. In moderate-to-severe disease obtain an ABG.

Viral studies with direct antigen or immunofluorescence testing of serologic or nasal secretions for RSV may be useful. Viral culture or PCR are employed less frequently due to time course to result.

Imaging: Chest x-ray may show hyperinflation and peribronchial thickening. Patchy atelectasis with volume loss may result from airway narrowing and mucus plugging. Look for flattened diaphragms and air-bronchograms which are indicative of disease.

Treatment

Supportive care.

Admission for toxic appearance, hypoxemia, cyanosis, moderate-to-severe respiratory distress, or caretaker is unable to care for patient at home.

Consider intubation and respiratory support. If suspicious of need, intubate earlier rather than later.

Give IV fluids.

Inhaled bronchodilators (albuterol) are routinely used; however, research does not lend them strong support. Oral bronchodilators have not been shown effective.

Nebulized epinephrine has been shown more effective than bronchodilators but should be tried after bronchodilators.

Corticosteroids have not been shown effective in mild-moderate disease in infants and children. However, younger infants, newborns, or those children with underlying lung disease may benefit from a short course.

Antiviral therapy such as ribavirin may be effective, but due to cost and impracticality should be reserved for sicker, younger patients with severe or complicating disease.

To help prevent flu virus-caused disease, vaccinate!

Take Home Points

- Eliminate other causes of wheezing in young children such as foreign body, pneumonia, or atopy before diagnosing bronchiolitis.
- Obtain pulse oximetry and consider ABG if indicated.
- Look for air-bronchograms and flattened diaphragms on x-ray.
- Consider admission in most patients.

Croup

A subacute, viral, upper respiratory tract infection causing inflammation of the larynx and subglottic regions leading to hoarseness, cough, and **stridor** in children. Croup is commonly caused by many different viruses including parainfluenza, paramyxovirus, influenza viruses, and others.

Symptoms

Often a disease of childhood, the patient presents with low-grade fever, "**barking**" or "seal-like" cough, **stridor**, fatigue, and possibly hypoxia and cyanosis in advanced cases. History may reveal recent URI.

Diagnosis

Largely a clinical diagnosis.

Physical exam: The most popular clinical tool is the Westley croup score.

TABLE 6.1 Westley Croup Score

Feature	Scale	Scale Explained
Level of consciousness	0–5	Normal, including sleep = 0; disoriented = 5
Cyanosis	0–5	None = 0; with agitation = 4; at rest = 5
Stridor	0–2	None = 0; with agitation = 1; at rest = 2
Air entry	0–2	Normal = 0; decreased = 1; markedly decreased =2
Retractions	0–3	None = 0; mild = 1; moderate = 2; severe = 3

The total score ranges from 0 to 17.

Mild croup is defined by a Westley croup score of ≤ 2. Typically these children have a barking cough and hoarse cry, but no stridor at rest. Children with mild croup may have stridor when agitated and either none, or only mild, chest wall/subcostal retractions.

Moderate croup is defined by a Westley croup score of 3 to 7. Children with moderate croup have stridor at rest, at least mild retractions, and may have other symptoms or signs of respiratory distress.

Severe croup is defined by a Westley croup score of ≥ 8. Children with severe croup have significant stridor at rest, although stridor may decrease with worsening disease and decreased air entry. Retractions are severe and the child may appear anxious, agitated, or fatigued. Prompt recognition and treatment of children with severe croup is very important.

Labs: CBC showing leukocytosis is common but not required. Lymphocytes in differential may be seen.

Rapid antigen testing is available in some centers.

PCR or viral culture is rarely used.

Imaging: Classic PA neck x-ray shows "**steeple chase**" sign indicating subglottic narrowing.

Order a lateral neck x-ray to exclude epiglottis.

Fiberoptic laryngoscopy if available and patient is stable.

Treatment

In mild cases, no treatment is necessary.

Outpatient monitoring in most, inpatient monitoring in severe cases.

Place patient on humidified oxygen.

Racemic, nebulized epinephrine for moderate-to-severe cases. Expect improvement within 30 minutes.

Corticosteroids are the standard treatment. These most commonly include dexamethasone or budesonide (Pulmicort) nebulizer. These generally show improvement within 6 hours. Oral prednisone may also be used but adjust dose to equal that of dexamethasone.

Follow up in 24 hours for confirmation of improvement.

Take Home Points

- The Westley croup score is commonly used to assess children with croup.
- The "steeple chase" sign is classic for croup on PA neck x-ray and represents subglottic narrowing.
- Consider corticosteroids for moderate to severe cases.

Pertussis

A highly contagious, respiratory bacterial infection that characteristically produces a high-pitched cough. Pertussis occurs in females more than males and generally strikes between 3 months and 6 years of age.

Symptoms

Characteristic "**whooping**" or "staccato" paroxysmal cough, mild fever, sore throat, rhinorrhea, anorexia, post-cough inspiratory gasp, or post-cough emesis.

Diagnosis

Labs: CBC for leukocytosis with marked lymphocytosis. Pertussis culture on special medium is rarely used due to timeframe to results.

PCR analysis is rapid, sensitive and specific. Different tests are available and are highly reliable.

Direct fluorescent antigen (DFA) testing is a rapid test although has relatively low sensitivity/specificity.

Antibody testing (ELISA serology assay) is available but generally used in combination with other methods (if at all).

Imaging: CXR is nonspecific and shows perihilar infiltrates, interstitial edema, or atelectasis.

Treatment

Immunize!

Antibiotics including macrolides. Erythromycin and azithromycin (Zithromax) are first line for children and adults. Give prophylactic doses of these antibiotics to household contacts.

Isolate patient until ≥ 5 days after antibiotics.

Admit very young children/infants if necessary.

Cough suppressant and symptomatic relief is warranted. Cough likely to persist after cure of disease.

Take Home Points

- Pertussis produces a characteristic "whooping" cough in children.
- Incidence has decreased dramatically due to widespread immunization.

Pneumonia

TABLE 6.2 Pneumonia by Etiology

Etiology	Symptoms	Diagnosis	Treatment
Community acquired (commonly *S pneumoniae*)	Moderate to high fever, productive cough, night sweats, chills, chest congestion, pharyngitis, wheezing, or chest pain.	Leukocytosis on CBC, often with left shift on differential. Elevated ESR, CRP. Obtain blood culture and sputum cultures to identify organism/susceptibilities. Chest x-ray is best way to diagnose. Opacity is often lobar or segmental. Make sure to check lateral chest x-ray to exclude retrocardiac opacities.	Treat supportively with oral hydration and routine inspiratory therapy as well as supplemental oxygen if O$_2$ sats < 93%. Consider admission. Give antipyretics to suppress fever as needed. Consider a mucolytic (guaifenesin) and/or chest percussion therapy to aid break up of consolidation. Antibiotics should be tailored to organism/setting but a **macrolide** (azithromycin, clarithromycin) is often first line. Respiratory flouroquinolone (levofloxacin, moxifloxacin, gemifloxacin) is second. Consider amoxicillin/clavulonate or cephalosporin in combination with above.
Viral	Low grade fever, mild cough, chest congestion, general malaise, headache, or wheezing. May be relatively asymptomatic.	Lymphocytosis on CBC without left shift on differential. Chest x-ray may show diffuse, patchy opacities throughout lung fields.	Supportive care that rarely needs admission. Fluids, mucolytics, inspiratory therapy, and antipyretics. Consider suppression of cough only late in disease course.
Atypical (*M pneumoniae, C pneumoniae, C psittaci, C burnetti*)	Moderate to high fever, productive cough, night sweats, chills, chest congestion, phayrngitis, wheezing, or chest pain.	Leukoytosis on CBC, Elevated ESR, CRP. If inpatient, obtain blood and sputum samples for culture and sensitivities. Labs positive **cold agglutinin** titer. Chest x-ray may show focal consolidation or diffuse interstitial pattern.	Treat with oral hydration and routine inspiratory therapy. Oxygen if sats < 93%. Consider admission especially in children. Antipyretics as needed. Antibiotics should include appropriate spectrum, commonly a macrolide (azithromycin, erythromycin, clarithromycin). Consider doxycycline or levofloxacin if of the appropriate age.

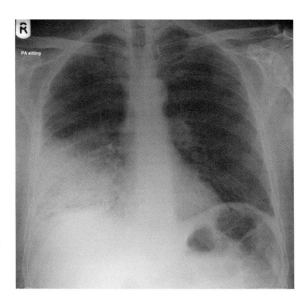

FIGURE 6.1 Opacity of right lower lobe indicating infiltrate in community acquired pneumonia. Reprinted with permission from Thomas J, Monaghan T. *Oxford Handbook of Clinical Examination and Practical Skills.* 2007, Oxford University Press.

TABLE 6.3 Pneumonia Associations

Aspiration (Alcoholic, sedated ospitalized)	*Klebsiella*, anaerobes, gram negatives
Elderly, exposed to indoor ventilation	*Legionella*
Klebsiella	"Currant jelly" sputum
Cystic fibrosis	*P aeruginosa, S aureus, H influenzae*
Immigrant or traveler	Tuberculosis
HIV/AIDS	PCP, fungal
Exposure to birds	*C psittaci, Histoplasmosis*
Bioterrorism	Anthrax
Prior active TB	Aspergillus or other fungus
Southwest US	Coccidioidomycosis

Influenza

An acute viral infection caused by influenza virus type A or B which is confined to the upper and lower respiratory tracks. Outbreaks occur annually with variants of these two viruses created by the process of antigenic drift.

Symptoms

Abrupt onset of fever, severe myalgias, anorexia, sore throat, headache, stuffy nose, arthralgias, cough, fatigue, chest congestion, and malaise. Clinically distinguish from a cold or URI. Influenza does not involve the GI tract (thus rarely causes associated symptoms).

Diagnosis

Labs: Nasal washings and direct antigen testing is the most accurate and convenient technique available. Several commercial testing kits are available but only one distinguishes between influenza types A and B. Viral culture, PCR, or antibody titers are possible but impractical. CBC may show mildly increased leukocytes, but if significantly high, consider secondary bacterial infection.

Chest x-ray is rarely needed but may be used if significant respiratory symptoms are present. Viral pneumonia appears as more diffuse, patchy infiltrates.

Treatment

Supportive outpatient care is often all that is needed.

Give NSAIDs or acetaminophen.

Antiviral agents include amantadine (Symmetrel), rimantadine (Flumadine), zanamivir (Relenza), and oseltamivir (Tamiflu). Amantadine and rimantadine are recommended for the treatment of influenza A only, zanamivir and oseltamivir work against both. Effectiveness depends on administration of antivirals within 48 hours of symptom onset.

Yearly vaccination still remains the best prevention.

Take Home Points

- Direct antigen testing of nasal washings is the most common technique for diagnosis.

- Influenza is a respiratory disease. It rarely involves the GI tract.

- To be effective, antiviral medications need to be started within 48 hours of symptom onset.

Chronic Obstructive Pulmonary Disease (COPD)

Chronic Bronchitis/Emphysema

COPD is a chronic, progressive disorder of airway limitation which is not fully reversible. COPD commonly refers to the two entities of chronic bronchitis and emphysema although others do exist, such as emphysema caused by genetic alpha-1-antitrypson deficiency. Both common forms may be seen in smokers. Incidence in the U.S. is at epidemic levels, which is why COPD remains the fourth leading cause of death.

Symptoms

Chronic bronchitis:

By definition, a productive cough for at least 3 consecutive months in two consecutive years. May also have dry cough, wheezing, smoking history, shortness of breath, dyspnea on exertion, and acutely progressive dyspnea at rest. Chronic bronchitis patients are called "**blue bloaters**" from the chronic, hypoxemic and hypercapnic state these patients are often in, giving a cyanotic appearance.

Emphysema:

Look for smoking history, exposure to noxious fumes or irritants, weight loss, wheezing, shortness of breath, dyspnea on exertion, and eventual dyspnea at rest. Emphysema patients are referred to as "**pink puffers**" due to their often emaciated appearance, higher than normal respiratory rate, and acyanotic appearance. These patients may also look plethoric due to possible polycythemia secondary to chronic hypoxemia.

Diagnosis

Physical exam: Rhonchi, wheezing, with often wet-sounding cough. Increased chest volume (barrel-chested), lower-than-expected diaphragm position, and prolonged expiratory phase. Pursed lip breathing may be observed along with use of accessory muscles and retractions.

Pulmonary function test (PFT) shows $FEV_1/FVC < 70\%$, increased total lung capacity (TLC) due to increased residual capacity. FEV1 may be normal or low.

Imaging: Chest x-ray shows **hyperexpanded lung fields, flattened diaphragms, narrowed mediastinum,** and possibly, superior segment **bullae**.

DL_{CO} (carbon dioxide diffusing capacity) is prolonged in emphysema.

ABG may show hypercapnia, hypoxia, and decreased pH, patients may have this state chronically so treat the patient, not the lab value!

CBC may show mild polycythemia due to chronic hypoxemia.

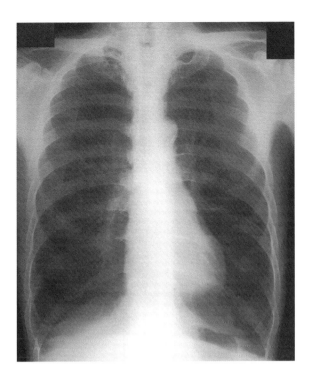

FIGURE 6.2 Chronic obstructive pulmonary disease. Reprinted with permission from Thomas J, Monaghan T. *Oxford Handbook of Clinical Examination and Practical Skills.* 2007, Oxford University Press.

Treatment

Oxygen and smoking cessation are the only treatments shown to reduce mortality.

Treatment guidelines come from those supported by the American College of Chest Physicians and by the Global Strategy for the Diagnosis, Management, and Prevention of Chronic Obstructive Pulmonary Disease. These groups support that β_2-agonists (albuterol), the long acting anticholinergic tiotropium (Spiriva), and the short acting anticholinergic iprotropium bromide (Atrovent) are mainstays of therapy. These may be used for chronic control of symptoms and acute exacerbations. Steroids, either IV or PO, may be given and show good effect in a short course. Also in acute setting, antibiotics (macrolide or fluoroquinolone) should be given and may decrease the course of exacerbations. Theophyline or the combination of inhaled steroids and β_2-agonist (Advair) may be considered for chronic disease (but are not a choice for acute exacerbations).

Consider bullectomy or lung volume reducing surgery in advanced cases. Lung transplant is reserved for optimal patients with advanced but isolated disease.

Vaccination against influenza and pneumonicoccal pneumonia (Pneumovax) should be given regardless of age.

Take Home Points

- Look for either chronic bronchitis (blue bloaters) or emphysema (pink puffers).
- Chest x-ray may show hyperexpanded lung fields, narrowed mediastinum, and flattened diaphragms.
- Be aware of the common comorbidity of cor pulmonale due to pulmonary hypertension.
- Supplemental oxygen and smoking cessation are the most important treatments.

Asthma

The disease state of reversible airway obstruction caused by the interplay between airway hyperresponsiveness, bronchospasm, and cellular response leading to airway inflammation. Asthma exacerbation may be incited by specific triggers including dust, pet dander, cold air, or acute exercise.

Symptoms

Patients may have wheezing, recurrent cough, decreased exercise tolerance, chest tightness, and shortness of breath. Asthma is usually diagnosed in children but may exist at any age. Look for frequency of rescue medication usage, accompanying conditions such as **eczema** and **allergic rhinitis**, environmental triggers (smoking in home), and family history.

Diagnosis

Physical exam: Wheezing (although may be absent if airways are totally constricted), prolonged expiratory phase, and tachypnea.

Lab: CBC most often normal. Differential may show eosinophilia.

Pulmonary function testing is the most accurate way of diagnosis with decreased FEV1 and peak expiratory flow (PEF). FEV1 classically improves ≥ **12%** after bronchodilator administration, which demonstrates **reversibility**.

Regular PEF measurement to monitor course of disease in known asthmatics is clinically useful.

Bronchoprovocation testing (methacholine challenge) is sometimes used, and shows greater response to common bronchoconstrictors in asthmatics. This challenge has a high negative predictive value.

Children who are too young for formal testing (< 5 years old) may clinically be given the diagnosis of reactive airway disease (RAD).

Imaging: Check chest x-ray at least once.

Consider skin allergen testing for common irritants which may illicit trigger identification.

Consider IgA, IgG testing for congenital abnormalities.

TABLE 6.4 Classification of Asthma

Degree of Disease	Symptoms	Nighttime Symptoms	Lung Function	Recommended Step for Initiating Treatment
Mild intermittent	Symptoms of asthma occurring ≤ 2 times per week.	≤ 2 nocturnal awakenings per month due to asthma symptoms	FEV1 or PEF ≥ 80% predicted	Step 1
Mild persistent	Symptoms ≥ 2 times per week but <once per day	≥ 2 times per month	FEV1 or PEF ≥ 80% predicted	Step 2
Moderate persistent	Daily symptoms with need of rescue medications, exacerbations affect activity and occur ≥ 2 times per week	≥ 1 time per week	FEV1 or PEF 60–80% predicted	Step 3
Severe persistent	Daily or continual symptoms that affect activity. Frequent exacerbations.	Frequent	FEV1 or PEF ≤ 60% predicted	Step 4 or 5

FEV1—Forced expiratory volume in one second
PEF—Peak expiratory flow

Treatment

In acute exacerbation, the mainstays are short-acting bronchodilators (albuterol, levalbuterol, and pirbuterol) and supplemental oxygen.

Add ipratropium (Atrovent) for synergism as needed acutely. No benefit, however, has been proven after admission to the hospital.

Give systemic corticosteroids (prednisone, methylprednisolone, prednisolone); although they are not short-acting, they are often helpful in the acute setting to speed recovery.

Consider epinephrine 1:1000 or terbutaline systemically or inhaled.

For severe exacerbations not responsive to initial therapy, consider IV magnesium sulfate or heliox.

Monitor patient for at least one hour after administration of medication to ensure effect.

The National Asthma Education and Prevention Program (NAEP) guidelines recommend a stepwise approach by starting with the most aggressive step first and then "stepping down" to achieve control.

TABLE 6.5 Stepwise Approach to Asthma Therapy for Patients ≥ 12 Years Old and Adults

Severity/Step	Treatment
Step 1	No daily medication needed Short acting bronchodilator PRN
Step 2	Short acting bronchodilator PRN Low dose inhaled corticosteroid Consider cromolyn, nedocromil (Tilade), zafirlukast (Accolate), montelukast (Singulair), or theophylline
Step 3	Short acting bronchodilator PRN Low to medium dose inhaled corticosteroid + long acting bronchodilator (combination=Advair) Consider addition of montelukast (Singulair), zafirlukast (Accolate), theophylline, or zileuton (Zyflo)
Step 4	Short acting bronchodilator PRN Medium dose inhaled corticosteroid + long acting bronchodilator (Advair), Consider addition of montelukast (Singulair), zafirlukast (Accolate), theophylline, or zileuton (Zyflo)
Step 5	Short acting bronchodilator PRN High dose inhaled corticosteroid + long acting bronchodilator (Advair), AND consider addition of omalizumab (Xolair)* for those with allergies
Step 6	Short acting bronchodilator PRN High dose inhaled corticosteroid + long acting bronchodilator (Advair) + oral corticosteroids AND consider addition of omalizumab (Xolair)* for those with allergies

Examples:
Short-acting bronchodilator—albuterol, levalbuterol, and pirbuterol
Long-acting bronchodilator—salmeterol (Serevent), formoterol (Foradil aerolizer)
Inhaled corticosteroids—budesonide, beclomethasone, flunisolide, fluticasone, mometasone, triamcinolone acetonide
Systemic corticosteroid—prednisone, methylprednisolone, prednisolone
Advair-Salmeterol/fluticasone
*Those placed on omalizumab should be educated and closely monitored for the rare but life-threatening side effect of anaphylaxis.

Educate patient and family with the "Asthma Action Plan," a color-coded written plan for taking medications at home.

Avoid triggers if identified.

Follow patient's home best peak flow recordings to be able to intervene early if needed.

Take Home Points

- The key feature of asthma is airway obstruction that is reversible.
- FEV1 classically improves ≥ 12% after bronchodilator administration which demonstrates reversibility.
- Approach treatment using a "step down" strategy for optimal control.
- When administering inhalational medications through metered dose inhaler (MDI) always use an aerochamber spacer.

Pneumoconiosis

Particulate inhalation leading to pulmonary inflammation and, over the long term, fibrosis of the interstitium. Also known as interstitial lung disease, this disease may be due to inhalation of many different inorganic dusts and thus presentation varies greatly. One of the most common inhaled particulates is asbestos, which leads to pulmonary plaques and markedly increased chance of mesothelioma.

Symptoms

May be asymptomatic or have severe shortness of breath, cough, weight loss, sputum production, wheezing, dyspnea on exertion, or hypoxemia. Look for a history that contains exposure to coal dust, silica, asbestos, mining, or berylliosis. Disease is worsened by smoking.

Diagnosis

Physical exam: Varied presentation of rhonchi and adventitial sounds.
Labs: No definite lab tests are indicative of disease. Rule out infectious process with proper labs.
Imaging: Chest x-ray is variable and may show patchy infiltrates throughout lung fields, hilar lymphadenopathy, miliary pattern, multiple small round opacities (pulmonary nodules), or larger single opacities (pulmonary plaques).

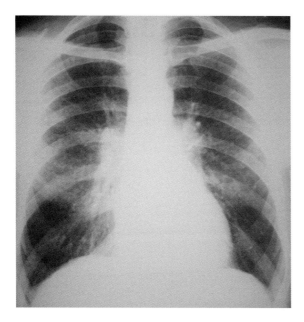

FIGURE 6.3 Pneumoconiosis showing extensive fibrosis. Reprinted with permission from Cox NLT, Roper TA. *Clinical Skills*. 2005, Oxford University Press.

Treatment

Prevention and avoidance is the only effective way to control disease. Otherwise, minimize symptoms.
Supplemental oxygen as needed.
Eventual lung transplant may be beneficial.

Take Home Points

- Pneumoconiosis may be caused by several forms of inorganic particles which eventually cause inflammation and scarring of lung tissue.

- Asbestosis is a very important form of pneumoconiosis. On CXR, linear opacities may appear at the lung bases along with pleural plaques.

- Mesothelioma is highly likely with prior history of asbestos exposure but chances of disease are exponentially compounded with a concurrent history of smoking.

Malignant Neoplasm of Bronchus and Lung

Malignancy originating in the lung. Bronchogenic carcinoma is the most common form and is made of two main types, small cell and non-small cell carcinoma. Histologically, non-small cell carcinoma is further subdivided into adenocarcinoma, squamous cell, and large cell. Other types include mesothelioma, carcinoid, sarcoma, and others. Lung carcinoma as a group is the leading cause of cancer deaths in the U.S.

Symptoms

Variable symptoms depend on histologic type and location but may include wasting, cough, **hemoptysis**, wheezing, fatigue, bone pain, fever, dysphagia, dyspnea, hoarseness (due to recurrent laryngeal nerve involvement), shortness of breath, chest pain, cachexia, loss of appetite, facial swelling, or **Horner syndrome (ptosis, miosis, and anhydrosis)**. Symptoms may also come from paraneoplastic syndromes seen commonly with lung malignancies. History often reveals smoking, exposure to asbestos, radon gas, or other irritant.

TABLE 6.6 Comorbid Conditions of Lung Malignancy

Syndrome	Association
Eaton-Lambert syndrome	Myasthenia gravis-like syndrome that spares ocular involvement.
Superior vena cava syndrome	Plethora and swelling of the face due to tumor compression of the superior vena cava.
Horner syndrome	Caused by Pancoast tumor (apical, posterior lung tumor that compresses spine). Produces classic triad of ptosis, miosis, and anhydrosis.

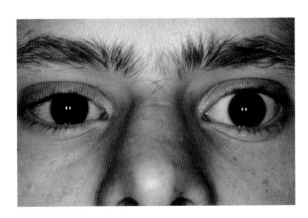

FIGURE 6.4 Horner syndrome. There is a partial ptosis as the right eyelid encroaches on the iris along with miosis of the right pupil. The left eye is normal. Reprinted with permission from Cox NLT, Roper TA. *Clinical Skills.* 2005, Oxford University Press.

Diagnosis

Physical exam: Lung exam may be normal or show dullness to percussion, rhonchi, rales, decreased breath sounds, increased tactile fremitus, or egophony. Look specifically for supraclavicular and infraclavicular lymphadenopathy.

Labs: CBC for leukocytosis or leukopenia, Basic chemistry including electrolytes and calcium, obtain ionized Ca if serum Ca is elevated, phosphate, magnesium, ACTH, thyroid hormone, parathyroid hormone, and parathyroid-related-peptide. Sputum sample or bronchoscopy with or without washings is useful in centrally located cancers and may reveal histologic type.

Imaging: CXR is often first indicator of a **nodule** or suspicious lesion. Look for location being either central or peripheral which may help with identification. If consolidation is seen in a single lobe or in one complete lung, consider the presence of a post-obstructive tumor (blocking bronchus).

CT scan is generally the next step and is useful in telling location and extent of disease. If positive, look for other tumors by scanning the rest of the body.

Bone scan may be useful in finding metastases.

Biopsy is the gold standard and may often be obtained transthoracically or bronchoscopically, depending on peripheral or central location, respectively. In patients whose disease is thought to be non-small cell histology and are surgical candidates, throracotomy may be used for diagnosis and treatment. In patients with suspected small cell or metastatic non-small cell cancers, a less invasive form such as thoracentesis of pleural effusion, lymph node biopsy, bronchoscopy, or transthoracic needle aspiration should be employed. In other tumors in which type and stage is less clear, modalities available are cytologic analysis of sputum, flexible bronchoscopy, and video assisted thoracoscopy (VATS).

TABLE 6.7 Classic Paraneoplastic Syndromes of Lung Malignancy Associated by Histologic Type

Histologic Cancer Type	Classic Paraneoplastic Syndrome
Small cell carcinoma	Cushing syndrome (ACTH production), hyponatremia (SIADH production)
Adenocarcinoma	Trousseau syndrome (hypercoagulable state)
Squamous cell carcinoma	Hypercalcemia, hypophosphatemia

Treatment

Small-cell lung cancers are usually found after the stage of metastasis, thus chemotherapy is the mainstay. Overall, however, small cell five-year survival rates are between 5% to 25%.

Non small-cell lung cancers are much more commonly found before metastasis and with localized disease, thus **surgical resection** is often effective. Local or regional disease may be treated with radiation or chemotherapy. Distant metastases are usually treated with chemotherapy or radiation but this is generally thought of as palliative.

Take Home Points

- Horner syndrome may be associated Pancoast tumors in the posterior apical lung field and causes the triad of ptosis, miosis, and anhydrosis.

- Paraneoplastic syndromes are common with lung cancers due to the common neuroendocrine derivation of cell types in the lung.

- The reason small-cell cancers have a poor prognosis is the common occurrence of finding them after the stage of metastasis.

- Generally, small-cell patients get chemotherapy, non small-cell patients undergo surgery.

Acute Respiratory Distress Syndrome (ARDS)

ARDS is on the severe end of the larger spectrum of acute lung injury (ALI) which is used to describe a unique respiratory reaction resulting in hypoxia; diffuse, non-cardiac infiltrates on x-ray; and low PaO_2/FiO_2 ratio, indicating poor oxygen exchange. Time course to onset is usually 4–48 hours. Three stages make up progression through ARDS: the acute **exudative** stage characterized by acute alveolar damage, the **proliferative** stage characterized by resolution of pulmonary edema and proliferation of type II alveolar cells, and in some patients, a **fibrotic** stage seen as development of pulmonary fibrosis and loss of lung compliance.

Symptoms

Fast labored breathing is the hallmark. Patients may demonstrate hypoxia-related mental status change beginning with agitation, then lethargy, progressing to obtundation. History often reveals an inciting event such as sepsis, aspiration, pneumonia, severe trauma/burns, massive blood transfusion, transfusion related lung injury (TRALI), or drugs and alcohol.

Diagnosis

Physical exam: Tachypnea, tachycardia, air hunger, use of accessory muscles for breathing, or cyanosis may be present. Rhonchi or rales may be heard throughout the lung fields. Hypoxemia is seen on pulse oximetry.

Labs: ABG is very important. CBC often reveals leukocytosis or leucopenia depending on cause. Basic metabolic panel may show electrolyte derangements or renal failure. B-type naturetic peptide (BNP) may be useful to evaluate for cardiac cause of pulmonary edema, which should be negative.

Echocardiography: Next step in determining cardiac cause of pulmonary edema.

Pulmonary artery catheterization: Last step in determining if cardiac cause; if pulmonary capillary wedge pressure exceeds 18 mmHg, cardiac cause is much more likely (although this does not exclude ARDS).

Criteria for diagnosis:

- Bilateral pulmonary infiltrates on CXR

- No evidence of cardiac cause (if measured, a pulmonary capillary wedge pressure of ≤ 18 mmHg)

- PaO_2/FiO_2 ratio derangement; when PaO_2 is expressed in mmHg and FiO_2 is a decimal between 0.21–1.00

  - 201–300 mmHg indicates ALI

  - ≤ 200 mmHg indicates ARDS

Treatment

Admit to the ICU!

Supplemental oxygen is very important.

Mechanical ventilation must be used in the vast majority of patients. Tidal volumes should be set low and positive end expiratory pressure (PEEP) should be optimized. In conjunction with PEEP, higher FiO_2 levels may be used. As well, increasing the inspiratory time (TI) and inspiratory:expiratory (I:E) ratio may improve oxygenation.

Place the patient on an appropriate antibiotic (tailored by cultures and sensitivities if available).

Manage multisystem needs as appropriate (enteral feeding, circulatory support, renal support, etc.)

Take Home Points

- Three stages comprise ARDS; exudative, proliferative, and fibrotic.
- PaO_2/FiO_2 ratio is key in determining the diagnosis along with exclusion of cardiac cause and presence of bilateral infiltrates on CXR.
- Intubate and start mechanical ventilation sooner rather than later.

Pulmonary Tuberculosis

A mycobacterial infection resulting from inhalation of typical bacilli, resulting in either active or latent (post-primary) disease. Primary exposure may result in active or latent disease that eventually becomes recrudescent, resulting in pulmonary infection or disseminated "miliary" disease.

Symptoms

Active disease: Cough, **hemoptysis**, fever, night sweats, weight loss, severe malaise, or pleuritic chest pain.

Miliary disease may show symptoms of distant organ system involvement and compromise. The classic example is Pott disease, which is TB of the spine. Detailed travel history and exposure history should be done to illicit possible transmission route.

Latent disease: Asymptomatic.

Diagnosis

Physical exam: Coarse sounding lungs, rhonchi, rales, decreased breath sounds, egophony, or tactile fremitus.

Labs: Three separate sputum samples stained for acid fast bacilli (AFB) may be used to give presumptive diagnosis. Culture is the gold standard but takes 2–6 weeks for results; sensitivities take longer. Direct nucleic acid amplification does exist although is used only if AFB stain is positive and the patient has had < 7 days treatment; it is very expensive. Also obtain CBC, Basic chemistry, liver panel for AST, ALT, bilirubin, alkaline phosphatase, serum creatinine, a platelet count, HIV, and Hep B and C. Obtain CD4 count if HIV+.

TABLE 6.8 Screening PPD (read 48–72 hours after placement)

Population	Positive Mantoux PPD Skin Test (induration)
HIV+ persons, chemotherapy patients, hepatitis C patients, recent exposure to active TB infected person, or immunocompromised	≥ 5 mm
Exposure risk factors such as health care workers, immigrants, homeless, diabetics	≥ 10 mm
Low risk of disease	≥ 15 mm

Confirm positive PPD with second test before diagnosing latent TB.

Steroids, anergy, recent live attenuated virus immunization, new (< 10 weeks) infection, chemotherapy, and immunocompromised states can cause a false negative screening PPD.

Boosted reaction: The positive PPD reaction caused by PPD sensitization in a patient with old latent TB conversion. In those individuals with recurrent testing, such as health care workers, a PPD skin test may appear to show recent conversion when the patient actually had waning immunologic reaction to old, latent disease. Thus, after exposure to the first dose of Mantoux antigen, the PPD is falsely negative, but after the second, the old antibody response is initiated. The test is still accurately read as positive, but infection is actually historic and does not represent recent conversion.

Imaging: Chest x-ray is the generally accepted imaging test which, in active disease, may show hilar lymphadenopathy (Ghon complex), cavitary lesions, opacity suggesting infiltrate, effusion, miliary pattern of opacities, or granulomas often in the apices. Reactivation TB tends to be in the superior, posterior lobes of the lungs. CT chest may also be used for confirmation of disease.

If extrapulmonary disease is suspected, imaging and/or biopsies may be needed.

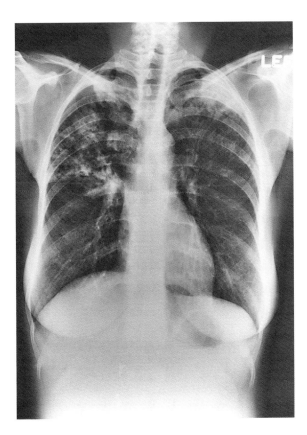

FIGURE 6.5 Tuberculosis in an HIV-infected female. Note upper lobe cavitary lesions. Reprinted with permission from Warrell DA, Cox TM, et al. *Oxford Textbook of Medicine*, 4th edition. 2003, Oxford University Press.

Treatment

The Joint Committee of the American Thoracic Society (ATS), the Infectious Diseases Society of America (IDSA), and the Centers for Disease Control and Prevention (CDC) recommend a two phase regimen of treatment of active disease to include an initial phase and continuation phase. The mnemonic **RIPE** summarizes the medications: **R**ifampin, **I**soniazid (INH), **P**yrazinamide, and **E**thambutol. These should be taken according to several regimens that include therapy lasting a total of six months. This therapy may be focused after cultures return sensitivities, although ethambutol should be included in the focused regimen. A baseline eye and visual examination should precede use of ethambutol and additional vitamin B6 should be given to prevent INH-associated neuropathy.

If treating latent TB (from positive PPD), recommendations are for a regimen of INH lasting 9 months (range 6–12 months). Give supplemental vitamin B6.

Monthly monitoring of treatment and lab testing is indicated.

Referral to infectious disease specialist may be necessary.

Take Home Points

- The PPD skin test is a delayed-type hypersensitivity reaction.
- Diagnosis with 3 separate sputum samples and chest imaging.
- Be aware of the reasons for false negative PPD, including the boosted reaction.
- Use the RIPE regimen for active TB, INH for latent TB. Consider that conversion is for life, even with treatment.

Sarcoidosis

Non-infectious, idiopathic, multisystem disease characterized by **noncaseating granuloma** formation and organ system infiltration. Most commonly seen in the lungs, genetic predisposition shows higher occurrence in African American females, Japanese, Irish females, and Scandinavians.

Symptoms

About half of patients are asymptomatic. Symptoms include cough, malaise, shortness of breath, fever, night sweats, skin lesions, Bell's palsy, weight loss, and arthritis. Often this disease is multiorgan, so look for extrapulmonary involvement (skin, cardiac, hepatic, renal).

Diagnosis

Labs: CBC often shows lymphopenia, anemia, or leukopenia. Liver and electrolyte panels may show increased ALT and infrequently hypercalcemia. Check urine for hypercalciuria (more common than hypercalcemia). Hypergammaglobulinemia may be seen. Angiotensin converting enzyme (ACE) level is often elevated (the value in using ACE level for monitoring disease is still unclear).

Imaging: Chest x-ray is most useful. **Bilateral hilar lymphadenopathy** is the key finding. CXR can be used to define stages by **Scadding's** classification:

TABLE 6.9 Scadding's Classification of Sarcoidosis

Stage	Findings on CXR
Stage 0	Normal
Stage 1	Hilar adenopathy alone
Stage 2	Hilar adenopathy and parenchymal infiltrates
Stage 3	Parenchymal infiltrates alone
Stage 4	Pulmonary fibrosis

CT scan is useful in demonstrating abnormalities in greater detail.

Positron emission tomography (PET) scan may localize disease to lungs, lymph nodes, etc.

PFTs reveal a **restrictive pattern** and are useful in following disease when done routinely.

Bronchoscopy with biopsy will demonstrate noncaseating granulomatous tissue. Bronchoalveolar lavage (BAL) may reveal characteristic CD4 positive lymphocytes.

Obtain routine ECG.

Obtain screening PPD.

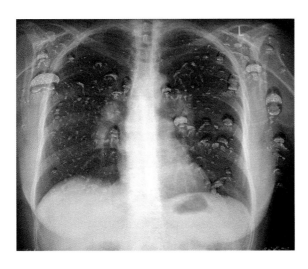

FIGURE 6.6 Bihilar lymphadenopathy due to sarcoidosis. Reprinted with permission from Thomas J, Monaghan T. *Oxford Handbook of Clinical Examination and Practical Skills.* 2007, Oxford University Press.

Treatment

If any treatment is necessary, **prednisone is the mainstay**. Other immunomodulating drugs such as methotrexate (Trexall), hydroxychloroquine (Plaquenil), and azathioprine may be used but require frequent monitoring.

Routine office visits are recommended while on prednisone and early in disease.

Refer patient for an ophthalmic exam.

Take Home Points

- Noncasseating granulomas are the pathognomonic pathologic finding.
- CXR shows bilateral hilar lymphadenopathy.
- Oral steroids and immunomodulators are the mainstay of therapy.

Cystic Fibrosis

CF is an autosomal-recessively inherited defect of the CFTR gene (ΔF508 area of chromosome 7), producing nonfunctional chloride exocrine channels. One of the top lethal genetic diseases in the U.S., with a Caucasian population incidence of 1/2500 births; less common in other races.

Symptoms

Most commonly seen affecting the pulmonary system. However, this disease may be seen in extrapulmonary systems before the lungs; classically, meconium ileus occurs at birth or intussusception occurs later in infancy. In the pulmonary system, patients often have recurrent lower respiratory infections, history of multiple pneumonias, chronic cough, wheezing, dyspnea, barrel chest, tachypnea, and other infections leading to symptoms of acute illness (fever, malaise, etc.). Malabsorption due to pancreatic insufficiency may be seen as steatorrhea, abdominal pain, vitamin deficiency, malnourishment, and failure to thrive. Pancreatic problems may progress to diabetes. In adults, males have infertility secondary to aspermia and females are prone to recurrent miscarriage.

Diagnosis

Physical exam: Focal loss of breath sounds, wet sounding cough, rhonchi, wheezing, tachypnea, or clubbing and cyanosis from hypoxemia.

Labs: Sweat chloride test (pilocarpine iontophoresis) is the gold standard (CF patients > 60 mEq/L). Confirm test with at least two positives. Genetic testing can also be done to confirm. Obtain screening labs for other abnormalities including Complete chemistry for electrolyte disorders and low albumin, CBC for acute infection or increased hematocrit. Transepithelial nasal potential difference, immunoreactive trypsin (newborn screening), fecal fat, and pancreatic enzyme secretion testing may be useful in some cases. Obtain periodic respiratory cultures as warranted.

Imaging: Chest x-ray may show consolidation, hyperaeration, hilar adenopathy, bronchiectasis, blebs, or rarely, pneumothorax.

PFTs for comparison and reference.

Exercise testing for respiratory function.

Echocardiogram for heart function.

Annual vitamin A and E levels and INR to evaluate clotting function.

Genetic testing of family and counseling on chances of disease/carrier state in future children.

Treatment

Oxygen as needed. Intubate if acutely necessary.

Give antibiotics acutely if warranted. Cover for *S aureus* and *Pseudomonas* as well as previously cultured bacteria per patient history. Ciprofloxacin, cephalexin (Keflex) for PO regimen or tobramycin plus ceftazidime (Fortaz), or vancomycin for IV regimen are good choices. Aerosolized tobramycin may be used for prophylaxis (one month on, one month off) if previously colonized with *Pseudomonas*.

Chest physiotherapy (percussion).

Therapeutic enemas or laxative therapy as needed.

BiPAP mechanical ventilation sometimes is used for nighttime hypoxia.

Bronchodilators if response has been demonstrated.

Dornase alfa (DNase) is the most widely used mucolytic.

Pancreatic enzyme replacement. Avoid high doses that may cause colonic strictures.

Vitamin supplements to replace fat soluble vitamins (vit A, D, E, K).

Treat diabetics with insulin as needed.

Annual flu vaccine.

High salt, protein, and calorie diet.

Surgery with lung or other solid organ transplant may be considered in end stage disease.

Take Home Points

- CF occurs due to a mutation of the CFTR gene at the ΔF508 area of chromosome 7.
- This is a multi-system disease.
- Diagnose with the sweat chloride test.

Pulmonary Embolism

The blockage of pulmonary vasculature from embolic phenomenon in the venous circulation. Thromboembolism from deep venous thrombosis (DVT) is most common but other sources of emboli are air, amniotic fluid (during C-section), and fat embolism (from long bone fracture or surgery).

Symptoms

Known as "the great masquerader," PE presents in many different ways. Common ones are pleuritic chest pain, shortness of breath, dyspnea, tachypnea, fever, anxiety, syncope, and hemoptysis; or it may be asymptomatic. Comorbid symptoms may include those of DVT, such as lower extremity swelling, pain, tenderness, and erythema. History may reveal Virchow's triad of risk factors.

TABLE 6.10 Virchow's Triad

Element	Risk Factor Examples
Stasis	Plane flight, immobility due to illness, obesity
Endothelial injury	Trauma, surgery, fracture
Hypercoagulable state	Pregnancy, smoking, OCP use, coagulation disorder, malignancy, burns

Massive PE is one that is much larger than most others and causes catastrophic lung injury, resulting in death 99% of the time. It has been defined as a PE associated with a systolic blood pressure < 90 mmHg or a drop in systolic blood pressure of 40 mmHg from baseline for a period > 15 minutes, which is not otherwise explained by hypovolemia, sepsis, or a new arrhythmia.

Diagnosis

Physical exam: Tachypnea, tachycardia, rhonchi, rales, decreased diaphragmatic excursion. DVT may be evident by lower extremity swelling, erythema, tenderness, and positive Homan's sign (pain on dorsiflexion of foot).

Labs: D-dimer is a popular test which may show coagulation but is only useful if negative. If positive, d-dimer is much too nonspecific to support almost any diagnosis. ABG is variable and may show an increased A-a gradient (although not reliable) or primary respiratory alkalosis due to hyperventilation or respiratory acidosis if massive PE.

Imaging: Spiral CT is becoming the study of choice although may miss small PEs in the periphery. CXR may be normal or show **Hampton hump** (wedge-shaped infarct), **Westermark's sign** (focal oligemia), atelectasis, consolidation, prominent central arteries, pleural effusion, or elevated hemidiaphragm.

Nuclear medicine V/Q scan is helpful if results are low probability (no PE) or high probability (PE). If intermediate probability then patient needs further workup. When ordering the V/Q scan consider the pre-test probability of PE and interpret the results accordingly.

Doppler ultrasound of the legs to evaluate for DVT.

Pulmonary angiography remains the gold standard but is invasive and expensive with a significant risk of morbidity/mortality.

ECG: Characteristic S wave in lead 1, Q wave in lead III, and T wave inversion in lead III (called the S1Q3T3). May otherwise show arrhythmia or sinus tachycardia, T wave inversion in V1-V3, right axis deviation, or right bundle branch block.

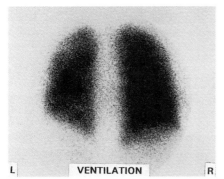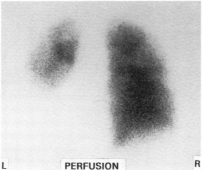

L   VENTILATION   R   L   PERFUSION   R

FIGURE 6.7 Ventilation and perfusion lung scan (posterior views). Ventilation scan shows nearly normal ventilation but the perfusion scan shows absent perfusion in the left lower lobe and mismatched perfusion defects in the left upper lobe. Perfusion defects (gray areas) are also shown in the right lung. This V-Q scan was read as high probability of pulmonary embolism. Reprinted with permission from Warrell DA, Cox TM, et al. *Oxford Textbook of Medicine*, 4th edition. 2003, Oxford University Press.

Treatment

Stabilize the patient as needed. Consider intubation if needed. Significant arrhythmias may be seen, thus cardiac monitoring is warranted.

Give oxygen.

Anticoagulate initially with heparin or low-molecular-weight heparin (enoxaparin (Lovenox)) then with warfarin (Coumadin). Overlap these two for a couple of days to avoid transient hypercoagulable state. Warfarin dose should be loaded, then the dosage adjusted to achieve **INR between 2–3**. Continue **warfarin for at least 6 months** in the uncomplicated patient and indefinitely in the patient with ongoing risk factors or history of multiple events.

If patient is not a candidate for anticoagulation, consider placement of IVC filters.

If patient has significant hypotension, saddle embolus is suspected, and situation is dire, consider embolectomy or tPA. Many contraindications to tPA and embolectomy, which have a mortality of 30%, so only attempt if extreme situation.

Place patient on "warfarin diet" if on warfarin.

Control risk factors.

Take Home Points

- Consider PE in almost all respiratory conditions.
- Order a spiral CT scan if PE is suspected. CXR may show "Hampton hump" or the "Westermark" sign. ECG shows S1Q3T3.
- Anticoagulation won't treat the existing clot but prevent further clot formation. Keep the INR between 2 and 3 with warfarin.

Pulmonary Hypertension (PH)

Primary and secondary disease types exist. Primary pulmonary hypertension (PPH) is generally idiopathic; secondary is most commonly caused by lung dysfunction including primary pulmonary disease (COPD, asthma, pneumonitis), pulmonary vasculature disease (CREST, sickle cell disease, PE, HIV) or thoracic diseases contributing to pulmonary dysfunction (obesity, sleep apnea, kyphoscoliosis). Generally, exclude secondary PH before diagnosing and treating primary.

Symptoms

Fatigue, dyspnea, syncope, chest pain, palpitations, hoarseness, hemoptysis, cough, or lower extremity edema. Look for symptoms of right heart failure (cor pulmonale). History may include causative drugs (such as fen-phen).

Diagnosis

Physical exam: Loud P2, right ventricular lift, tachypnea, murmur of tricuspid insufficiency or pulmonic insufficiency, increased jugular venous pulsations, hepatomegaly, pulmonic ejection click, right ventricular S3 or S4, or lower extremity edema.

Labs: Test for suspicious causes of secondary pulmonary hypertension (autoantibody tests, HIV, hepatic function tests). ANA is positive in upper $1/3$ of PPH patients. ABG may show arterial hypoxemia, reduced diffusion capacity (DLCO), and hypocapnia.

Imaging: CXR shows enlarged central pulmonary arteries, right ventricular enlargement, or increased interstitial markings.

Doppler echocardiography may show right ventricular enlargement, valvular abnormalities including insufficiencies, and is the most accurate non-invasive way to estimate pulmonary artery pressure.

Consider CT or V/Q scan to evaluate for causative emboli. Pulmonary angiography if these are reasonably positive, but caution is advised due to the possibility of hemodynamic collapse.

ECG: May be helpful and show rightward axis deviation, right bundle branch block, and/or increased P wave in leads II, III, and aVF.

Pulmonary exercise testing.

Cardiac catheterization: Catheter placement to measure pulmonary artery pressure and hemodynamics is the gold standard and is used if Doppler echocardiography is inadequate.

Treatment

Oxygen therapy is the only proven strategy to improve mortality.

All types of PH should be given other therapies for control of disease and symptoms. This includes diuretics, anticoagulation with warfarin, and exercise. Digoxin is still controversial and unproven.

Otherwise, guidelines depend on subtype of disease. These may include vasodilators, calcium channel blockers, prostanoids, endothelian receptor antagonists, corticosteroids, and PDE inhibitors (Sildenifil).

Surgical candidates may benefit from lung transplant.

Take Home Points

- PH is either primary (idiopathic), or secondary due to other disease.

- Look for cor pulmonale which is a major comorbidity in PH.

- Give oxygen along with other treatments.

Pneumothorax

The trapping of air between the visceral and parietal pleura of the lungs. This may occur most commonly by injury to the chest wall and compromise of the pleural cavity such as in a penetrating injury. Spontaneous pneumothorax (that which occurs due to lung injury) also occurs and is either idiopathic (more common in young males) called primary, or due to underlying lung disease such as COPD or CF, termed secondary. Tension pneumothorax occurs when the air in the pleural space has no exit and positive pressure develops, often causing shifting of pleural cavity contents.

Hemothorax—Blood between the visceral and parietal lung pleura. Blood tends to accumulate in the dependant, inferior pulmonary cavity. This may occur in concomitance with pneumothorax, especially in a multiple trauma patient.

Symptoms

Often due to direct trauma; however, primary symptoms include pleuritic chest pain, shortness of breath, air hunger, tachycardia, and tachypnea. Main risk factor for tension or open pneumothorax is blunt or penetrating trauma. Primary spontaneous pneumothorax may be associated with risk factors such as smoking; being tall, thin, and male; or having a positive family history. Secondary spontaneous pneumothorax may carry risk factors of underlying lung disease such as COPD, cystic fibrosis, TB, or *Pneumocystis carinii* (HIV).

Diagnosis

Physical exam:

Tension pneumothorax—Tracheal deviation, distended neck veins, decreased/absent breath sounds over one lung field, hyperresonance/tympany to percussion, hypotension, decreased tactile fremitus, and shallow/fast breathing.

Open pneumothorax—Chest wall defect with direct communication to the pleural cavity resulting in paradoxical air movement with respiratory effort (sucking chest wound). If occurring with trauma such as a gunshot wound, search for accompanying entrance/exit wound that may prevent treatment.

Spontaneous pneumothorax—Exam may reveal decreased or absent breath sounds in one lung field, show tachypnea, tachycardia, or respiratory distress. Clinically, spontaneous pneumothorax may also be impossible to detect.

Labs: Pulse oximetry and ABG may show hypoxia and hypercapnia.

Imaging: CXR will reveal retracted lung with identifiable border, lung markings that do not extend to the periphery, hyperlucent lung field, depressed diaphragm, deviated trachea, and shifted mediastinum (if tension exists, shift will be away from the affected side).

Ultrasound (FAST exam) may be used in significant trauma patients and is proving a very sensitive testing modality.

CT chest if other modalities of imaging do not show clear pneumothorax and clinical suspicion is still high.

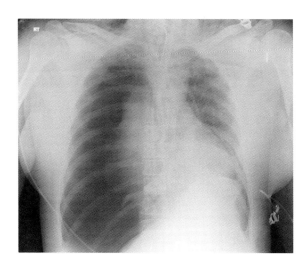

FIGURE 6.8 Chest x-ray showing a right-sided tension pneumothorax. Note lack of right sided lung markings, left shifted mediastinum, and right hemithorax overinflation. Reprinted with permission from Thomas J, Monaghan T. *Oxford Handbook of Clinical Examination and Practical Skills.* 2007, Oxford University Press.

Treatment

Give oxygen!

If you suspect tension pneumothorax by symptoms and exam, do not wait for chest x-ray; treat immediately.

Tension pneumothorax—Needle decompression by inserting a large gauge needle through the inferior 2nd intercostal space at the midclavicular line should be considered immediately. Listen for a rush of air. Place a three-way stopcock valve on the needle and close the valve after decompression (alternatively, remove the needle and perform needle decompression every time pressure builds up).

Open pneumothorax—Seal the chest wall and pleural cavity with one of several commercial chest sealing devices such as the Asherman Chest Seal. This allows pressurized air out but not in. Make sure to seal all pleural cavity wounds.

Insert a chest tube:

Give heavy analgesia and narcotic pain medications and insert 16 to 22 French **chest tube** through the 4th, 5th, or 6th intercostal spaces at the midaxillary line. Confirm placement with a CXR and place the tube to an underwater seal. Keep the seal in place 24 hours or until bubbles cease.

For primary spontaneous pneumothorax, catheter air aspiration using an 18 gauge needle and catheter attached to a 60 mL syringe can be used to draw out the excess air in the pleural cavity. Enter the chest wall through the 4th, 5th, or 6th intercostal spaces in the midaxillary line as if placing a chest tube. Aspiration may take several attempts to evacuate the entire air volume. However, if ≥ 4 liters are removed without re-expansion of the lung, consider the presence of a lung surface leak which necessitates chest tube placement or thoracoscopy. When air is successfully evacuated, especially in the setting of multiple occurrences, consider pleurodesis with talc or other agent.

For secondary spontaneous pneumothorax, direct chest tube placement is considered more effective and reliable.

Surgery should be considered for recurrence or refractory events with thoracoscopy or video-assisted thoracoscopy (VATS).

If the patient is stable with a small, non-recurrent, primary spontaneous pneumothorax they may be safely discharged home with a follow up chest x-ray in 24–48 hours.

Take Home Points

- Pneumothorax may occur due to chest wall injury or lung injury.
- If penetrating trauma exists, search for an exit wound which may prevent treatment.
- Consider needle thorocostomy to buy time in a trauma situation. Insert a chest tube to treat.
- In spontaneous pneumothorax, consider catheter aspiration or chest tube placement for primary occurrences and chest tube placement for secondary occurrences.

Wegener Granulomatosis

A multi-system autoimmune granulomatous vasculitis that classically affects the triad of **upper airway, lung,** and **kidneys.**

Symptoms

Depends on the systems affected. Common symptoms include fever, cough, arthralgias, nasal congestion, chest congestion, chest pain, hemoptysis, weight loss, skin rash, epistaxis, or symptoms of renal failure.

Diagnosis

Physical exam: Lung exam may reveal rhonchi, egophony, tachypnea, and cough. Destructive nasal lesions may produce "saddle nose" deformity. Skin ulcers may be present from peripheral vascular involvement.

Labs: CBC shows leukocytosis, anemia, and thrombocytosis. ESR is markedly elevated. Basic metabolic panel may show renal failure or renal insufficiency. Rheumatoid factor increased in 50% of cases. UA may show hematuria, cellular casts, or protein. Classic lab is **C-ANCA** (cytoplasmic antineutrophilic cytoplasmic antibody) which shows excellent specificity for this disease.

Imaging: CXR may show localized infiltrates or discrete nodular densities consistent with central necrosis and cavitation. CT of chest or sinuses shows indicative findings in these areas.

Biopsy of affected kidney, lung, or mucous membrane of upper airways may show most definitive evidence of disease.

Treatment

Consider admission even for mild disease.

Initially, cyclophosphamide-corticosteroid combinations should be used to induce remission. Corticosteroids should then be tapered off at 2–4 weeks. Methotrexate in mild cases or in conjunction with cyclophosphamide or corticosteroids may be used. Cyclophosphamide (Cytoxan) is most successful but also most toxic of therapies. Monitor these patients with weekly CBCs for leukopenia and bone marrow suppression.

Recommend high fluid intake while on cyclophosphamide.

Take Home Points

- The classic triad of Wegener is the involvement of the upper airway, lung, and kidneys.
- Test for C-ANCA which is characteristic of Wegener disease.
- Treat with steroids and immunosuppressants.

7   Gastroenterology

Cancer of the Esophagus

Esophageal cancer occurs most commonly in the distal esophagus, which contributes to its common late discovery. Risk factors include long standing gastroesophageal reflux disease (GERD), smoking, EtOH use, achalasia, male sex, diet high in nitrates, history of head/neck cancer, and age > 50 years. The histologic type of **adenocarcinoma** is associated with history of **Barrett's esophagus**.

Symptoms

This disease usually presents later in its course, with progressive dysphagia especially to solids, weight loss, regurgitation, aspiration, hiccups, cough, hoarseness, or anemia.

Diagnosis

Physical exam: Cachexia, cervical lymphadenopathy.
Labs: CBC for anemia. Basic chemistry for electrolyte abnormalities. Once confirmed, evaluate hepatic function for possible metastasis.

Esophagoscopy with biopsy or brushing is the gold standard and determines histologic type.
Imaging: Barium swallow for a constricting lesion. Use CT scan for local disease and visualization. Endoscopic ultrasound is useful in determining local spread.

Treatment

Therapy is often palliative due to advanced disease at the time of diagnosis.

Surgery is the mainstay. Radiation may be adjunctive. Chemotherapy, stricture dilation, photocoagulation, and endoluminal stent placement are generally palliative.

Control risk factors and maintain surveillance of those at high risk, especially with Barrett's esophagus.

Take Home Points

- Esophageal carcinoma may be adenocarcinoma or squamous cell in type.
- Adenocarcinoma is associated with Barrett's esophagus.
- Late presentation is common, thus, palliative treatment may be the only option.

Esophageal Varices

Pathologic enlargement of the submucosal veins in the esophagus and proximal stomach that connect the portal venous system with the superior vena cava. These veins enlarge and become engorged due to increased portal venous pressure and are prone to rupture, commonly are a source of upper GI bleeding.

Symptoms

Painless upper GI tract bleeding may present with hematemesis, weakness, pallor, or melena. Symptoms of liver cirrhosis are commonly comorbid and may include ascites; large, hard liver; and uncommonly noticeable splenomegaly. History is often positive for chronic excessive EtOH consumption or hepatitis.

Diagnosis

Physical exam: Signs of liver sclerosis may include ascites, multiple spider angiomatas, caput medussa, jaundice, hepatomegaly, splenomegaly, etc.
Labs: CBC for anemia. Stool may show occult blood (beware false negatives); PT/aPTT/INR may be increased due to decreased liver function; hepatic transaminases may be increased if liver damage is present (although may be normal in the advanced liver sclerosis patient).
Imaging: First line is esophagoscopy, which may demonstrate large, tortuous, bleeding varices often in the lower third of esophagus. Simultaneous treatment is possible if active bleeding is present. Doppler sonography may demonstrate patency of large vessels. Other imaging includes MRI, endoscopic ultrasound, or venous phase angiography.

Treatment

Stabilize the patient if needed. Consider transfusion.

For acute bleeding, give systemic **octreotide (Sandostatin)**.

Endoscopy may be used to inject octreotide or vasopressin to control acute bleeding. If these fail, proceed to endoscopic **sclerotherapy** or **ligation**.

Lastly, consider **TIPS** (transjugular intrahepatic portacaval shunt).

If no acute bleeding, place patient on β-blockers, specifically propanolol (Inderal). If bleeding recurs, add isosorbide mononitrate.

Monitor with repeat blood work and repeat endoscopies to ensure stability.

Surgery includes TIPS, portocaval shunt placement, esophageal transection, or liver transplantation.

Take Home Points

- Esophageal varices occur in the presence of increased portal venous pressures and are a common source of upper GI bleeding.

- Comorbid liver damage is often present.

- For acute bleeding, give octreotide (Sandostatin) and consider endoscopy.

Dysphagia

Difficulty or painful swallowing, dysphagia is divided into several types including: oropharyngeal (transfer dysphagia) or esophageal. Specific etiologies differ by adult or pediatric state but may include two categories: neuromuscular or structural.

Symptoms

Take age into account. Symptoms may include choking, coughing with swallowing, weak voice, weight loss, pressure sensation in mid-chest, heartburn, or longer eating time. Ascertain if the severity is worse with solids or liquids, smoking, EtOH use, or long standing GERD.

If symptoms occur with both **solids and liquids** → neuromuscular problem.

If symptoms occur only with **solids** → likely a structural problem.

Diagnosis

Physical exam: Evaluate for external source such as thyroid tumor, etc. Cachexia seen in advanced cases. In infants or newborns attempt to pass NG tube to stomach and through nose to evaluate for esophageal and choanal atreasias.

Imaging: Barium swallow studies are first line. These may include videofluoroscopy with various viscosities of barium material. Endoscopy or nasolaryngoscopy with biopsy may be useful if stricture or tumor is suspected. Chest x-ray may be useful. CT scan helpful if tumor is suspected. Targeted testing includes esophageal manometry or 24 hour pH testing.

Treatment

For structural problems, surgery is the mainstay and is effective. Tumors may be excised and radiation may help (see above).

Neuromuscular causes (achalasia, multiple sclerosis, myasthenia gravis, etc.) may respond to underlying treatment of condition.

Complications caused by GERD may respond to acid reducers or fundoplication surgery.

Referral to gastroenterologist may be warranted.

Take Home Points

- Dysphagia may be neuromuscular or structural.
- Barium swallow studies with videofluoroscopy is first line.
- Biopsy via endoscopy or nasolaryngoscopy may be indicated if malignancy is suspected.

Malignant Neoplasm of the Stomach

Gastric carcinoma is overwhelmingly histologically adenocarcinoma and is commonly classified as intestinal type or diffuse type. Both these types may be associated with *H pylori* infection but intestinal type tends to be more predictable and less aggressive. Up to the early 1980s, gastric cancer was one of the most common cancers in the world until it was overtaken by lung cancer. The next few decades saw a marked decrease in incidence, although worldwide it still remains one of the most common cancers found.

Symptoms

Often asymptomatic, although may present as decreased appetite, early satiety, and weight loss. Risk factors include chronic gastritis, *H pylori* infection, and diet high in nitrates (smoked fish) and salts.

Diagnosis

Physical exam: Classically, Virchow's node (palpable supraclavicular lymphadenopathy) is present. Dermatologic associations include appearance of diffuse and many seborrheic keratoses (called the Leser-Trelat sign) or acanthosis nigricans.

Labs: CBC may show anemia due to ulcerated tumor bleeding. Consider hepatic function panel and alkaline phosphatase for possible metastasis.

Imaging: EGD with biopsy is the best test for evaluation, even initially if gastric carcinoma is suspected. Barium swallow studies may also be useful. Evaluate other areas of the body for metastasis (sometimes seen in the ovaries, called a Krukenberg tumor) with CT which also provides info on staging. Consider endoscopic ultrasound if available.

Treatment

Surgery is the mainstay and may involve partial resection of the stomach. Postoperative adjuvant chemotherapy can be added. Since disease is often advanced at presentation, prognosis is commonly poor.

Take Home Points

- *H pylori* is a major risk factor for gastric carcinoma.
- EGD with biopsy is the best single test for evaluation.
- Surgery is the mainstay but carcinomas are often advanced when discovered.

Peptic Ulcer Disease

A common disease of ulcer formation in the stomach or duodenum. The most significant risk factors include presence of *H pylori* infection and use of NSAIDs. Other risk factors include smoking, family history of ulcers, HLA-B12 positive status, or rarely, Zollinger-Ellison (ZE) syndrome.

Symptoms

Gnawing, burning, epigastric pain. Belching, bloating, abdominal distention or food intolerance may accompany. May present with nonspecific symptoms or be asymptomatic until bleeding occurs, causing symptoms of anemia.

Gastric ulcer pain is classically worsened by meals.

Duodenal ulcer pain is relieved by meals with exacerbation hours later.

Diagnosis

Labs: *H pylori* testing is essential. This can be done by urea breath test, serum antibody, stool antigen, or biopsy during endoscopy. CBC for hematocrit. Serum gastrin levels along with further workup indicated if ZE suspected.

Imaging: Endoscopy with biopsy is the gold standard. Barium meal may be alternative and is less invasive. If rupture is suspected, obtain upright plain x-ray and evaluate for air under the diaphragm.

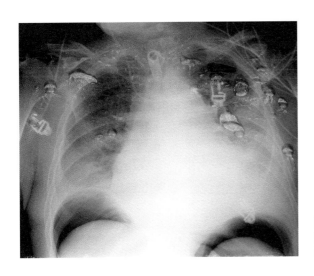

FIGURE 7.1 Chest x-ray showing pneumoperitonium. Reprinted with permission from Cox NLT, Roper TA. *Clinical Skills.* 2005, Oxford University Press.

Treatment

Stop NSAID use.

Control acid environment with antacids, sucralfate, H_2 blockers (ranitidine (Zantac), famotidine (Pepcid), etc), or proton pump inhibitors (rabeprazole (Aciphex), omeprazole (Prilosec), etc.). Monitor for liver enzyme metabolism alteration with some H_2 blockers such as cimetidine (Tagamet). Proton pump inhibitors are generally most effective although must be taken every day.

Test for and eradicate *H pylori* with triple therapy: Proton pump inhibitor + amoxicillin + clarithromycin for 14 days. Quadruple therapy includes a PPI + metronidazole (Flagyl) + tetracycline + bismuth. Test for cure after treatment.

Surgery may be a viable option for those ulcers producing acute complications such as bleeding or perforation, or are extensively refractory to medical treatment.

Take Home Points

- NSAIDs and *H pylori* infection are the major risk factors for PUD.

- Triple therapy may be used for eradication of *H pylori*. Different regimens exist but commonly include a PPI and two different antibiotics. Quadruple therapy adds bismuth to this regimen.

Gastritis and Gastropathy

A disease of inflammation of the stomach lining causing a characteristic syndrome. Gastropathy, or injury to the mucosal stomach lining, is a term commonly used to describe damage to the endothelial lining of the stomach without inflammation. The two terms will not be distinguished here due to the similarity of the clinical presentation and treatments. Acute gastritis is most commonly due to an infectious agent while chronic gastritis/gastropathy is often due to chemical, medication, or disease specific cause.

Symptoms

Nonspecific epigastric pain, burning, or discomfort, anorexia, **nausea/vomiting**, or hiccups. History may reveal *H pylori* diagnosis, recent viral exposure, alcohol use, or NSAID use.

Diagnosis

Physical exam: Diffuse abdominal tenderness, decreased bowel sounds, and guarding.
Labs: CBC for leukocytosis, Basic chemistry for BUN and electrolyte levels, K is often low after vomiting.

Treatment

Stop NSAIDs.

Often supportive with antacids, H_2 blockers, and proton pump inhibitors. Misoprostol (Cytotec) may help protect gastric mucosa from damage.

Test for and eradicate *H pylori* infection.

After the acute phase (in acute disease) educate the patient to return to normal food by starting slowly with the BRAT (bananas, rice, apple sauce, toast) diet.

Take Home Points

- Acute gastritis is commonly from infectious etiology.

- Stop NSAIDs, eradicate *H pylori*, and reduce acid to control.

Acute Pancreatitis

Acute inflammation of the pancreas due to many different etiologies including gallstones, alcohol use, trauma, steroids, autoimmune mechanisms, scorpion venom, hypercalcemia, hyperlipidemia, drugs (azathioprine (Imuran), pentamidine (Pentam), mercaptopurine (Purinethol)), and pregnancy. A self perpetuating cycle is started with inflammation of pancreatic tissue which leads to activation of pancreatic enzymes within pancreatic tissue causing a spectrum of injury from edema to necrotizing tissue loss.

Symptoms

Abdominal pain commonly in the epigastrum, right or left quadrants, which may radiate to the back or shoulder. Nausea/vomiting, anorexia, weight loss, low grade fever, restlessness, steatorrhea, and myalgias are common.

Diagnosis

Several clinical prognostic scales exist for predicting mortality and severity of acute pancreatitis. The most established of these is the Ranson criteria (presented in Table 7.1) although research has not supported its being the best scale for positive and negative predictive value. The Acute Physiology and Chronic Health Evaluation II (APACHE II) score has been shown to be more accurate in severity prediction and has the advantage of being useful before the 48 hour evaluation point that other scales require. However, APACHE II remains cumbersome (requires addition of multiple factors and adding of point scores) which limits its practical use. Other scales include the Imrie (Glasgow) and CT severity index.

A common clinical tool is the Ranson criteria which predicts severity of disease:

TABLE 7.1 The Ranson Criteria

Presentation	
Age	> 55 years
WBCs	> 16,000 mm³
Blood glucose	> 200 mg/dL
LDH	> 350 U/L
AST	> 250 U/L
48 hours	
Hematocrit	Fall by ≥ 10%
BUN	Increase of ≥ 5 mg/dL despite fluids
Serum calcium	< 8 mg/dL
pO2	< 60 mm/Hg
Base deficit	> 4 MEq/L
Fluid sequestration	> 6000 mL

One point for each factor in table.
Score 0 to 2: 2% mortality
Score 3 to 4: 15% mortality
Score 5 to 6: 40% mortality
Score 7 to 8: 100% mortality

Physical exam: Tenderness to epigastric region, diaphoresis, mildly increased temperature, dry mucous membranes, and possibly jaundice (depending on cause). Grey-Turner sign (flank discoloration) or Cullen's sign (umbilical discoloration) may herald extreme disease or rupture.

Labs: See table of Ranson criteria. Other classic labs include lipase (most specific) and amylase (less specific), elevated billirubin, and elevated alkaline phosphatase.

Imaging: Plain abdominal x-ray may show signs of ileus (air fluid levels, etc.) and "sentinel loop" in loop of bowel adjacent to inflamed pancreas.

CT scan with contrast is the test of choice. Look for **pseudocyst** or abscess formation. Ultrasound or MRI may also be used. ERCP (endoscopic retrograde cholangiopancreatography) or MRCP (magnetic resonance cholangiopancreatography) may evaluate for otherwise unseen blockage of pancreatic or common bile duct but is less practical unless already admitted.

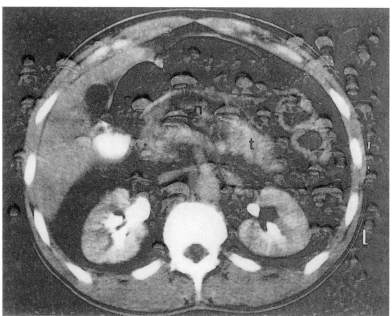

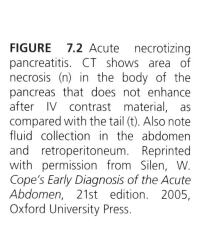

FIGURE 7.2 Acute necrotizing pancreatitis. CT shows area of necrosis (n) in the body of the pancreas that does not enhance after IV contrast material, as compared with the tail (t). Also note fluid collection in the abdomen and retroperitoneum. Reprinted with permission from Silen, W. *Cope's Early Diagnosis of the Acute Abdomen*, 21st edition. 2005, Oxford University Press.

Treatment

Give aggressive IV fluid replacement until urine output is adequate.

Make NPO immediately. This is the treatment of choice.

Consider NG tube if vomiting.

Pain control with IV pain medications such as meperidine (Demoral).

Consult surgery if indicated for complication of pseudocyst or abscess.

Monitor blood sugars and place on sliding scale insulin as needed.

Maintain NPO status until pain resolves, then return to regular diet slowly.

Prophylactic antibiotics are unproven and controversial. If started should only be in moderate-severe disease.

If not improving, consider CT scan and/or fine needle aspiration. Necrosis may develop.

Chronic pancreatitis may develop, especially with those patients with recurrent acute pancreatitis. If possible, treat etiology. As exocrine and endocrine pancreatic function fails, these patients will need dietary pancreatic enzyme replacement, vitamin B12 replacement, and insulin therapy.

Take Home Points

- Pancreatitis has many etiologies but the most common is EtOH use and gallstones.
- Imaging may show a "sentinel loop" or a pseudocyst.
- Give IV fluids aggressively and make the patient NPO. Consider an NG tube if vomiting.

Malignant Neoplasm of the Pancreas

Pancreatic carcinoma is most commonly adenocarcinoma in type and the vast majority of these arise from the exocrine cells (ductal and acinar cells) of the pancreas. This disease remains the fourth leading cause of cancer related death in the U.S. largely due to its typically late discovery and therefore dismal prognosis. Risk factors include occupational exposures, **smoking**, and lack of physical exercise and high body mass index (BMI).

Symptoms

Most cancers are found at late stages, thus have advanced presentations. Pruritus, weight loss, pain, jaundice, anorexia, diabetes, referred pain to the shoulder, malnutrition, hepatomegaly, palpable mass, abdominal tenderness, or ascites.

Diagnosis

Physical exam: Abdominal exam may reveal tenderness in epigastrium, hepatomegaly, jaundice, or mass. A nontender gallbladder may be felt (Courvoisier's sign) in patients with jaundice. Left sided supra-clavicular lymphadenopathy (Virchow's node) may be palpable.

Labs: CBC may show anemia. Alkaline phosphatase elevation, billirubin level increased due to obstruction, occult blood in stool. Specific enzymes such as gastrin or insulin may be elevated. Biomarker **CA19-9** used in pancreatic cancer but has low sensitivity and specificity.

Imaging: Helical CT scan has high sensitivity and specificity and is currently the test of choice. Transabdominal ultrasound is also useful for screening but not in staging. Endoscopic ultrasound is emerging as a very accurate test that shows smaller tumors and is used in staging. ERCP, MRI, MRCP (magnetic resonance cholangiopancreatography) are also useful and may be able to obtain biopsy at the time of the procedure.

Biopsy is essential whether done endoscopically or percutaneously.

Treatment

Surgery is the only option that has been shown to decrease mortality. However, most tumors are found too late to be resectable. Surgery may be done by the Whipple procedure (pancreaticoduodenectomy) or total pancreatectomy.

Chemotherapy and directed radiation therapy are palliative but may extend life. Other procedures such as celiac plexus block and biliary decompression may provide symptom relief.

Diabetes mellitus is often comorbid and requires insulin control.

Take Home Points

- Pancreatic cancer is most commonly adenocarcinoma of the exocrine (ductal or acinar) cells.
- Diagnosis is usually dismal due to advanced stage of discovery.
- Surgery may be useful but prognosis is still relatively poor.

Gallstones

Gallstones occur due to supersaturation of the bile in the gallbladder most commonly with cholesterol causing precipitation of stones. These stones form a "sludge" which may or may not contain calculi that become obstructive when secreted into the cystic duct. The ones that become obstructive commonly cause symptoms and can lead to cholecystitis.

Definitions:

Cholelithiasis—Formation and presence of stones in the gallbladder.

Cholecystitis—Inflammation of the gallbladder wall, usually due to obstruction of the cystic duct by gallstones.

Choledocholithiasis—Presence or obstruction of the bile ducts by gallstones.

Symptoms

Cholelithiasis is often asymptomatic especially if stones are large and unobstructing. Choledocholithiasis often leads to cholecystitis, which presents with colicky abdominal or right upper quadrant pain, worsened with meals, nausea/vomiting, fever/chills, clay colored stool, or jaundice. History may reveal 5 F's-"Female, Fat, Forty, Fertile, and Febrile." Rapid weight loss, pregnancy, or total parenteral nutrition (TPN) use are all prominent risk factors.

- Charcot's triad—RUQ pain, jaundice, fever/chills.
- Reynold's pentad—Charcot's triad *plus* shock and altered mental status. Seen with suppurative **cholangitis**.

Diagnosis

Physical exam: RUQ tenderness, positive **Murphy's sign** (pain on RUQ pressure with inspiration), jaundice, and increased temperature.

Labs: CBC shows leukocytosis, CMP shows increased billirubin (increased direct/conjugated bili), alkaline phosphatase, and GGT. Slightly elevated AST and ALT. Take blood cultures before starting antibiotics.

Imaging: Ultrasound is the classic first test for disease. If negative but strong clinical evidence exists, obtain hepato-iminodiacetic acid (HIDA) scan (if this test does not show a gallbladder, it indicates obstruction). CT may also be helpful and show dilation of ducts, abscess, or pancreatitis if present. ERCP, MRCP, or PTC shows status of biliary duct system and presence of stones, but is usually limited by availability and cost.

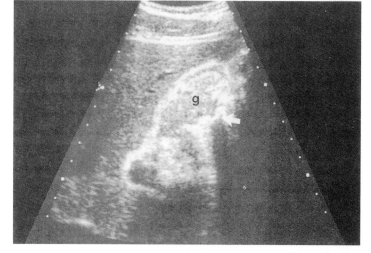

FIGURE 7.3 Ultrasound showing slightly distended gallbladder (g) with thickened wall. Variably echogenic lumen indicates presence of debris or sludge and presence of acoustic shadowing (arrow) is demonstrated. Reprinted with permission from Silen, W. *Cope's Early Diagnosis of the Acute Abdomen*, 21st edition. 2005, Oxford University Press.

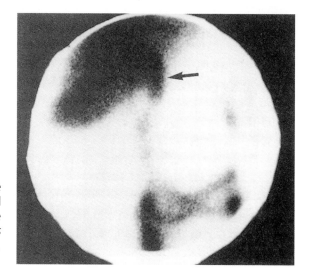

FIGURE 7.4 Normal HIDA scan virtually excluding acute cholecystitis. Note filling of the gallbladder (arrow) and excretion of the radioisotope (Technetium 99m) into the bowel. Reprinted with permission from Silen, W. *Cope's Early Diagnosis of the Acute Abdomen*, 21st edition. 2005, Oxford University Press.

Treatment

Start antibiotics, IV fluids, electrolyte repletion, and narcotic pain control.

Antibiotics should cover gram negative gut bacteria: Piperacillin-tazobactam (Zosyn), ampicillin-sulbactam (Unasyn), or ticarcillin-clavulanate (Timentin).

Surgery with laproscopic or open **cholecystectomy** is the most common and effective treatment. At time of surgery, intraoperative cholangiogram should be done to evaluate for further duct stones. Surgery is often delayed for 48–72 hours to wait for resolution of acute attack. In acute cholangitis (inflammation of the bile duct itself), decompressive surgery or ERCP sphincterotomy and stent placement may be needed.

Consider using ursodiol (Actigall) prophylactically to prevent gallstone formation in those patients attempting rapid weight loss.

Take Home Points

- Clinically, determine if the patient's symptoms are caused by or coincidental to the presence of gallstones.

- Ultrasound is often the best first test for disease.

- Surgery for cholecystectomy is often delayed in the acute phase to aid in reduction of local inflammation.

Primary Sclerosing Cholangitis

Primary sclerosing cholangitis (PSC) is characterized by progressive inflammation, fibrosis, and stricturing of the intrahepatic and extrahepatic bile ducts. Destruction of bile ducts may lead to eventual end stage liver disease and portal hypertension, thus, early detection is crucial.

Symptoms

Often presents with RUQ pain, fever/chills, jaundice, fatigue, and pruritus. History commonly reveals age < 45 years, male sex, and history of inflammatory bowel disease (IBD) (especially ulceractive colitis).

Diagnosis

Physical exam: RUQ pain, positive Murphy's sign, jaundice, and increased temperature.
Labs: CBC may show leukocytosis, CMP shows elevated GGT (gamma-glutamyl transferase), alkaline phosphatase, increased bilirubin (direct/conjugated). **P-ANCA positive**.
Liver biopsy may show characteristic "onion skin" and fibrotic appearance to tissue.
Imaging: ERCP is the test of choice and shows serial dilations/constrictions of the bile ducts "beads on a string" appearance. MRCP is also helpful.

Treatment

Supportive care and antibiotics for acute attacks.

ERCP is often used for stent placement over duct constrictions but is generally a temporary measure.

Ursodeoxycholic acid (URSO) may reduce pruritus and have positive effects on liver tests.

Corticosteroids, azathioprine (Imuran), penicillamine (Cuprimine), methotrexate (Trexall), and cholestyramine have all shown variable results.

Ultimately, liver transplantation is the only cure.

Think of **cholangiocarcinoma,** which has a strong association with PSC and is often fatal.

Take Home Points

- Ulcerative colitis and PSC are strongly correlated.
- Diagnosis classically shows positive P-ANCA, "onion skin" liver biopsy, and "beads on a string" on ERCP.
- Cholangiocarcinoma is strongly associated with PSC and may be fatal.

Malignant Neoplasm of Liver

Hepatocellular carcinoma (HCC) is a primary cancer of the hepatocyte and may result in liver failure or metastasis. HCC commonly occurs in the setting of alcoholism, cirrhosis, hepatitis B or C, hemochromatosis, alpha-1-antitrypsin deficiency, smoking, NASH (nonalcoholic steatohepatitis) or exposure to vinyl chloride. It should be noted, however, most cancer in the liver is of metastatic origin.

Symptoms

RUQ and vague abdominal pain, weight loss, nausea/vomiting, and low-grade fever commonly in an unexplained deterioration in a stable cirrhosis patient. Paraneoplastic symptoms such as feminization, osteoarthropathy, or carcinoid syndrome may be present.

Diagnosis

Physical exam: Hepatomegally, RUQ mass, hepatic friction rub, or bruit.

Labs: CBC may show polycythemia, CMP shows elevated calcium, low glucose, elevated AST and ALT and other nonspecific liver function derangements. Tumor markers include **alpha-fetoprotein** (AFP > 400 µg/L), des-gamma-carboxyprothrombin, GGT, and carcinoembryonic antigen (CEA).

Imaging: Ultrasound is the most widely used scan and may be used for surveillance after treatment. CT scan is important in finding extrahepatic spread. MRI shows greater detail of the tumor margins and features. Lipoidal angiography with CT is very good at delineating small tumors and may be used for a chemotherapeutic or radioactive vehicle.

Liver biopsy with/without US or CT guidance is essential to diagnosis and may confirm histologic type.

Treatment

Prevent disease with control of risk factors! Monitor high risk and prior disease patients with periodic AFP and ultrasounds.

   Surgery is the mainstay for primary disease. However, prognosis is still often grim due to late presentation. Liver transplant in more extensive but non-metastatic disease can be successful.

   Palliative techniques include: X-ray-guided radiofrequency ablation, alcohol injection, or chemotherapeutic embolization.

Take Home Points

- Major risk factors for HCC include cirrhosis of any type, hepatitis infection, and toxin (such as EtOH) exposure.
- AFP may be used for detection in high risk populations and surveillance after resection.
- Surgery is the cornerstone of treatment.

Appendicitis

Appendicitis involves inflammation of the appendiceal wall followed by localized ischemia and abscess formation eventually leading to perforation and the development of a contained or generalized peritonitis. Obstruction is the most common cause and may occur from adjacent hypertrophy of lymphatic tissue, fecolith impaction, neoplasm, or fibrosis.

Symptoms

Abdominal pain classically starts in the generalized or peri-umbilical area then localizes to the right lower quadrant (RLQ). This disease may be associated with fever, nausea/vomiting, anorexia, diaphoresis, or myalgias.

Diagnosis

Physical exam: Elevated temperature, abdominal muscle guarding, and **rebound tenderness** over McBurney's point.

- Rovsing's sign—RLQ pain on palpation of LLQ.
- Psoas sign—pain with extension of hip.
- Obturator sign—pain with internal rotation of flexed right thigh.

Labs: CBC shows leukocytosis with left shift.

Imaging: CT scan with oral contrast is becoming the standard and may show thickened appendiceal wall, appendolith, or surrounding fat stranding. CT is better to evaluate for abscess or other cause of pain. Ultrasound is also used although is more operator dependent. Plain x-ray may be suggestive of appendicitis but is not used in diagnosis.

Barium enema may show lack of filling of the appendix but is uncommon unless another indication is present.

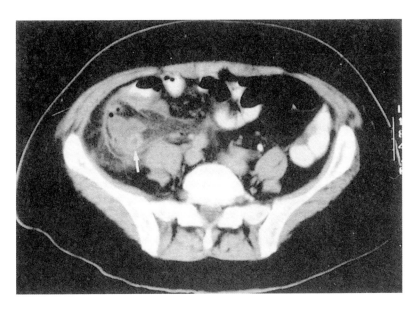

FIGURE 7.5 CT scan indicating acute appendicitis. Note thickened appendiceal wall (arrow) and surrounding "dirty fat" indicating inflammation. Reprinted with permission from Silen, W. *Cope's Early Diagnosis of the Acute Abdomen*, 21st edition. 2005, Oxford University Press.

Treatment

Consult surgery for appendectomy.

Consider giving a dose a broad spectrum antibiotic such as a fluoroquinolone or metronidazole (Flagyl) before surgery.

Take Home Points

- Obstruction of the appeniceal opening is the most common etiology.
- Look for generalized abdominal pain that localizes to the RUQ.
- Classic signs are rebound tenderness, Rovsing's, psoas, and obturator signs.
- Treatment is surgical.

Intestinal Obstruction

Obstruction of the intestines occurs when there is a block to normal fecal flow through the gut tract; it most commonly occurs in the small bowel. Causes are most commonly adhesion formation after surgery and hernias but others include tumors, intussusception, volvulus, congenital obstruction, meconium obstruction, inflammatory stricture, radiation enteritis, etc.

Symptoms

Diffuse abdominal pain, nausea/vomiting, anorexia, and obstipation. History may reveal lack of or infrequent stooling or risk factors including history of obstruction, meconium ileus, Meckel's diverticulum, volvulus, colon cancer, recent surgery, etc. Constipation in the elderly is a common cause.

Diagnosis

Physical exam: Distended abdomen, decreased bowel sounds or high pitched sounds, cessation of flatus, tenderness to direct palpation. Rectal exam may reveal fecal impaction or mass.

Labs: Screening CBC may show leukocytosis if strangulation of hernia or infectious cause is present. Hepatic function panel often shows increased bilirubin.

Imaging: Plain upright x-ray may reveal distended haustra and air-fluid levels.

Barium enema may reveal colonic obstruction or mass. Enema may be therapeutic in intussusception.

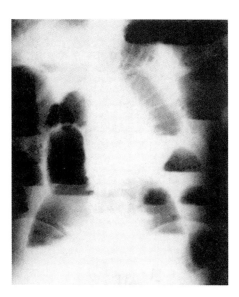

FIGURE 7.6 Erect film of bowel obstruction demonstrating multiple "step ladder-like" air fluid levels accompanied by distended bowel. Reprinted with permission from Silen, W. *Cope's Early Diagnosis of the Acute Abdomen*, 21st edition. 2005, Oxford University Press.

Treatment

Correct electrolytes.

Consider nasogastric tube if emesis is significant problem.

Attempt correction of stool impaction if this is clinically appropriate.

Surgical consultation if other causes thought likely; these may include adhesions, volvulus, incarcerated hernia, foreign body, obstructing malignancy (amongst others).

Surgery may include: lysis of adhesions, reduction of hernia, bowel resection, intestinal bypass, colostomy, or cecostomy. Attempt at intussusception reduction may be made by hydrostatic/pneumatic enema.

Take Home Points

- Plain abdominal x-ray may show distended haustra and air fluid levels in a "step ladder-like" pattern.

- Prompt surgical consultation should be initiated.

Diverticular Disease

Diverticulosis—Commonly right-sided intestinal wall herniation that, because of vascular supply to location, tends to bleed.

Diverticulitis—Inflammation and infection of commonly left-sided colonic wall herniations that tend to cause acute illness.

Prevalence of diverticulosis in the general population increases with age, and recent estimates indicate 40–50% of the U.S. population have some form by the 7th decade of life, with diverticulitis having an annual incidence of about 2,700 cases/100,000 per year.

Symptoms

Diverticulosis often causes painless bleeding. Diverticulitis may cause abdominal pain, cramping, diarrhea, anorexia, and fever/chills. Complications include perforation, abscess, and fistula formation with symptoms including acute peritoneal signs, mass, or pneumaturia, fecauria, etc.

Diagnosis

Physical exam: Diverticulosis may show blood on occult testing. Diverticulitis may show LLQ tenderness, high pitched or absent bowel sounds, or abdominal distention.

Labs: CBC shows leukocytosis in diverticulitis and low hemoglobin/hematocrit in diverticulosis. Obtain blood and urine cultures.

Imaging: Diverticulosis may be seen with barium enema or colonoscopy. Bleeding sites may be evaluated with radio-labeled RBC scan or angiography. Diverticulitis is commonly demonstrated with **CT scan** with and without rectal contrast. CT is also useful in diagnosis of abscess, perforation, or fistula formation if present. Obtain upright CXR and abdominal x-ray to evaluate for free air in the abdomen if clinical presentation is indicative. Barium enema is less helpful in inflammatory state since uptake into diverticulae is not reliable.

Colonoscopy for diverticulosis is the procedure of choice as it allows for direct therapy at the same time as visualization.

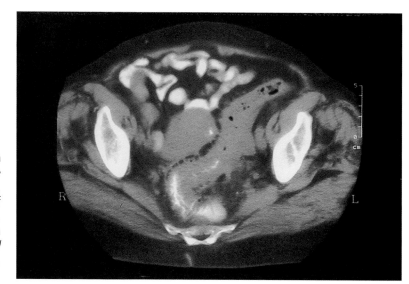

FIGURE 7.7 CT of the pelvis in a patient with acute diverticulitis. The sigmoid colon is grossly thickened, the lumen narrowed, and pockets of air are seen in the diverticular disease. Reprinted with permission from Warrell DA, Cox TM, et al. *Oxford Textbook of Medicine, 4th edition.* 2003, Oxford University Press.

Treatment

High fiber diet for prevention. Some controversy exists on trigger foods such as popcorn, strawberries, raspberries, and poppyseed muffins.

Diverticulosis bleeding stops without therapy in a very high proportion of patients. If needed, local injection of epinephrine or electrocaudery may be used. If bleeding is profuse, consider surgical consultation.

Diverticulitis may be treated outpatient unless complications exist. Antibiotics include ciprofloxacin (Cipro) + metronidazole (Flagyl) for 7 days.

If complications such as abscess, perforation, or fistula are found, immediate surgical consultation is indicated.

Recurrent attacks of uncomplicated diverticulitis are an indication for segmental bowel resection.

Take Home Points

- Diverticulitis may cause an acute abdominal illness while diverticulosis commonly causes bleeding.
- Order a CT scan in the emergency department setting if suspected diverticulitis is the cause of symptoms. Colonoscopy may be used in the non-acute setting.
- Treat diverticulitis attacks with oral antibiotics, pain control, and gradual change to high fiber diet.
- Segmental bowel resection may be considered if attacks of diverticulitis are significant.

Inflammatory Bowel Disease

TABLE 7.2 Comparison of Crohn Disease and Ulcerative Colitis

Characteristic	Crohn Disease	Ulcerative Colitis
Typical population	Those of Caucasian or Jewish descent. Bimodal age distribution in 20s then in 50–70s.	Often young women in mid-30s of Caucasian or Jewish descent
Location	Classically occurs in terminal ileum but my arise **anywhere from the mouth to the anus**	Typically in distal colon and rectum

TABLE 7.2 continued

Characteristic	Crohn Disease	Ulcerative Colitis
Clinical features	**Non-bloody diarrhea**, abdominal (RLQ) pain, wt loss, anorexia, low-grade fever.	**Bloody diarrhea**, cramping, abdominal pain, wt loss, fatigue, bowel urgency, low-grade fever, tachycardia, and heme-positive stools.
Associations	Pyoderma gangrenosum, erythema nodosum, fatty liver, iritis, episcleritis, gallstones, kidney stones, and arthritis.	**Primary sclerosing cholangitis**, pyoderma gangrenosum, erythema nodosum, arthritis, ankylosing spondylitis, and iritis. Beware of toxic megacolon (obtain x-rays).
Pathology	Transmural involvement commonly with **"skip lesions."** Cobblestoning may be seen on colonoscopy. Fissures, abscess, granuloma, or **fistula** formation are common.	Mucosal or submucosal involvement only. Ulcers and erosions possible. Barium enema may show lead-pipe colon with loss of haustra. Biopsy reveals **crypt abscesses**.
Labs	CBC shows normocytic-macrocytic anemia, increased ESR, normal LFTs.	CBC shows normocytic anemia, increased ESR, low albumin, positive p-ANCA.
Treatment	Mild cases: 5-aminosalicylic acid (5-ASA) compounds such as mesalamine (Pentasa, Asacol) and sulfasalazine (Azulfidine) ± oral steroids. Moderate cases: 5-ASA compounds + oral steroids and addition of azathioprine (Azasan), 6-mercaptopurine (Purinethol), or methotrexate. Consider addition of steroid enemas. Severe cases: Admission to hospital, NPO status, IV steroids, steroid enemas, metronidazole (Flagyl) and consider TPN. Consider anti-TNF antibody-infliximab (Remicade). Surgery: May be helpful in UC but is often ineffective and possibly harmful in uncomplicated Crohn disease.	

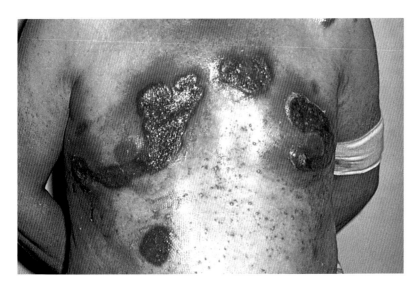

FIGURE 7.8 Pyoderma gangrenosum associated with inflammatory bowel disease. Reprinted with permission from MacKie, RM. *Clinical Dermatology*, 5th edition. 2003, Oxford University Press.

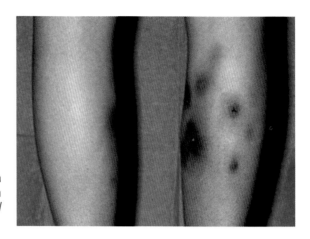

FIGURE 7.9 Erythema nodosum associated with inflammatory bowel disease. Reprinted with permission from Flynn JA. *Oxford American Handbook of Clinical Medicine*. 2007, Oxford University Press.

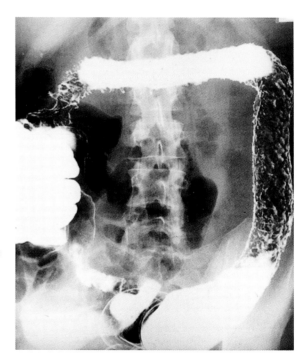

FIGURE 7.10 Barium enema showing Crohn disease of the colon and terminal ileum. Distal sigmoid, rectum, and a segment of ascending colon are normal. The diseased segments show loss of haustration, shortening, and fissure ulcers. Reprinted with permission from Warrell DA, Cox TM, et al. *Oxford Textbook of Medicine, 4th edition*. 2003, Oxford University Press.

Irritable Bowel Syndrome

Irritable bowel syndrome (IBS) is a disorder characterized by chronic abdominal pain and altered bowel habits in the absence of any organic diagnosable cause. Pathophysiology is complex and likely reflects a mix of influencing factors including: abnormal gastrointestinal motility, intestinal tract flora alteration, post-infectious reactivity, microscopic inflammation, gut tract hypersensitivity, psychological dysfunction, and emotional stress.

Symptoms

Several subtypes include: IBS with diarrhea, IBS with constipation, mixed IBS, and untypable IBS. Abdominal pain and change in bowel habits are prominent features. History often reveals coexisting anxiety or psychologic disorder, history of childhood sexual abuse, or prior autonomic nervous system abnormality.

"Red Flag" Symptoms that Should Prompt Further Urgent Investigation

Age of onset > 50 years
Fever
Nocturnal symptoms
Blood in stools
Anemia
Weight loss > 10% body weight
Profuse or large volume of diarrhea
Family history of inflammatory bowel disease or cancer
Fever
Organomegaly
Jaundice
Peritoneal signs or focal abdominal tenderness

Diagnosis

The most common and researched criteria for clinical assessment include the **Manning criteria:**

- Pain relieved by defecation
- More frequent stools at the onset of pain
- Looser stools at the onset of pain
- Visible abdominal distention
- Passage of mucous
- Sensation of incomplete evacuation

Symptoms should be present for at least 3 months before IBS is diagnosed.

Labs: Evaluate for other causes of symptoms as appropriate with stool studies (ova/parasites, fecal leukocytes, culture, etc.), serum markers for inflammatory bowel disease, TSH, etc. In IBS, these studies are generally negative.

Imaging: Evaluate for other causes and obtain plain radiograph or CT as appropriate.

Colonoscopy is often negative but may be appropriate to eliminate other causes of disease.

Treatment

Detailed diet history to eliminate or reduce modifiable contributors such as high fat diet, etc.

Strong physician-patient relationship is essential.

Trial of increasing fiber in diet and increased daily exercise is reasonable. Add bulk forming agents such as psyllium (Metamucil) or fiber supplements.

Antispasmodics may be helpful including dicyclomine (Bentyl), hyoscyamine (Levbid), or chlordiaz-epoxide-clidinium (Librax).

Diarrheal predominant type may be treated with loperimide (Imodium) or diphenoxylate-atropine (Lomotil) after each loose stool.

Antibiotics, rifaximin (Xifaxan) may be helpful in diarrheal type but research is not totally conclusive.

Serotonin receptor antagonists including alosetron (Lotronex) and tegaserod (Zelnorm) have both been shown somewhat effective in IBS but currently have restricted prescribing status in the U.S. These should only be used in severe refractory cases due to possible side effects.

Simethicone (Mylicon) may be helpful for bloating and *Lactobacillus* supplements have shown subjective success.

TCAs such as amitriptyline (Elavil) have shown good response. SSRIs are still being investigated for this indication.

Alternative therapies such as biofeedback, bowel training, herbal medications, and hypnosis have been used although evidence showing benefit is lacking.

Take Home Points

- The etiology of IBS is yet unknown. Comorbidity with psychosocial stressors is prominent.

- Treatment is aimed at symptom control with some psychoactive medications showing benefit.

Acute Peritonitis

The disease state of acute inflammation of the parietal or visceral surfaces within the peritoneal cavity. Commonly occurs in conjunction with peritoneal cavity violation in penetrating external injury, visceral perforation, or disease to the internal organs. Internal injury may be intestinal gangrene, perforated ulcer, ischemic colitis, etc. The entity of spontaneous bacterial peritonitis (SBP) is associated with the presence and infection of ascitic abdominal fluid.

Symptoms

Acute abdominal pain (made worse with movement), fever/chills, nausea/vomiting, constipation, and abdominal distention. History may reveal ascites from cirrhotic liver disease, penetrating injury, perforated bowel, abdominal surgery, or inflammatory intra-abdominal organ disorder.

Diagnosis

Physical exam: Tenderness to palpation/percussion of all four quadrants of the abdomen (may be rebound). Tachycardia, tachypnea, and increased temperature.

Labs: CBC for leukocytosis, increased ESR/CRP. Obtain blood cultures. Peritoneal fluid culture is the gold standard. Also analyze for ascitic fluid for cell count and differential, albumen, and total protein concentration. Consider obtaining LDH concentration, glucose, and cytology.

Imaging: Upright CXR and abdominal x-ray are indicated for free air below the diaphragm. **CT scan** of the abdomen may show perforation site or abscess. Ultrasound may demonstrate ascites or mass.

Treatment

IV fluids as indicated.

Control pain with IV opioids.

Empiric antibiotics should be started before culture results known. Ampicillin/sulbactam (Unasyn), piperacillin/tazobactam (Zosyn), or ticarcillin/clavulanate (Timentin) are good choices. Narrow spectrum according to peritoneal culture results.

Prevention of spontaneous bacterial peritonitis (SBP) in patients with known chronic ascites with SMX-TMP DS (Bactrim, Septra) or ciprofloxacin significantly reduces episodes of disease.

Take Home Points

- Peritonitis often occurs as a result of peritoneal cavity or visceral perforation.
- If ascitic fluid is present, a "diagnostic tap" is indicated for possible SBP. Analyze the fluid.
- Broad spectrum parenteral antibiotics with good gram negative organism coverage is indicated before cultures return. Use Unasyn or Zosyn.

Gastrointestinal Bleeding

Bleeding occurring into the gut tract coming from a source of the gut tract itself.

Upper GI bleeding—Proximal to the ligament of Treitz.

Lower GI bleeding—Distal to the ligament of Trietz.

Finding the source of bleeding, which can be elusive, is the most important aspect of the workup. Remember the phrase "the most common source of lower GI bleeding is upper GI bleeding."

Symptoms

Regardless of location of bleeding, the patient may suffer from lightheadedness, vertigo, fatigue, orthostatic hypotension, noticeable blood loss in stools, pica, melena, or weight loss. If upper GI in origin, the patient is more likely to notice hematemesis and have a history of peptic ulcer disease (PUD), recent vomiting, or risk factors for varices. Lower GI bleeding may present with bright red blood per rectum, history of diverticulosis, hematochezia, or diarrhea. Look for historical NSAID use, EtOH use, smoking, sick contacts, or anticoagulant use. Recent change in bowel habits, narrowed caliber of stools, hematochezia, and abdominal pain should prompt evaluation for colorectal cancer.

Diagnosis

Physical exam: Pallor, tachycardia, tachypnea, or hypotension, if severe. Rectal exam and possible anoscopy is indicated to check for rectal/anal source.

Labs: CBC may show anemia, leukocytosis if infectious, thrombocytopenia. Check coagulation studies (PT/aPTT/INR), and LFTs.

NG tube placement may reveal flecks of coagulated blood indicating upper GI origin.

Endoscopy, initially EGD, is the most common way to find bleeding. See individual sections for varices, Mallory-Weiss tears, etc.

Radio labeled red blood cell (99Tc-tagged RBC) scan may be used if colonoscopy is not useful. Angiography or exploratory laparoscopy are options but only if brisk and bleeding source is not found.

Treatment

Apply ABCs as necessary.

Consult surgery as indicated.

Address volume status deficiencies with fluid replacement then consider blood transfusion needs.

Vast majority of non-brisk GI bleeding ceases without treatment. Other therapy depends on diagnosis but may include octreotide (Sandostatin), local endoscopic injection therapy, TIPS, band ligation, β-blockers, or embolization. See individual sections for treatment modalities of different etiologies.

Take Home Points

- Most mild to moderate GI bleeding halts without treatment.
- Location is the key.
- Long term bleeding may lead to anemia—don't miss it because you're looking for hemorrhage.

Hernia

TABLE 7.3 Types of Hernias

Hernia	Protrusion of visceral contents through facial defect in containing wall. Often in abdomen and commonly inguinal, umbilical, ventral, femoral, or incisional.
Reducible hernia	Herniation of most often visceral contents which is either manually or spontaneously reduced.
Incarcerated hernia	Herniation which is not reducible externally but blood supply is preserved.
Strangulated hernia	Herniation in which blood supply is acutely compromised causing eminent ischemia of the tissues. A surgical emergency.
Indirect inguinal hernia	Herniation through the internal inguinal ring, lateral to the inferior epigastric artery.
Direct inguinal hernia	Herniation through the wall of the inguinal canal, specifically through structures forming Hesselbach's triangle.

Symptoms

Depending on location and degree of herniation, often a bulge is felt, pain, pain with lifting, or extreme pain at bulge site or groin indicating strangulation. Males may feel a fullness of scrotum or increase in scrotal size.

Diagnosis

Physical exam: The most reliable means of diagnosing a hernia is physical exam which may reveal palpable mass, spontaneous reduction, palpable fascial defect, fullness of scrotum, or in the case of strangulation, extreme pain on palpation with surrounding erythema and swelling.

Imaging: CT may be useful but is often unneeded.

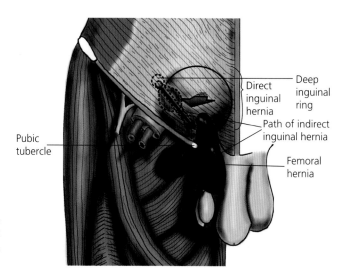

FIGURE 7.11 The relationship of indirect, direct, and femoral hernia. Reprinted with permission from Cox NLT, Roper TA. *Clinical Skills.* 2005, Oxford University Press.

Treatment

Surgery is the mainstay and only effective treatment. Hernioplasty with mesh placement is most common with simple closure of defect less common.

If asymptomatic without danger of strangulation, may elect to not treat.

Prevent hernias by avoiding heavy lifting or with proper lifting technique (avoid high intraperitoneal pressures).

Take Home Points

- Hernia is basically a hole in the containing wall allowing contents to extrude through.
- Treatment is surgical; strangulated hernias require emergent surgery.

Colorectal Cancer

Malignant neoplasm most commonly of the adenocarcinoma type arising from the luminal wall of the colon, rectum, or anus. Genetic factors such as the presence of the RAS oncogene and suppression of tumor suppressor genes are found in many cases.

Symptoms

Vague abdominal pain, abdominal enlargement, change in bowel habits/appearance, hematochezia/melena, weakness, anemia, or weight loss. History may indicate risk factors including:

- Colorectal cancer in first degree relative aged < 60 years or two first degree relatives of any age.
- Family or personal history of familial adenomatous polyposis (FAP) or other genetic colon cancer disease.
- Adenomatous polyps on prior evaluations.
- Inflammatory bowel disease.
- Cancer of other areas.
- Age > 50 years.

Diagnosis

The American Cancer Society recommends screening average risk patients for colorectal cancer beginning at age 50 years by one of the following methods:

- Fecal occult blood testing (FOBT) annually.
- Flexible sigmoidoscopy every 5 years.
- Annual FOBT plus flexible sigmoidoscopy every 5 years.
- Double-contrast barium enema every 5 years.
- Colonoscopy every 10 years.

Performed on 2–3 consecutive stools at home. In-office single FOBT inadequate.

These recommendations are supported by the United States Preventive Services Task Force (USPSTF) and American Academy of Family Physicians (AAFP).

Increased risk and high risk patients generally should obtain colonoscopy every 1–3 years.

Labs: CBC for possible anemia. CEA (carcinoembryonic antigen) provides disease surveillance after treatment but is not used for screening.

Imaging: As discussed above, best visualization with endocoscopy (coloncopy, flexible sigmoidoscopy, or anoscopy). Virtual colonoscopy and "pill colonoscopy" are emerging technologies. CT scan may be used for staging or evaluating possible metastatic spread.

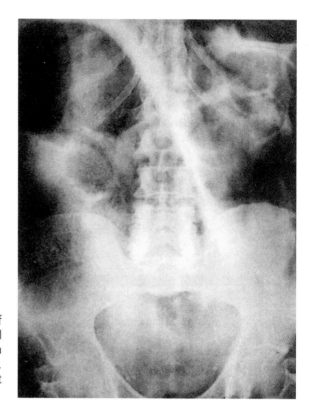

FIGURE 7.12 Obstruction of the colon by carcinoma of the sigmoid. Note massive distention of the large bowel from the cecum to the sigmoid where the obstruction was situated. Reprinted with permission from Silen, W. *Cope's Early Diagnosis of the Acute Abdomen*, 21st edition. 2005, Oxford University Press.

Current staging is with the American Joint Committee on Cancer (AJCC) TNM staging system. This system uses characteristics of the tumor, nodal involvement, and metastasis to classify the cancer. The Duke criteria has historically been used for staging but has been modified and improved and is now no longer widely employed.

Treatment

Prevention with high fiber, low fat diet, smoking cessation, and scheduled health maintenance.

Resection of the bowel segment and regional lymph nodes is the standard. Radiation and chemotherapy may be adjutants based on TNM stage and location (rectal, anal more common). The classics are 5-fluorouracil (5-FU) and leucovorin.

Refer to gastroenterologist.

Take Home Points

- Start screening at age 50 years.
- Staging is with the TNM staging system.
- Resection with consideration of chemotherapy and radiation is the mainstay of treatment.

Perirectal and Perianal Abscess

Abscesses in the perirectal or perianal area are commonly caused by obstruction and infection of an anal gland with mixed flora including staphylococci, streptococci, *E coli*, etc. The fluid cavity formed may follow several planes of dissection in the rectal area depending on the location. Types include: perianal, ischiorectal, intersphinchteric, supralevator, and horseshoe.

Symptoms

Perianal or perirectal swelling, redness, tenderness, throbbing pain, pain on defecation, and possibly fever. History may reveal risk factors including IBD, injection of internal hemorrhoids, foreign objects, prolapsed hemorrhoids, and anal intercourse/trauma.

Diagnosis

Physical exam: Palpable, tender, fluctuant mass in the anal or rectal region.
Labs: CBC often shows leukocytosis. Anemia from bleeding is uncommon.

Treatment

Incision and drainage is the mainstay. Perianal abscesses are often treated with local anesthetic while higher ones require general anesthesia and surgery. Iodoform packing for 1–4 days is often needed.

Primary fistulotomy is preferred during incision/drainage for horseshoe abscesses.

Antibiotics including TMP/SMX DS (Bactrim, Seprtra) or ciproflocacin/levofloxacin, *plus* metronidazole (Flagyl).

Give stool softener for first 1–2 weeks.

Monitor for common complication of fistula formation.

Take Home Points

- Most commonly caused by obstruction and infection of anal glands.
- Superficial abscesses may be drained in the office or ER but deeper ones or those difficult to access require referral and surgery.

Hemorrhoids

Varicosities of the hemorrhoidal venous plexus, which, depending on location, become symptomatic in various ways. Risk factors include pregnancy, age, prolonged sitting, chronic constipation, liver disease, and portal hypertension. A common grading system exists (see table below).

TABLE 7.4 Grades of Classification of Hemorrhoids

Grade	Characteristics
Grade I	May be visualized on anoscopy and may bulge into the lumen but do not extend below the dentate line.
Grade II	May prolapse out of the anal canal with defecation or with straining but reduce spontaneously.
Grade III	May prolapse out of the anal canal with defecation or straining and require manual reduction into their normal position.
Grade IV	Are irreducible and may strangulate.

Symptoms

Depending on location, may present with feeling of incomplete evacuation, painless bleeding, prolapse, pruritus, palpable mass, pain associated with a thrombosed hemorrhoid, or fecal soilage. Internal hemorrhoids (those proximal to the dentate line) classically are the source of bleeding while external hemorrhoids (those distal to the dentate line) are more sensitive and painful.

Diagnosis

Anoscopy is the mainstay of diagnosis.
Sigmoidoscopy may be useful for more proximal disease.

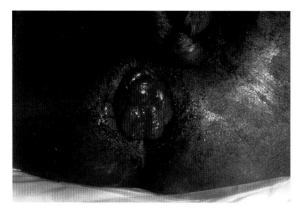

FIGURE 7.13 Thrombosed hemorrhoid. Reprinted with permission from Cox NLT, Roper TA. *Clinical Skills.* 2005, Oxford University Press.

Treatment

Prevent them with high fiber diet, increased fluid intake, weight loss, and avoiding straining.

Topical corticosteroids (Cortifoam), anesthetics (Nupercainal, Anusol, Proctofoam), astringent suppositories (Preparation H), and sitz baths for early symptom control. Mixes of these conservative treatments are common (such as Proctofoam-HC). However, avoid use of these topical preparations, especially steroid containing ones, for more than 2 weeks to avoid side effects such as mucosal atrophy and contact dermatitis.

Nonoperative techniques for ablating non-thrombosed, internal hemorrhoids include injection sclerotherapy, heat/laser coagulation, and rubber band ligation.

Surgical excision should only be used in severe cases or thrombosis/strangulation. Effectiveness of surgery is higher than other techniques but recurrence is common.

If thrombosed, external hemorrhoids are present, surgical excision techniques vary but common practice is to use a "wedge" removal technique where a wedge of overlying skin is excised and the clot removed.

Take Home Points

- Hemorrhoids are one of the most common sources of lower GI bleeding.
- Hemorrhoids proximal to the dentate line classically cause bleeding, those distal to the dentate line classically cause pain.
- Treat conservatively unless very painful and thrombosed or strangulated.

8 Gynecology

Malignant Neoplasm of the Breast

Breast cancer is the most common cancer occurring in women and the second leading cause of cancer death in this group. Two basic types of breast malignancy exist, ductal and lobular. Ductal is more common and visible on mammography. Lobular is usually incidentally discovered by biopsy of other abnormalities and is generally less visible on mammography. In situ lesions (DCIS, LCIS) are those showing malignant potential but have not invaded beyond the surrounding breast duct or lobule. Sometimes referred to as "pre-cancer," they make up the majority of malignant breast disease. Other types include Paget disease (carcinoma involving the nipple) and inflammatory carcinoma.

Risk Factors

Age

Caucasian race

Benign breast disease with cytologic atypia

Personal history of breast cancer

Higher socioeconomic status

Lack of physical activity

High dietary fat intake

Lifetime exposure to endogenous estrogens (influenced by age of menarche, parity, age of menopause, etc.)

Family history and genetic factors

Exposure to ionizing radiation

Symptoms

Often asymptomatic but commonly presents as a breast lump felt either by the patient or physician. Cancers are hard and mobile in surrounding tissue but all lumps need to be investigated. Other symptoms include *peau d'orange* (skin of the orange) skin change, regional lymphadenopathy, and nipple bleeding or non-milky discharge. Classically, cancer occurs in the upper outer quadrant (tail of Spence).

Diagnosis

Current Recommendations

Authoritative bodies differ on recommendations for screening, especially for women under the age of 50. The American Medical Association (AMA), the American College of Radiology (ACR), and the American Cancer Society (ACS), all support screening with mammography and clinical breast exam (CBE) beginning at age 40. The American College of Obstetricians and Gynecologists (ACOG) supports screening with mammography beginning at age 40 and clinical breast exam (CBE) beginning at age 19. The American Academy of Family Physicians (AAFP) recommends beginning mammography for average-risk women at age 50 with mammography in high-risk women beginning at age 40. The AAFP recommends that all women aged 40–49 be counseled about the risks and benefits of mammography before making decisions about screening.

Organizations also differ on their recommendations for the appropriate interval for mammography. Annual mammography is recommended by the AMA, ACR, and ACS. Mammography every 1–2 years is recommended by the AAFP. Finally, ACOG recommends mammography every 1–2 years for women aged 40–49 and annually for women aged 50 and older.

TABLE 8.1 BI-RADS Scoring System for Screening Mammography

BI-RADS Category	Recommendation
0: Need additional imaging	Spot compression and magnification (diagnostic) views or ultrasonography as soon as possible
1: Totally negative	Routine follow-up
2: Benign findings	Routine follow-up
3: Probably benign finding	Diagnostic evaluation of breast with suspicious lesion within six months

TABLE 8.1 Continued

BI-RADS Category	Recommendation
4: Suspicious	Biopsy as soon as possible
5: Highly suggestive of malignancy	Biopsy as soon as possible
6: Biopsy-proven carcinoma	

BI-RADS = Breast Imaging Reporting and Data System.

Imaging: After screening raises suspicion, further evaluation should be performed. Generally, mammography can be used for older women with less dense breasts and ultrasound for younger women with denser breasts or those with suspected cystic masses. Contrast enhanced MRI may be used if mammography or ultrasound is not considered optimal, carcinoma has already been found and occult malignancies are in question, or for screening purposes in those considered high risk. If positive, fine needle aspiration or excisional biopsy can be performed on palpable masses. Stereotactic biopsy can also be used to localize the lesion if not felt. Incisional biopsy and core biopsy may also be chosen. Remember, mammography, physical exam, or aspiration cannot tell if cancer exists: **"If the rumor is tumor, tissue is the issue!"**

Labs: Obtain screening CBC, renal function, and LFTs. If family history suggests a high incidence of breast or gynecologic cancer, obtain genetic analysis for BRCA 1 and 2.

Upon positive biopsy, obtain estrogen, progesterone, and HER-2 status of the tumor to guide treatment.

Treatment

Surgery: Several procedures exist and are progressively decreasing the amount of tissue taken.

TABLE 8.2 Surgical Treatment Types for Breast Cancer

Procedure	Definition/Associations
Radical mastectomy (Halsted)	Complete en bloc removal of anterior chest wall including breast tissue, skin, nipple/areola, axillary lymph nodes, and pectoralis major/minor. Rarely used today.
Modified radical mastectomy	Removes breast tissue, skin, nipple/areola, axillary lymph nodes, and pectoralis fascia.
Simple mastectomy	Removes breast tissue, nipple/areola, and skin but spares lymph nodes, muscles, and fascia. Often used with radiation for DCIS, LCIS.
Local excision/lumpectomy/ segmental mastectomy	Lesion specific removal of tumor and surrounding breast tissue. Often frozen sections are used to assure clear margins in the OR. May/may not be accompanied by node dissection. Appropriate for tumors less than 4 cm without surrounding tissue fixation, skin involvement, or fixed node involvement. Often used with radiation therapy.
Sentinel node biopsy	Biopsy of main lymph node(s), draining area suspicious of lesion. Newest approach to avoid side effects of complete node dissection.

Chemotherapy:

Estrogen receptor status of tumor must be assessed. Treatment for estrogen receptor positive tumors may include selective estrogen receptor blockers (SERBs) such as tamoxifen and raloxifene (Evista).

Aromatase inhibitors (anastrozole [Arimidex], letrozole, and exemestane) work by reducing androgen conversion to estrogen, thus reducing estrogen effect on responsive cancers. Side effects tend to be less than those with SERBs and therefore are becoming more commonly used.

Trastuzumab (Herceptin) may also be used in HER-2 receptor positive cancers.

Other traditional chemotherapy regimens can be used for metastatic or likely metastatic disease.

Radiation: Can improve survival rates after newer breast sparring procedures. Generally side effects are mild but a classic one is unilateral arm lymphedema.

Take Home Points

- Breast cancer involves ductal, lobular, and in situ tumors. The most common location is the upper outer quadrant (tail of Spence).
- Mammography is the most common screening strategy.
- If breast malignancy is found, estrogen, progesterone, and HER-2 status may be used to guide therapy decisions.
- Surgical treatment should be guided by stage but focus is on breast-conserving procedures.

Benign Masses of the Breast

Several types of benign breast masses exist including fibroadenoma, fibrocystic changes, intraductal papilloma, fat necrosis, and mammary duct ectasia. Most common, especially in younger, premenopausal women, are fibroadenomas and fibrocystic change.

Symptoms

Many present with breast mass but several types present with overlying skin inflammation, bloody nipple discharge, breast enlargement, pain, and cyclic response to menstrual cycle.

Diagnosis/Treatment

Commonly, the history and physical exam are used to assess the need for biopsy. Ultrasound can be used to evaluate for cystic structures and mammography if the mass is thought to be suspicious for malignancy. Ultimately, excision, biopsy, or aspiration is the standard. OCPs (oral contraceptive pills) can help symptoms by regulating periods until benign lesion is confirmed. NSAIDs can help discomfort. Advise patient to quit smoking and caffeine use. Vitamin E and evening oil of primrose have also been used as alternative treatments.

Take Home Points

- Young women often have benign masses in the breast attributable to fibrocystic changes or fibroadenoma.
- Biopsy may be needed to determine benign vs. malignant status depending on other characteristics.

Mastitis/Breast Abscess

Mastitis and breast abscess may complicate postpartum breastfeeding. Although congestive mastitis is common, especially in the postpartum woman who chooses not to breastfeed, only infectious disease needs care beyond simple measures. Retrograde colonization and infection starting at the nipple is often the mechanism.

Symptoms

Unilateral, swollen, warm, and exquisitely painful breast often with nipple retraction. Mastitis may have accompanying fever and signs of systemic infection although full progression to sepsis is rare. Purulent nipple discharge can be present in advanced cases. Abscess may form. Both abscess and mastitis are strongly associated with breast feeding but may also accompany breast surgery, implants, and radiation therapy.

Diagnosis

Physical exam and history are highly suggestive.
Labs: Culture of drainage (usually shows *Staph* or *Strep*), CBC shows leukocytosis.
Imaging: Ultrasound may show fluid pocket.

Treatment

Mastitis: Continue breastfeeding and give *Staph* active **antibiotics** such as dicloxacillan or cefazolan. Conservative treatments such as heat application, frequent warm showers, and breast support may reduce pain.

Breast abscess: As with any abscess, **I/D** (incision and drainage) is mandatory. Stop breastfeeding (although continue manual milk expression) and give antibiotics such as nafcillan or oxacillan.

Take Home Points

- Mastitis is not a contraindication to breast feeding. Only breast abscess should prompt cessation of breast feeding (on the affected side).

- The causative bacteria are overwhelmingly *Staph* and *Strep* skin species.

- Give antibiotics aimed at the appropriate organism.

Malignant Neoplasm of the Ovary

Many histologic types exist, including epithelial, germ cell, sex cord-stromal, unclassified, and metastatic. Epithelial tumors are the most common and the most likely to be malignant. Risk factors include: uninterrupted menstruation, breast cancer, late menopause, delayed childbearing, and family history/BRCA-1 gene mutation. Factors that lessen risk are multiparity, breastfeeding, and hormonal birth control. Associated syndromes:

Krukenberg tumor—Metastasis from stomach to the ovaries.

Meigs syndrome—Presence of ovarian tumor, ascites, and right hydrothorax. Seen in sex cord-stromal tumors.

Symptoms

Often, abdominal mass is the first indication of a tumor. After advancement and tumor size increases, GI complaints, urinary frequency, dysuria, and pelvic pressure can ensue. Since presentation is often after mass effect is felt, stage is usually advanced at diagnosis.

Diagnosis

Suspected by physical exam and presence of negative **pregnancy test**. Exam will show solid, fixed, nodular pelvic mass; with/without ascites or pleural effusion.

Labs: CA-125 tumor marker can be used to follow progression/regression of disease but is not used as screening (yet) because it is very non-specific. Other markers such as alpha fetoprotein (AFP), β-HCG, LDH, estrogen, and testosterone can also be elevated characteristically with subtype of malignancy.

Staging is surgical and follows the American Joint Committee on Cancer (AJCC) and International Federation of Gynecologic Oncologists (FIGO) joint staging system. Pathology is very important to diagnosis and prognosis.

Genetic testing for BRCA 1/2 is appropriate.

Imaging: Ultrasound is the mainstay of evaluation although tumor is usually visible on CT/MRI. Other imaging should be completed to exclude metastasis or extra ovarian tumors including CT scan, CXR, and mammography.

Treatment

Surgery is first line treatment. May include TAH/BSO (total abdominal hysterectomy with bilateral salpingo-oopherectomy), omentectomy, or tumor debulking.

Some pathologic types respond well to chemotherapy and some respond well to radiation. In either case, a specialist should be involved.

Take Home Points

- Epithelial ovarian cancer is the most common type.
- Definitive diagnosis is surgical excision which also determines stage. Specific tumor markers and characteristic findings on U/S may raise suspicion.
- Surgery with or without adjuvant chemotherapy and radiation is the treatment.

Ovarian Cyst

Ovarian cysts are a common source of menstruation-related abdominal pain. Several types of functional cysts exist including follicular, corpus luteal, and theca luteal. Most commonly, cysts form by either failure of the follicle to rupture properly during menstruation or failure of the corpus luteum to regress normally after rupture.

Symptoms

Cysts can be asymptomatic but commonly cause vague lower abdominal pain, disturbances in menstruation timing/flow, and dyspareunia. Ovarian torsion is a rare complication that may occur in conjunction with a persistent cyst.

Diagnosis

Ultrasound is the best technique to evaluate ovarian cysts but they may be discovered incidentally on other imaging of abdomen such as CT/MRI. Tumor markers are generally not useful.

Treatment

Given the low chances of malignancy, treatment is based on the menses state of the patient. Premenarchal and postmenopausal patients need exploratory laparotomy with biopsy as relation to menstruation and therefore existence of the cyst is not explained.

Observe others for **6–8 weeks** and repeat ultrasound to evaluate for regression. If the cyst persists without regression or is ≥ 8 cm at diagnosis, consider laparotomy and biopsy.

Give NSAIDs for pain control as needed.

Take Home Points

- Ovarian cysts are a common source of abdominal pain in menstruating women.
- Observation and reevaluation commonly confirms the diagnosis of benign ovarian cyst.

Polycystic Ovarian Syndrome (PCOS)

A syndrome comprising a constellation of endocrinologic derangements including elevated estrogen, androgen levels, and LH/FSH ratio. PCOS is thought to be due to a mechanism resulting from multiple derangements including adrenal hypersecretion of androgens, peripheral hormone conversion by adipose tissue, and insulin resistance. Ovaries often have multiple simple cysts.

Symptoms

Patients present with any combination of **infertility, amenorrhea, irregular menses, hirsutism, and obesity**. Physiologically, symptoms of increased androgen levels are common. Concomitantly, increased BMI, insulin resistance, hypertension, and type II diabetes are common.

Diagnosis

The National Institutes of Health (NIH) proposed guidelines to diagnose PCOS which include:

- Menstrual irregularity due to oligo or anovulation.
- Evidence of hyperandrogenism, whether it is clinical (hirsutism or male pattern balding) or biochemical (high serum androgen concentrations).
- Exclusion of other causes of hyperandrogenism and menstrual irregularity, such as congenital adrenal hyperplasia, Cushing syndrome, androgen-secreting tumors, and hyperprolactinemia.

Another later, international conference proposed the Rotterdam criteria. After the exclusion of other possible disorders, these consist of:

- Menstrual irregularity due to oligo or anovulation.
- Evidence of hyperandrogenism, whether it is clinical (hirsutism or male pattern balding) or biochemical (high serum androgen concentrations).
- Measured polycystic ovaries on ultrasonography.

However, these criteria also only require two of the three for diagnosis. The best criteria for diagnosis are still debated today.

Labs to evaluate for hyperandrogenism include: total and free testosterone level (although physiologically variable), androstenedione, and DHEA.

Labs that support PCOS but are not evidence of hyperandrogenism include: LH/FSH ratio ≥ 2.5–3.0:1, increased serum estrone, and decreased sex hormone binding globulin (SHBG). Testing for insulin resistance with fasting glucose or fasting glucose:insulin ratio (< 4.5 supports insulin resistance) is warranted.

Labs to evaluate for other endocrinologic disorders include: DHEA-S (increased in androgen producing tumors), dexamethasone suppression test (for Cushing syndrome), 17α-OH progesterone (increased in non-classic adrenal hyperplasia), TSH, and prolactin.

Imaging: Ultrasound demonstrating polycystic ovaries is only required in the Rotterdam criteria for the diagnosis of PCOS.

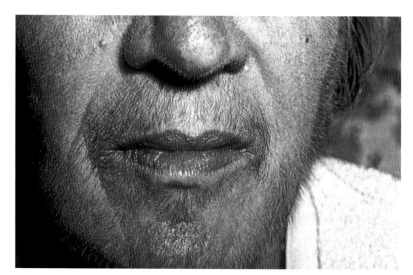

FIGURE 8.1 *Facial hirsutism seen on the cheeks and chin of a female. Reprinted with permission from MacKie, RM. Clinical Dermatology, 5th edition. 2003, Oxford University Press.*

Treatment

Consider child bearing desire of the patient. If no desire for children: Metformin (Glucophage), weight loss, finasteride, flutamide, spironolactone (Aldactone), and OCPs (particularly drospirenone/ethinyl estradiol (Yasmin)) are the mainstay.

If desire for children: Clomiphene (Clomid), metformin (Glucophage), and weight loss.

Weight loss alone can often be used to treat disease.

Take Home Points

- PCOS requires the presence of menstrual irregularity, hyperaldosteronism (clinical or biochemical), and the exclusion of other causes of symptoms. Depending on criteria set, ultrasonographic polycystic ovaries may be present.

- Comorbid state including diabetes mellitus type II and hyperlipidemia commonly exist.

- Treat with weight loss, increasing insulin sensitivity, induction or suppression of ovulation (depending on fertility desire), and androgen suppression.

Acute Parametritis and Pelvic Cellulitis (Pelvic Inflammatory Disease)

Acute infection of the upper female genital tract, involving any or all of the uterus, fallopian tubes, and ovaries which may be accompanied by infection of neighboring pelvic structures. PID is most commonly caused by STDs, especially *N gonorrhea* and *Chlamydia*. The presence of an intrauterine device (IUD) is a major risk factor for PID.

Symptoms

Sexually active females with PID often present with abdominal pain, adenexal tenderness, dyspareunia, and fever. The patient may also have upper right quadrant abdominal pain/vomiting/hepatic symptoms by Fitz-Hugh-Curtis mechanism (perihepatitis from infectious fluid traveling in the posterior peritoneal gutter to the hepatic membranes). Unusual vaginal discharge is often present.

Diagnosis

Physical exam: Adnexal tenderness, abdominal tenderness, **cervical motion tenderness** (Chandelier sign), and purulent cervical discharge.

Labs: Obtain pregnancy test, CBC for leukocytosis, and STD cultures or DNA probe from cervix. Consider HIV and syphilis workup.

Imaging: None specific but in the acute setting consider ultrasound to evaluate for ovarian torsion or abscess.

The decision must be made to admit or not. Consider presence of fever, degree of leukocytosis, IUD presence, adolescent patient, primigravid patient, and likelihood of sepsis.

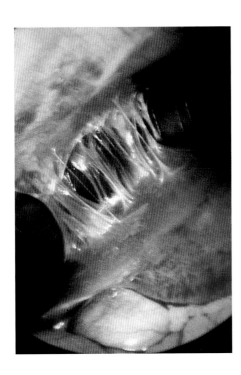

FIGURE 8.2 Laparoscopic views of adhesions in perihepatitis due to Fitz-Hugh-Curtis syndrome from *C trachomatis*. Reprinted with permission from Warrell DA, Cox TM, et al. *Oxford Textbook of Medicine, 4th edition.* 2003, Oxford University Press.

Treatment

Always treat with more than one antibiotic.

Outpatient regimen: Ofloxacin/levofloxacin + metronidazole × 14 days *OR* ceftriaxone IM × 1, metronidazole + doxycycline × 14 days.

Inpatient regimen: Cefotetan/cefoxitin IV + doxycycline IV *OR* clindamycin IV + gentamicin IV then doxycycline IV.

Remove IUD if present.

Treat partner if STD is etiology of infection.

Take Home Points

- PID is commonly caused by bacterial STDs.
- Remove IUD to lessen the chance of significant scarring.
- Treat with more than one antibiotic.

Endometrial Cancer

Histologically, endometrial cancer consists of adenocarcinoma that spreads locally or by lymphatics. Two types exist; type I consists of estrogen-related carcinomas and type II, which are estrogen independent. Risk factors, which most commonly apply to type I cancer, include: obesity, PCOS, nulliparity, late menopause, family history, diabetes, estrogen secreting malignancy, tamoxifen (Soltamox) use, hereditary nonpolyposis colorectal cancer (HNPCC), or estrogen replacement therapy without progesterone.

Symptoms

Vaginal bleeding after menopause is the most common presentation and is a red flag for malignancy.

Diagnosis

Physical exam: Bleeding from the uterus, uncommonly a palpable mass on bimanual exam.
Labs: Tumor marker CA-125 may be elevated (although not as useful as in ovarian cancer). Routine CBC, U/A, stool guaiac, LFTs, BUN, creatinine, and fasting glucose are helpful.
Imaging: Transvaginal ultrasound of the uterus evaluating for endometrial stripe thickness (≤ 5 mm is normal; 20 mm is considered highly suspicious). Caution: Only useful in postmenopausal women since endometrial stripe thickness varies greatly in the ovulating female. Chest x-ray may be indicated for possible metastasis.
Endometrial biopsy is the next step. If endometrial biopsy is negative but suspicion still exists, hysteroscopy with directed biopsy or dilation and curettage (D&C) are the next steps. Estrogen and progesterone receptor assays should be performed on the biopsies which help in treatment guidance.

Treatment

Total abdominal hysterectomy with or without removal of ovaries (TAH-BSO) is the most common treatment. Radiation may be used locally if spread is suspected. Chemotherapy is not effective as primary treatment but may be attempted if metastatic disease is present, doxorubicin (Adriamycin) or cisplatin is most common.

In advanced cases, administration of progesterone or tamoxifen (Soltamox) may prolong life.

Take Home Points

- Endometrial cancers are either estrogen related (80%) or estrogen independent (20%).
- Ultrasound may be the first diagnostic step, then biopsy.
- Treatment is mainly surgical with radiation and is commonly effective.

Leiomyoma of Uterus (Fibroids)

Benign tumor arising from the uterine smooth muscle. These tumors are classified based on the area within the uterine wall they originate from and thus are submucosal, intramural, or subserous, although other anatomic features may be present including pedunculated tumors, intraligamentous location, or vaginal protrusion.

Symptoms

Often these tumors are asymptomatic early in their course but can cause menorrhagia, menometrorrhagia, pain, pressure, urinary or bowel problems, and may complicate pregnancy especially with increased size.

Diagnosis

Physical bimanual exam usually gives suspicion.

Imaging: Ultrasound confirms diagnosis. CT or MRI will also show bulky tumors. After imaging confirms diagnosis, follow for 4–6 months to assess if they are stable or growing. Stable fibroids may be followed annually.

Endometrial biopsy in the uncomplicated patient or hysteroscopy with directed biopsy or dilation and curettage (D&C) in the complicated case may help identify malignant lesions.

Treatment

For minimally symptomatic patients consider iron supplements, close follow up, and/or progestin supplementation (norethindrone, medroxyprogesterone) which may reduce bleeding.

Consider luteinizing hormone releasing hormone (LHRH) agonists (nafarelin, goserelin, leuprolide) before surgery to shrink the tumor as much as possible.

Resection is the mainstay. Myomectomy or hysterectomy are options but have disadvantages associated with major surgery. Thus, asymptomatic stable fibroids should just be monitored without treatment.

For younger patients, alternative surgical options include hysteroscopic or laparoscopic cautery or laser myomectomy.

Take Home Points

- Fibroids are common benign tumors of the myometrium.
- Ultrasound is the preferred imaging study.
- Treatment is conservative unless symptoms are persistent, in which case hysterectomy or myomectomy is the mainstay.

Endometriosis

Hormone-responsive endometrial tissue outside the uterus. Theories of endometrial spread vary, including retrograde menstruation, lymphatic/vascular metastasis, and direct implantation.

Symptoms

The cardinal symptom of endometriosis is cyclic abdominal or pelvic **pain** of unclear etiology; other symptoms include dyspareunia, dysmenorrhea, pain on defecation, abdominal bloating, suprapubic pain on urination, and rarely, rectal bleeding with menses. Classically, the extent of disease does not correlate with severity of symptoms.

Diagnosis

A clinical diagnosis made by detailed history and physical exam with screening labs such as CBC and Chem 7. Expect labs to be normal.

Laparoscopic visualization with biopsy is the gold standard.

Treatment

At the time of visualization, electrocautery, laser ablation, or local removal are usually tried.

Medical treatment includes consideration of child-bearing desire.

If patient does not desire children: **Oral contraceptive pills (OCPs)** are the mainstay. GnRH agonists have been used, but long term treatment (> 6 months) is contraindicated due to bone mineral loss.

Danazol, an antigonadotropin, can also be used but hyperandrogenic side effects limit its use in the vast majority of patients.

Hysterectomy (with estrogen therapy afterward) can be used as last resort.

Pregnancy and menopause alone usually improve symptoms.

Take Home Points

- Endometriosis is a disease of ectopic hormonally-responsive endometrial cells outside the uterus which causes symptoms.

- Medical therapy may include hormonal medications; surgical treatment is that of finding the islands of endometrium and eliminating them.

Abnormal Uterine Bleeding

Abnormalities in vaginal bleeding with respect to amount or timing outside the normal menstrual cycle. Bleeding can be classified as ovulatory, nonovulatory, or nonuterine in source.

Symptoms

TABLE 8.3 Definitions for Abnormal Uterine Bleeding

Oligomenorrhea	Cycle length > 35 days
Polymenorrhea	Cycle length < 21 days
Amenorrhea	Complete absence of menses for 3 cycles or 5 months (whichever is first)
Menorrhagia	Regular cycles with excessive flow or duration
Metrorrhagia	Irregular vaginal bleeding outside the normal cycle
Menometrorrhagia	Irregular cycles with excessive flow and duration
Dysfunctional uterine bleeding	A **diagnosis of exclusion** after ruling out an anatomic lesion
Contact (postcoital) bleeding	Bleeding in conjunction with sexual contact

Diagnosis

Decide if ovulatory, anovulatory or nonuterine based on history. Physical exam may be warranted and may reveal obvious cervical source, vaginal source, or cervical motion tenderness (indicating infection).

Labs: Do a **pregnancy test** on everyone! Order CBC and coagulation profile to assess for anemia and clotting disorders. Consider pap smear or colposcopy if the patient is at risk for cervical pathology (especially if postcoital bleeding is present).

Ovulatory bleeding: Consider hysteroscopy, U/S, endometrial biopsy, or D&C (gold standard).

Anovulatory bleeding: Complete an endocrine workup with TSH, FSH, LH, and prolactin. Consider a trial of progesterone to evaluate unopposed estrogen presence. If bleeding ceases during the trial, the test is positive. Proceed to ultrasound/endometrial biopsy to evaluate for endometrial hyperplasia or cancer, especially in the postmenopausal woman.

Treatment

Acute bleeding: ABCs, high dose IV estrogen, D&C, or endometrial ablation. Extreme cases may require uterine artery embolization or hysterectomy. Make sure the patient is hemodynamically stable with volume expansion, etc.

Chronic treatment is generally OCPs (estrogen, progesterone, or combination) or endometrial ablation. Regimens of ethinyl estradiol/norethindrone have been developed and include a "hormone burst" vs. 9 day taper designed to treat abnormal uterine bleeding. Clomiphine may be considered in patients who desire pregnancy.

Take Home Points

- Decide if bleeding is uterine and if ovulatory or nonovulatory in nature.
- Obtain β-Hcg.
- OCPs may be used to regulate cycles with a regular daily dosing or in a burst/taper regimen.

Malignant Neoplasm of the Cervix

The majority of cervical cancer is squamous cell in type with the remainder (25%–30%) consisting of adenocarcinoma, adenosquamous, and undifferentiated type. The role of HPV in the malignant transformation of cervical cells cannot be overstated. Thus, high risk HPV type testing is becoming part of the routine pap smear laboratories.

Symptoms

Vast majority of cases are asymptomatic and found by pap smear. Classic presentation is of patient with postcoital bleeding. Other symptoms may include: menometrorrhagia, abnormal vaginal discharge, with possible presentation of advanced cases with obstructive uropathy, foul-smelling vaginal discharge, and pelvic pain.

Risk factors include:

- HPV infection (serotypes 16, 18, 31, et al)
- Multiple sexual partners
- Immunocompromised state
- History of multiple STDs
- Early onset of sexual activity
- Tobacco use

Diagnosis

Pap smear is the best screening tool and catches 90% of cases early on. Investigation should proceed to colposcopy with biopsies if Pap smear is positive (see algorithm). If the entire lesion or the transformational zone cannot be visualized, a cone biopsy via LEEP (loop electrosurgical excision procedure) or cold knife may be performed.

Remember, invasion usually occurs locally and lymphatically. Death is commonly by urosepsis.

Pap Smear Screening

Different groups have slightly different recommendations on when/how often to begin screening. The American College of Obstetrics and Gynecology (ACOG) recommends starting at age 21 and then every 2 years until age 30. After age 30, screen every 3 years if the patient has had three consecutive negative paps (and if risk factors are minimal). The United States Preventative Services Task Force (USPSTF) recommends screening at least every 3 years and makes no distinction after age 30. The American Cancer Society (ACS) recommends starting within 3 years of sexual activity or age 21 and annually until age 30 if using the conventional pap or every 2 years if with cytologic-based technique. After age 30, every 2–3 years if the patient has had three negative paps.

TABLE 8.4 Bethesda System of Cytologic Classification

Result	Treatment
ASC-US (atypical squamous cells of undetermined significance)	See figure below for ASC-US algorithm.
ASC-H (atypical squamous cells—cannot exclude HSIL)	Colposcopy/biopsies
AGC (atypical glandular cells)	Colposcopy /biopsies
LSIL (low-grade squamous intraepithelial lesions)	Colposcopy/biopsies without HPV testing (since most are high risk type). May treat with ablation or biopsy. In patients that are postmenopausal, pregnant, or adolescent, consider repeat Pap in 4–6 months without colposcopy.
HSIL (high-grade squamous intraepithelial lesions)	Colposcopy/biopsies. If satisfactory colposcopy, consider excisional biopsy. If unsatisfactory colposcopy (incomplete visualization of transformational zone) consider cone biopsy.

Adapted from American Society of Colposcopy and Cervical Pathology.

TABLE 8.5 Histologic Results (from Biopsy)

LSIL	HSIL	
CIN I	CIN II	CIN III
Mild dysplasia	Moderate dysplasia	Severe dysplasia
Disordered growth in the lower third of the epithelial lining	Disordered growth in up to two-thirds of the epithelial lining	Disordered growth in more than two-thirds of the epithelial lining

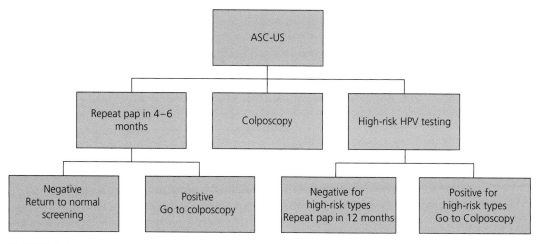

FIGURE 8.3 ASC-US algorithm.

Treatment

Can be treated at time of colposcopy with **cryotherapy**, LEEP, or excisional biopsy. If advanced disease, consider hysterectomy with removal of cervix. If invasive, lymph node dissection and staging with further imaging such as CT and MRI are indicated. Radiation therapy has shown benefit both pre and post surgically; however, can have adverse effects on local tissues such as rectum and urinary system. Chemotherapy is reserved for metastatic cases but may be considered palliative.

Take Home Points

- Cervical cancer exists as one end of the cervical dysplasia spectrum. Most cytologic dysplasia is caught with Pap smear before reaching this point in transformation.
- The start and interval of Pap screening is variable amongst authoritative bodies.
- Most abnormal results of Pap smear should be further investigated with colposcopy and biopsies; ASC-US has further options.

Cervicitis/Endocervicitis

Most commonly caused by infection, cervicitis denotes inflammation of the uterine cervix. Common infectious agents are sexually transmitted and include: *C trachomatis, N gonorrheae*, herpes simplex, HPV, *Trichomonas*, HIV, and *Mycoplasma* species. Chronic cervicitis may be due to the above infectious agents or cervical atrophy (postmenopausal patients), cervical dysplasia, or local trauma, among other etiologies.

Symptoms

Pelvic pain, unusual vaginal discharge, bleeding (usually spotting), or dyspareunia. Risk factors include sexual promiscuity, low socioeconomic status, early onset of sexual activity, and non-married state, which may increase the risk of multiple sexual partners.

Diagnosis

Diagnosis is aided by physical exam that shows cervical motion tenderness (chandelier sign), cervical discharge, unusual vaginal odor, or cervical bleeding.

Labs: Techniques include:

- Cervical culture
- GC/*Chlamydia* DNA probe
- KOH (potassium hydroxide) slide preparation to look for branching/budding hyphae and perform "whiff test" for bacterial vaginosis
- Wet mount slide to look for trichomonades or "clue cells"
- Viral culture of lesions

Treatment

Elect to treat gonorrhea and chlamydia together since they are commonly seen in co-infection.
Regimens vary but memorize the classic (see table below).

TABLE 8.6 Common Treatment of Typical Etiologies of Cervicitis/ Endocervicitis

	Classic	Alternate
N gonorrhea	Ceftriaxone IM × 1	Ciprofloxacin PO
C trachomatis	Doxyclycline PO × 7 days	Azithromycin PO × 1

Others:

- *Trichomonas*: Metronidazole (Flagyl)
- *Gardnerella* spp: Metronidazole (Flagyl)
- HSV: Acyclovir (Zovirax), valacyclovir (Valtrex)
- HPV: Cryotherapy, acid, electrocautery
- *Candida*: Fluconazole (Diflucan)
- Chronic cervicitis due to atrophy may respond to topical estrogen creams

Remember: Treat the partner!

Take Home Points

- Acute cervicitis is most commonly caused by STDs.
- Screen and treat the partner.

Malignant Neoplasm of the Vagina

Vaginal malignancy, like cervical cancer, occurs along a spectrum, from vaginal intraepithelial neoplasia (VIN) to confirmed vaginal carcinoma. VIN represents carcinoma in situ without invasion of the basement membrane. Basically there are two types of carcinoma: squamous cell carcinoma (SCC) and adenocarcinoma (Clear cell type is seen in female offspring of women exposed to diethylstilbestrol (DES)).

Symptoms

Most commonly these cancers are asymptomatic but can present with increasing vaginal discharge, bleeding, and pruritus.

Diagnosis

Physical exam: Suspicious lesion may be seen at time of Pap smear.
Biopsies of suspicious lesions are appropriate. Metastasis from other primary sites is possible although uncommon.
If cancer is found, further surveillance imaging should be completed such as CXR, abdominal CT, intravenous pyelogram, etc.

Treatment

Treated according to stage. If low stage (I or II), can treat with excision, local fluorouracil (Efudex), hysterectomy, vaginectomy, laser ablation, or lymph node biopsy. If higher stage, radiation is generally used with/without surgery. Chemotherapy is classically ineffective for vaginal carcinoma.

Take Home Points

- Female offspring of mothers exposed to diethylstilbestrol (DES) may develop clear cell adenocarcinoma of the vagina.
- VIN represents malignant cellular change toward vaginal cancer.

Vulvovaginitis

A condition that involves infection and inflammation of the vagina and vulva.

Symptoms

Vaginal pain, unusual discharge, unusual vaginal odor (musty or fishy), dyspareunia, or pruritus.

Diagnosis/Treatment

Physical exam is invaluable.

TABLE 8.7 Typical Findings by Etiology of Vulvovaginitis

Cause	Diagnostic Clues	Treatment
Gardnerella/Bacterial vaginosis (polymicrobial)	Clue cells on Saline mount, fishy smell on KOH "whiff test," increased pH (> 4.5)	Metronidazole; **no need to treat partner**
Candidiasis	Branching pseudohyphae on KOH prep, "cottage-cheese" like discharge, history of pregnancy, diabetes, or recent antibiotics	Fluconazole (Diflucan) 150 mg PO × 1. Investigate underlying cause if recurrent
Trichomonas	Wet mount reveals trichomonade organism. Discharge is green, often frothy; pH (> 4.5)	Metronidazole; **treat partner**

Prolapse of the Vaginal Walls

Damage or weakening of any of the network of muscles and ligaments that make up the vaginal vault leading to local collapse.

TABLE 8.8 Types of Vaginal Prolapse

Anterior wall	Cystocele (bladder), urethrocele (Urethra)
Upper posterior vaginal wall (rectovaginal septum)	Enterocele (bowel)
Lower posterior vaginal wall (rectovaginal septum)	Rectocele (rectum)
Cardinal ligaments	Uterine prolapse

Symptoms

Pelvic pressure, backache, dyspareunia. Urinary symptoms such as incontinence, frequency, hesitancy, recurrent infection or rectal symptoms such as constipation, painful defecation, or incomplete defecation. Vaginal atrophy from lack of endogenous estrogen is often seen.

Diagnosis

Primarily diagnosed by physical exam and visualization of defect. Correlate with history.

Treatment

Strengthening of pelvic muscles is essential. Kegel exercises and possibly weighted vaginal cones can be used.

If atrophic vagina, give estrogen cream.

Nonsurgical removable pessaries are often effective to support the internal vaginal walls.

Last resort is surgery and includes hysterectomy, anterior/posterior colporrhaphy, and several types of sling and suspension techniques.

Take Home Points

- Vaginal prolapse may be associated with urinary incontinence, bowel habit changes, or uterine prolapse.

- Strengthen vaginal musculature with Kegel exercises etc. as first line.

Bartholin Duct Cyst/Abscess

Bartholin glands reside at 4 and 8 o'clock positions at the opening of the vagina. For unclear reasons, the ducts can become obstructed and normal lubricating secretions may accumulate, forming a cyst. Infection of this fluid becomes an abscess.

Symptoms

Cystic lesion located on inside of the vaginal opening, which is usually nonpainful although may become symptomatic during coitus. If abscess has formed, patient may have exquisite pain, dyspareunia, and local irritation.

Diagnosis

Physical exam reveals a rubbery mass at the corresponding position of the introitus. Lesions are typically 0.5–4 cm. The nature may be confirmed by ultrasound but this is usually not necessary.

Treatment

For simple cyst of 1–2 cm in size, conservative treatment with repeated Sitz baths is appropriate. Spontaneous regression is the norm.

For abscesses, incision and drainage are the mainstay. Culture any fluid expressed. Pack the abscess and change daily.

Recurrence is common and necessitates permanent treatment which may consist of "marsupialization" of the cavity, which basically indicates sewing the two lips of the incision open and allowing to close after healing becomes apparent. Thus there is no closed space for recurrence of the infection.

Placement of a Word catheter is an alternative to marsupialization and consists of sewing a specifically designed drain in the abscess cavity.

Give antibiotics based on culture results.

Take Home Points

- Bartholin duct cysts may become infected and form an abscess. Treat like any abscess with incision and drainage (closure is what differs in this case).
- Marsupialization or Word catheter placement until healed is most commonly needed due to recurrence.

Dysmenorrhea

Defined as pain associated with the premenstrual or menstrual state. Classification includes primary (most common) and secondary due to structural abnormality of the genital tract. Primary dysmenorrhea has long been known to be associated with much higher than normal levels of prostaglandins and other mediators in the uterus. These factors likely act to produce localized platelet aggregation, vasoconstriction, and dysrhythmic contractions of the myometrium.

Symptoms

Cyclic abdominal cramping and lower abdominal pain that occurs in relation to menses. Begins in days preceding menses. Not related to GI or other disturbances. History reveals strong correlation to menses, and physical exam generally shows no further abnormalities to point toward other physical defect.

Diagnosis

Imaging: May rule out gynecologic abnormalities with ultrasound. Dysmenorrhea is often difficult to separate from endometriosis.

Treatment

Mainstay of therapy is NSAIDs and acetaminophen (Tylenol).
Hormonal birth control often better regulates menses and thus provides relief.
Nonpharmacologic therapy such as local heat application and exercise may help.
Very rarely, hysterectomy may be used for severe, debilitating symptoms.

Take Home Points

- Dysmenorrhea is caused by local actions of prostaglandins and other mediators upon the uterus.
- NSAIDs and acetaminophen are the cornerstones of therapy.

Premenstrual Dysphoric Disorder (PMDD)

Premenstrual dysphoric disorder is made up of an ill-defined constellation of symptoms occurring before menses. PMDD is also thought to be made of dominantly emotional symptoms, although this disorder, by definition, interferes significantly with one's life.

Symptoms

Symptoms of dysmenorrhea and related headache, bloating, breast tenderness, back/abdominal pain, irritability, fatigue and others. A difference in PMDD from premenstrual syndrome (PMS) is the further presence of 5 of the following 11 symptoms: depressed mood, affective lability, concentration difficulties, decreased interest in daily activities, lack of energy, change in appetite, sleep disturbance, feeling of being overwhelmed, or anxiety. In addition, some patients may have suicidal thoughts. These make a significant impact on the patient's quality of life.

Diagnosis

History and symptoms must be recorded for at least two menstrual cycles in a home "diary." This record should show symptom activity only in the luteal phase. It is important to consider degree of effect on life activities.
Check TSH and hemoglobin/hematocrit to eliminate organic systemic disease.

Treatment

Often SSRIs are effective and comprise adequate treatment. Fluoxetine (Prozac) and sertraline (Zoloft) are mainstays and may be given continuously or only during the luteal phase of the menstrual cycle. Start with a low dose and titrate up. TCAs such as clomipramin (Anafranil) and nortryptyline (Pamelor) have also proven effective. Otherwise, partially effective treatment to help reduce symptoms includes calcium replacement, vitamin B_6 in moderate doses, NSAIDs/acetaminophen, vitamin E, spironolactone, danazol, and evening oil of primrose (alternative treatment).
Always screen for suicidal ideations.

Take Home Points

- PMDD is a significant source of morbidity in patients with the disorder.
- Treatment with psychoactive medications is the mainstay of therapy.

Amenorrhea

Causes are many and varied and may include: pregnancy (most common), hypothalamic dysfunction, PCOS, congenital adrenal hyperplasia, thyroid disorders, premature ovarian failure, menopause, hyperprolactinemia (galactorrhea), Müllerian dysgenesis, imperforate hymen, Asherman syndrome, Kallmann syndrome, anorexia nervosa, testicular feminization, and others.

Primary: Absence of menses by age 16 years or age 14 years in the absence of other secondary sexual characteristics.

Secondary: Cessation of menses for ≥ 3 cycles or 6 months (whichever comes first).

Symptoms

The state of no menses. Often accompanied by lack of other symptoms such as periodic cramping, irritability, bloating, etc. associated with normal menstruation.

Diagnosis

Labs: β-HCG! Then obtain TSH and prolactin level to evaluate hypothalamic pathways.

If primary, evaluate for existence of a patent vagina, then for a uterus and ovaries, then for sexual maturation and secondary sexual characteristics such as breast development/pubic hair growth. If all is normal, workup for secondary amenorrhea (see below). If abnormal, consider karotype or anatomic abnormality.

If secondary, do a **progestin challenge** (progestin 10 mg PO × 7–10 days after which monitor for withdrawal bleeding; if present the test is negative because of appropriate response). Then follow the algorithm in figure below.

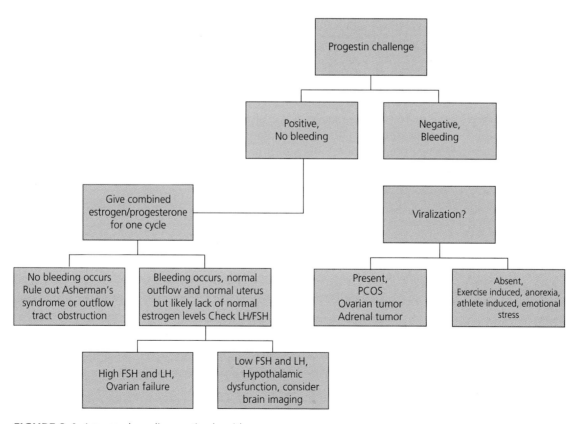

FIGURE 8.4 Amenorrhea diagnostic algorithm.

Treatment

Treat the underlying cause.

Correct thyroid dysfunction if present; if prolactin dysfunction, consider bromocriptine (Parlodel). For ovarian failure consider OCPs to regulate endometrial shedding. Clomiphine (Clomid) may be used to induce ovulation if pregnancy is desired. Treat PCOS as above. For women with hypothalamic dysfunction, GnRH analogs have been used for ovulation. Refer eating disorders to psychiatry.

Take Home Points

- Amenorrhea is 1) lack of menses by age 16 or 14 without secondary sexual characteristics or 2) lack of menses for ≥ 3 cycles or 6 months.

- Diagnosis is the most important step. Treat according to findings.

Menopause

Menopause is the physiologic cessation of the ovulatory and menstrual cycle. In the U.S., the average age is 50–51 years.

Symptoms

Symptom onset is usually in the perimenopausal period defined as age 48–52 years. Hot flashes are generally the first symptom noticed but are often accompanied by fatigue, irritability, insomnia, depression, memory loss, headache, anxiety, vaginal dryness, labial atrophy, and, by definition, cessation of menses. If these symptoms occur before age 40, investigation of cause should be completed.

Diagnosis

Diagnosis is based on a history of 12 months of amenorrhea in the perimenopausal period (in absence of other medical reasons for amenorrhea).

Common practice is to test for FSH, which is usually high in ovarian failure. It is a myth that FSH is of any value during the perimenopausal period. In this period, the production of FSH is physiologically far too variable to be relied upon as an indicator of menopause. However, it may be of use in younger patients to investigate premature ovarian failure. **Menopause is a clinical diagnosis!**

Treatment

A recent very large, multi-center, long-term study, **The Women's Health Initiative**, recently suggested adverse effects of hormone replacement therapy (HRT) particularly when combined with estrogen/progesterone therapy, which produced dramatic increases in cardiovascular effects such as heart disease and stroke, as well as breast cancer rates. The estrogen-only arm showed increased risk of stroke and DVT. The study did, however, support protective effects of hormone therapy on osteoporosis and lessening of symptoms attributable to menopause. Several limitations of the study exist however, not the least of which was that the results and adverse events were only seen with 4 or more years of HRT. Further investigations are ongoing.

Therapies that may help symptoms are many but include short term HRT (unproven), clonidine, SSRIs, SSNRIs, and vitamin E. Herbal remedies have been tried and show anecdotal evidence including black cohosh and soy-containing foods (presumably for phytoestrogen content).

For protection against osteoporosis, place most patients on a bisphosphonate such as alendronate (Fosamax), risedronate (Actonel), or ibandronate (Boniva); or calcitonin, as well as supplementation of calcium and vitamin D. Weight-bearing exercise is also an effective lifestyle change. See Chapter 12: Orthopedics and Rheumatology for the section on osteoporosis.

Control risk factors for heart disease and stroke.

Take Home Points

- Menopause is defined as 12 consecutive months without menses in the perimenopausal age.
- Treatment is a combination of symptom-based medications.

Female Infertility

Female infertility factors are thought to account for 40–50% of causes of infertility, 30–40% due to male factors, 10–20% are unknown. Female etiologies for infertility include ovulatory factors (hypothalamic insufficiency, gonadal dysgenesis, ovarian tumor, premature ovarian failure, thyroid, liver, or renal disease), pelvic factors (endometriosis, infection such as PID, uterine adhesions (Asherman syndrome)), and cervical factors (surgical treatment, infection).

Symptoms

Defined as inability to conceive after 12 months of regular unprotected sexual intercourse.

Diagnosis

Assess **ovulation status**. Have the patient keep a diary of menstrual cycles and predicted ovulation. Evaluation of basal body temperature may be taken to assess timing and predict most fertile days. Patient should take oral temp as soon as she awakens every day and graph this data on paper. A rise of only tenths of degrees should be noted in the luteal phase and thus reveal time of ovulation. Home ovulatory urine tests may also accomplish this same goal and have been shown to be more accurate than basal body temperature.

Labs: TSH/prolactin should be taken to rule out related disorders. Androgen levels may be used to evaluate for PCOS.

History and physical should direct the physician to investigate other disorders such as endometriosis, scarring s/p PID, scarring s/p IUD, fibroids, Asherman syndrome, and anatomic abnormalities.

Hysterosalpingogram may be considered to evaluate for scaring of the tubes/uterus. Asherman syndrome can be ruled out. This also evaluates anatomic abnormalities, including fallopian tube agenesis, bicornate uterus, fibroids, foreign body, etc.

Endometrial biopsy may be done to assess viability of stroma and endometrial lining. Pelvic ultrasound at the correct time in cycle may be done to assess thickness of endometrial lining. Cervical mucous studies may be indicated to assess density and functionality.

Treatment

Depending on the problem, different solutions are needed.

Timing may be adjusted if this is the problem.

Clomiphine citrate (Clomid) for induction of ovulation. However, consider the side effects including multiple gestation.

GnRH analogs to regulate FSH/LH production and encourage ovulation.

Surgery with ligature of adhesions or removal of fibroids.

Implantation therapy may be tried in the receptive uterus as a last resort.

Take Home Points

- Female infertility factors account for the majority of infertility cases.
- The first step of diagnosis is assessment of ovulation.
- Diagnosis should include evaluation of hormonal and structural factors.

9   Pregnancy and Childbirth

Supervision of Normal Pregnancy

TABLE 9.1 Maintenance Schedule*

At every visit	Assess weight gain
	Ausciltate fetal heart tones
	Screen fundal height
	Screen for HTN
	Breastfeeding education
	Assess flu shot status if in season
	Counsel on family planning
	Screen for domestic abuse
	Educate regarding preterm labor
	Tobacco/EtOH screening

(continued)

TABLE 9.1 Continued

Weeks 6–8	Blood type and Rh factor/antibody screen Rubella titer Varicella Hemoglobin/hematocrit, platelet count Hepatitis B surface antigen Syphilis with RPR/VDRL Urinanalysis/urine culture HIV testing (obtain written consent) Sickle cell carrier screen (if high risk) PPD for TB (if high risk) Tetanus booster if needed Flu shot if indicated
Weeks 10–12	Screening Pap smear Testing for gonorrhea/chlamydia Test for cystic fibrosis
Weeks 16–20	Triple acreen (estriol, β-hCG, MSAFP) or quadruple screen (estriol, β-hCG, MSAFP, inhibin A) Routine ultrasound
Week 26–28	Gestational diabetes screen (50 g GTT) Iron supplements if needed Rh-negative patients receive RhoGAM
Week 36	Culture for group B *strep* Assess fetal position with Leopold maneuvers and/or ultrasound
Week 41	Induction and augmentation if not contraindicated Biweekly non-stress tests

*Start visits at 6–8 weeks and have patient return every 4–6 weeks until 36 weeks. Then every 1–2 weeks until delivery.

TABLE 9.2 Physiologic Changes During Pregnancy

Complaint	Brief Description
Ptyalism (sialism)	Excess salivation
Pica	Ingestion of non-food items
Urinary frequency	Frequent need to urinate
Varicose veins	Varicosities of vulva or legs
Edema	Mild generalized or dependent edema
Backache, pelvic pressure, joint pain	Hormonal change may soften ligaments leading to pain localized to several joints
Acrodysesthesia	Numbness or tingling of the fingers
Muscle cramps	Muscular cramps thought due to lack of diffusible calcium and excess phosphorus
Breast soreness	Tenderness or soreness of the breasts
Hemorrhoids	Anal hemorrhoidal tissue development
Nausea/vomiting (morning sickness)	Common early in pregnancy due to high hormone levels

TABLE 9.2 Continued

Complaint	Brief Description
Carpal tunnel syndrome	Commonly thought due to swelling of wrist tendon sheaths where they transit through the carpal tunnel
Heartburn	Increased incidence of GERD, especially late
Round ligament pain	Generally described as a sharp, laterally-located pain in the lower abdominal quadrants
Spider telangiectases, palmar erythema, linea nigra, striae, and chloasma (mask of pregnancy)	Normal skin changes thought due to hormonal changes

Delivery and Labor with Minor or No Complications

Labor is defined as the physiologic state of uterine contractions that produce cervical dilation. When a patient presents to the labor and delivery deck, diagnosing labor is often the pivotal clinical decision at hand. In conjunction with the existence of labor, the physician should determine if membrane rupture has occurred. To do this, three clinical tests are employed:

Nitrazine (pH paper) paper test will demonstrate change from normal acidic vaginal secretions to alkaline amniotic fluid. A swab from the posterior fornix should be used to transfer mucous to the nitrazine paper and if positive, blue color change will occur.

Ferning often occurs when amniotic fluid is placed on a glass microscope slide and allowed to dry quite well. This test is low specificity as many substances also cause ferning.

Pooling of fluid in the vaginal vault lends the greatest sensitivity and specificity of the three tests and lends a great deal of evidence to membrane rupture if present.

Symptoms

Contractions can be felt differently for many women. Some are felt as back pain, some with lower abdominal pressure. Most patients feel contractions as tightening or pain in the lower abdomen. Patients may also describe ROM (rupture of membrane) with anywhere from a rush to a trickle of amniotic fluid leakage. Subjectively, labor can be subtle.

Diagnosis/Treatment

If labor is confirmed (a clinical decision), progress should be followed by physical exam.

Bishop score is a scale which adds cervical consistency and cervical position to those elements in table below.

TABLE 9.3 Physical Exam of the Cervix

Cervical Dilation	Measured in centimeters. 0–10 cm corresponds to "long and closed" to "complete"
Cervical effacement	Percentage of thinning of cervix
Station	Assesses position of head in relation to ischial spines, estimated in centimeters -5 (superior to spines) to 0 to +5 (inferior to spines). An alternative scale is to use -3 to 0 to +3 although this refers to thirds of the birth canal; not centimeters

Labor progression follows the stages in table below.

TABLE 9.4 Stages of Labor

Stage	Definition/Association
Stage 1	Latent: Dilation of 0 to 3–4 cm. Longest lasting stage which may be 6–12 hours.
	Active: Dilation of 3–4 cm to complete (10 cm). Nulliparous should maintain ≥ 1.2 cm/hour dilation. Multiparous, ≥ 1.5 cm/hour.
Stage II	From complete dilation to delivery. If lasts longer than 2 hours in nulliparous or 1 hour in multiparous it's considered prolonged (add 1 hour to this if epidural given).
Stage III	Delivery of infant to delivery of placenta.

External monitoring includes uterine contraction monitor and continuous fetal heart rate monitor. Reading fetal strips is much like reading ECGs; it's an art. Here are the basics:

Reactivity:

Baseline is between 110 and 160 beats per minute with good variability.

Variability denotes at least two accelerations above baseline of at least 15 bpm lasting 15 seconds or more on a 20-minute strip.

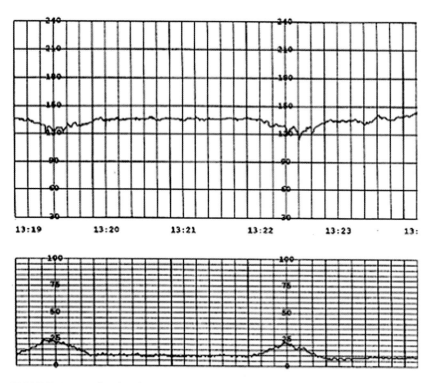

FIGURE 9.1 Early deceleration: Mirrors contractions. Caused by increased vagal tone secondary to head compression.

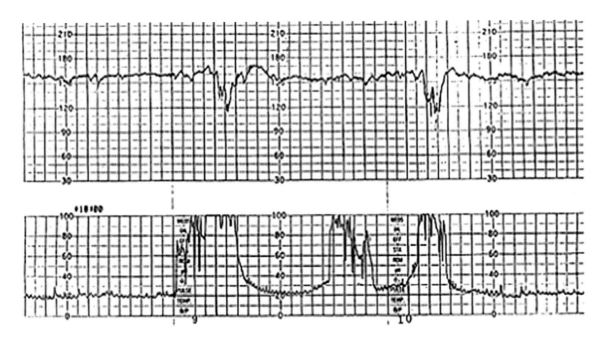

FIGURE 9.2 Variable deceleration: Deceleration uncorrelated to contraction that drops fairly precipitously then sharply returns to baseline. Caused by umbilical cord compression and is of concern.

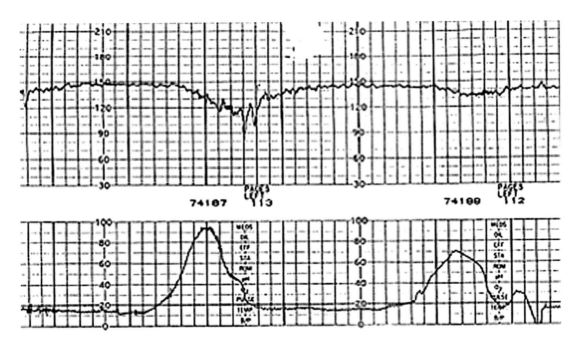

FIGURE 9.3 Late deceleration: Deceleration that starts and ends after the beginning and ending of contractions, respectively. They result from uteroplacental insufficiency and are very worrisome. Repeated lates may indicate need for Cesarean.

Delivery occurs after completion of dilation and usually with controlled pushing by the mother.

Cardinal movements are: **Engagement, descent, flexion, internal rotation, extension, external rotation (restitution), and expulsion.**

Perineal Trauma

From the physician's point of view, controlling the descent and supporting the perineum may help control any lacerations that could occur. Episiotomy can also be used if more room for the physician's hands is needed. Shoulder dystocia cannot be relieved by episiotomy.

Lacerations types:

- 1st Degree—Through the skin or mucosa
- 2nd Degree—Extending to and involving the perineal body
- 3rd Degree—Extending through the anal sphincter
- 4th Degree—Extending through the anal mucosa into the rectum

Repair with absorbable suture.

Follow up: Generally new mothers should stay in the hospital at least 24–48 hours. Diminishing lochia and pain should be noted with absence of prolonged fever (although some increased temperature is normal with delivery). Pelvic rest for 6 weeks and nonestrogen birth control should be prescribed.

Research shows breastfeeding is best for both mother and infant.

Take Home Points

- Labor is the onset of contractions which produce cervical dilation.
- Test for rupture of membranes upon admission to labor and delivery deck.
- External fetal monitoring should assess for variability and timing of decelerations.
- Laceration of the perineum should be graded and repaired.

Postpartum Hemorrhage (PPH)

Hemorrhage that is often just after delivery of the fetus or placenta and is estimated to be > 500 mL after vaginal delivery or > 1000 mL after Cesarean delivery. By definition, < 24 hours from delivery is early onset PPH, ≥ 24 hours is late onset.

Common causes of PPH include:

Uterine atony

Cervical lacerations

Vaginal lacerations

Retained products of conception (POCs)

Uterine inversion

Uterine rupture

Placenta accreta

Symptoms

Signs or symptoms of acute blood loss are the same as if due to another cause. The patient may exhibit signs of lightheadedness, weakness, fatigue (overt), or orthostatic hypotension. Risk factors for PPH may include: Overdistention of uterus (multiple fetuses, polyhydramnios), coagulation disorders, exhausted myometrium, chorioamnionitis, placental abnormalities (previa, accreta, abruption), forceps delivery, and others. After delivery, PPH is associated with Sheehan syndrome (pituitary infarction).

Diagnosis

Physical exam: Pale, clammy skin. Vital signs may show increased heart rate. In extreme cases, decreased blood pressure (non-orthostatic).

Labs: Pre-delivery CBC will give a hemoglobin/hematocrit baseline, post-delivery CBC will show change.

Treatment

If patient is unstable, use volume expansion agents and treat possible hypovolemic shock. Consider blood products if needed.

Manual uterine sweep (exploration) should be one of the first maneuvers performed upon diagnosis of PPH.

In general, the most common cause of PPH is uterine atony. For this etiology, start fundal massage and consider the following treatments (see table below).

TABLE 9.5 Treatment Options for PPH

Agent	Dose	Associations
Oxytocin	Dose 10 units IM or 10–40 units in 1 L NS at a rate which controls atony	Increases uterine smooth muscle contraction
Methylergonaovine (Methergine)	Dose 0.2 mg IM. Max 5 doses	Contraindicated in hypertension
Carboprost tromethamine (Hemabate)	Dose 250 mcg IM. Max 2 mg total dose	Contraindicated in asthmatics. Diarrhea is a common side effect
Misoprostol (Cytotec)	Dose varies but generally 800–1000 mcg rectally	Route varies from PO to intravaginally to rectally

If cervical or vaginal lacerations are present, surgical repair is required.

Retained POCs may be treated with manual uterine sweep maneuvers or D&C if persistent.

Extreme measures include uterine artery embolization or emergent hysterectomy.

Take Home Points

- PPH is defined as blood loss > 500 mL in vaginal delivery or > 1000 mL in Cesarean.
- The most common cause is uterine atony, thus, use oxytocin, Methergine, or Hemabate to control this type of PPH.

Placental Disorders

TABLE 9.6 Placental Disorders

Abnormality		Definition
Placenta previa		Implantation or extension of the placenta over the cervical os. Painless bleeding may occur.
Placenta	Accreta	Villi adhere to superficial myometrium.
	Increta	Villi invade the myometrium.
	Percreta	Villi penetrate the entire myometrium.
Placental abruption		Premature separation of the placenta from the uterine wall. May be associated with uterine tenderness, bleeding, fetal distress, or contractions.

Chorioamnionitis

Infection of the amniotic fluid and membranes surrounding the fetus. Most infections of the chorion and amnion are caused by ascension of vaginal bacteria, including group B and D strep and anaerobes.

Symptoms

Intrapartum fever with no other obvious source. This is often associated with fetal or maternal tachycardia, uterine tenderness, foul smelling amniotic fluid, and/or leukocytosis. Risk factors include prolonged rupture of membranes (≥ **18 hours**), untreated vaginal infection including GBS (group B *strep*), and multiple exams during labor.

Diagnosis

Most commonly, chorioamnionitis is a clinical diagnosis based on increased temperature, maternal (consistently > 90 bpm) or fetal tachycardia (> 160 bpm), and uterine tenderness.

Labs: The gold standard is amniotic fluid culture, although culture is much too slow to base clinical decisions on in labor. Other amniotic fluid studies including Gram stain, glucose concentration, WBC concentration, leukocyte esterase level, and measurement of cytokines (e.g., IL-6), ceramide lactoside, or short-chain organic acids have been used in several studies but sensitivity and specificity are still lacking at this time. CBC shows leukocytosis.

Treatment

Prevent cases with extensive risk factors with prophylactic antibiotics including ampicillin or penicillin.

Treatment with broad spectrum antibiotics is the standard. Commonly, ampicillin/gentamicin covers for typical bacteria very effectively. Alternatively, clindamycin may be used. Regimens commonly vary. Continue treatment until patient is > 24 hours afebrile.

Take Home Points

- Chorioamnionitis may involve any of the following signs/symptoms: Maternal or fetal tachycardia, uterine tenderness, fever, leukocytosis, or foul smelling amniotic fluid.

- Treat with IV ampicillin and gentamicin.

Intrapartum Group B Streptococcus (GBS)

Colonization of group B strep (*S agalactiae*) is an occasional finding in the normal pregnant patient. The risk of infection is not particularly concerning for the mother but that of vertical transmission to the infant during vaginal delivery could lead to sepsis and death.

Symptoms

Most commonly colonization is asymptomatic but may present during pregnancy as urinary tract infection, pyelonephritis, chorioamnionitis, bacteremia, or post-partum endomyometritis. After delivery, neonate is at risk for signs/symptoms of sepsis, bacteremia, or respiratory distress.

Diagnosis

Pre-partum risk factor assessment is often done to determine need for intrapartum antibiotic prophylaxis (IAP). Some main risk factors requiring prophylaxis during labor include: Previous child with invasive GBS infection, GBS bactiurea during current pregnancy, unknown GBS status during current pregnancy, and labor < 37 weeks.

Labs: Commonly, screening cultures of vagina/rectum are taken at 35–37 weeks gestation. If positive, sensitivities should be done to find the most potent antibiotic for prophylaxis (especially if penicillin-allergic patient).

Treatment

Penicillin G, 5 million units IV × 1 then 2.5 million units IV q4 hours is the classic first line for prophylaxis. Ampicillin, 2 grams IV × 1 then 1 gram IV q4 hours may also be used as first line. Loading doses are used in both cases followed by q4 hour dosing. Most common practice in the U.S. is to consider the patient "adequately treated" if ≥ 4 hours pass between the first dose and the delivery of the infant. Penicillin-allergic patients should receive clindamycin or erythromycin IV.

No prophylactic treatment after delivery is warranted for the mother.

Standard of care of the infant varies with locale. However, "adequate treatment" status indicates a low level of acuity and concern for further lab investigation of the infant. Most institutions regard infants born to adequately treated mothers virtually equivalent to those born to GBS-negative mothers. Infants born to mothers who are not adequately treated often have blood cultures, C-reactive protein, and CBC with differential (for I/T ratio) drawn to evaluate for GBS sepsis. See section on Neonatal Sepsis in Chapter 14: Neonatal Medicine.

Take Home Points

- GBS cultures are taken as part of normal pregnancy care, if positive, the patient should be placed on intrapartum prophylactic penicillin or ampicillin.

- If the baby is delivered to an inadequately treated mother, neonatal sepsis should be strongly considered.

TORCHES Infections of Pregnancy

TABLE 9.7 TORCHES Infections of Pregnancy

Disease	Sequelae
Toxoplasmosis	Retinitis, intracranial calcifications, mental retardation, jaundice, stillborn.
Other (hepatitis B, coxsackie, varicella)	Specific for disease. Varicella may cause limb hypoplasia.
Rubella	Deafness, cataracts, microphthalmia, cardiovascular defects such as VSD and patent ductus.
Cytomegalovirus (CMV)	Deafness, microphthalmia, cerebral calcifications, mental retardation, still birth.
HErpes	Skin lesions, encephalitis, conjunctivitis.
HIV	Transmission to infant
Syphilis	Rhinitis, saber shins, Hutchinson teeth, interstitial keratitis, and skin lesions.

Postpartum Fever

TABLE 9.8 Seven Ws of Postpartum Fever

Womb	Endomyometritis
Wind	Atelectasis, pneumonia, pulmonary embolism
Water	Urinary tract infection
Walking	DVT
Wound	Incision, lacerations, hematoma
Weaning	Breast engorgement, mastitis, breast abscess
Wonder drugs	Drug fever

Complications of Labor and Delivery

TABLE 9.9 Definitions of Labor and Delivery Complications

Term	Definition	Diagnosis/Associations	Treatment
Premature rupture of membranes (PROM)	Rupture of amniotic membranes before onset of labor.	Physical exam to include sterile speculum. Test cervical secretions for nitrazine paper positivity, pooling in post vagina, ferning under microscope.	If > 36 weeks, induce and augment labor, < 36 weeks, antibiotics, steroids, and bed rest.
Preterm rupture of membranes	Rupture of amniotic membranes before 37 weeks' gestation.	Signs as above. By definition, labor is progressing.	If > 36 weeks, deliver baby. < 36 weeks, consider steroids, and deliver.

TABLE 9.9 Continued

Term	Definition	Diagnosis/Associations	Treatment
Prolonged rupture of membranes	Ruptured or suspected rupture > 18 hours.	Signs as above. Monitor closely for development of chorioamnionitis.	Start antibiotics (ampicillin or penicillin), deliver.
Post-term pregnancy	Pregnancy > 42 weeks.	Complications from macrosomia are increased.	Induction and augmentation with special attention to possible complications. Usually offered at 41 weeks' gestation to avoid complications.

Shoulder Dystocia

Shoulder entrapment during delivery of the fetus against the bony pelvis. The anterior shoulder may become impacted behind the pubic symphysis, causing an arrest of descent. Incidence is 0.15–1.7% of vaginal births with direct correlation to birthweight. Risk factors include fetal macrosomia, gestational or other diabetes mellitus, history of shoulder dystocia, prolonged second stage of labor.

Symptoms

Arrest of descent of the fetus during labor. Note ineffective contractions and pushing. The "turtle" sign refers to the head retracting back up the birth canal after a contraction/push.

Diagnosis

Clinical diagnosis at time of delivery. Estimation of fetal weight should be done in those patients who are at high risk for shoulder dystocia; however, ultrasound has limited accuracy at term.

Treatment

Shoulder dystocia is a true obstetric emergency.

Several maneuvers are outlined in the table below and should be performed in order of appearance in table.

TABLE 9.10 Treatment of Shoulder Dystocia

Maneuver	Definition
McRobert's	Elevation of legs and extreme flexion of hips. Have assistant help with pushing back maternal knees.
Suprapubic pressure	Sharp pressure just superior to pubic symphysis. Meant to dislodge fetal anterior shoulder.
Episiotomy	May be cut at any point in delivery to make room for the operator's hands.
Rubin's	Pressure to the accessible shoulder to push it toward the anterior chest, which decreases the bisacromial diameter.

(continued)

TABLE 9.10 Continued

Maneuver	Definition
Wood's screw	Pressure behind the posterior shoulder to try to turn the infant and dislodge the anterior shoulder. "Screwing the baby out."
Delivery of post arm	Decreases diameter of shoulder.
Intentional fracture of clavicle/humorous	Decreases bisacromial diameter. Associated with good postnatal outcomes.
Zavanelli's	Pushing the head and fetus back into the birth canal and performing a stat Cesarean section.

Take Home Points

- Shoulder dystocia is a fetal shoulder vs. bony pelvis problem.
- Suprapubic pressure and McRobert's maneuver relieve 95% of dystocias.

Cesarean Delivery

TABLE 9.11 Indications for Cesarean Delivery

Maternal/Fetal	Maternal	Fetal	Placental
• Cephalopelvic disproportion (CPD) • Failed induction • Severe shoulder dystocia (Zavanelli's maneuver)	• Eclampsia/severe preeclampsia • Cervical cancer • Prior C/S • Prior uterine rupture • Prior myomectomy • Fibroids • Ovarian tumor	• Nonreassuring fetal monitoring • Bradycardia • Absence of FHTs • Loss of fetal heart variability • Scalp pH < 7.20 • Cord prolapse • Fetal malpresentation • Multiple gestation • Hydrocephalus • Osteogenesis imperfecta	• Placenta previa • Placental abruption

Pregnancy Loss

Causes of pregnancy loss are many and include chromosomal abnormalities (nondysjunction, etc.), teratogenic factors, genetic abnormalities, trauma, placental nonviability, Rh incompatibility, and maternal factors. Of those clinically and biochemically recognized pregnancies, estimates of $1/3$–$1/2$ end in spontaneous abortion.

Symptoms

TABLE 9.12 Definitions of Pregnancy Loss

Term	Definition
Abortus	Fetal loss < 20 weeks, < 500 g, or < 25 cm (varies by state)
Complete abortion	Complete expulsion of all POCs
Incomplete abortion	Partial expulsion of POCs
Inevitable abortion	Bleeding and cervical dilation without expulsion of any POCs
Threatened abortion	Any uterine bleeding before 20 weeks WITHOUT cervical dilation or expulsion of POCs
Missed abortion	Death of fetus without expulsion of any POCs or cervical dilation

Diagnosis

Diagnosis is made by history of bleeding or expulsion of products of conception (POCs) coupled with physical exam and assessment of cervical dilation. Other signs may include low symphysis-fundal height for gestational age.

Labs: Before 10 weeks, serial quantitative β-hCGs may be obtained (which should approximately double every 48 hours in the viable pregnancy). These may show less than doubling in a 48-hour period indicating non-viable pregnancy or very high results indicating molar pregnancy.

After confirmed abortion, quantitative β-hCG should be followed until 0.

Imaging: Doppler ultrasound often does not register a fetal heart beat which should lead to a pelvic or vaginal ultrasound showing either no heart beat or an ectopic pregnancy.

Treatment

Initially stabilize the patient then complete a pelvic/vaginal ultrasound.

Treatment then depends on the type of abortion. Complete abortions may be followed for temperature elevation or signs of infection (septic abortion). Incomplete abortions may be allowed to complete on their own.

Dilation and evacuation (D&E) may be completed, although this is more commonly done for inevitable or missed abortion after significant amount of time has passed. Any recovered POCs should be sent for genetic analysis. Threatened abortions should be followed closely for cessation of bleeding or advancement of abortion, status should be strict "nil per vagina" status. Rh-immunglobulin, RhoGAM, should be given to all women with vaginal bleeding who are Rh-negative.

Second trimester:

Treatment is as above but with consideration of later pregnancies (about 16–24 weeks) that cervical ripening and induction of labor may be tried before D&E. Care should be taken to make sure all POCs are expelled. The possibilities of preterm labor or cervical incompetency should then be assessed and may be treated during future pregnancies.

Take Home Points

- Pregnancy loss is extremely common and due to many factors, most of which go undiscovered in individual patients.

- Generally, treatment consists of watchful waiting or surgical (D&E).

Ectopic Pregnancy

Implantation of a fertilized ovum outside the uterus. Sites include fallopian tubes (55% ampullary), ovarian, abdominal, intraligamentary (broad ligament), and cervical. By definition, these pregnancies are nonviable and may pose mortal threat to the mother. Risk factors include previous tubal surgery/pregnancy, previous or current PID, pelvic adhesions, previous uterine surgery, use of IUD (especially in conjunction with an STD), previous STD, history of infertility, history of endometritis, or recipients of assisted reproductive techniques.

Symptoms

The most common symptom is lower abdominal pain. Other symptoms include vaginal bleeding, secondary amenorrhea, passage of a **"decidual cast,"** referred shoulder pain, GI symptoms such as constipation or diarrhea, or possibly syncope.

Diagnosis

Physical exam: Lower abdominal tenderness may be diffuse or localized. Sterile speculum exam may show adnexal mass and cervical/uterine changes of pregnancy.

Labs: Check CBC for rise of WBC count or fall of hemoglobin/hematocrit. β-hCG is perhaps the most important lab test and is virtually always positive in this disorder. Quantitative β-hCG may not always show the pathopneumonic doubling in the 48-hour period.

Imaging: Ultrasound is the best imaging test for ectopic pregnancy. In early ectopic pregnancy, U/S should be used in conjunction with quantitative β-hCG. Transvaginal U/S should find an intrauterine pregnancy at a level of 1500 mIU/mL, transabdominal at 1800–3600 mIU/mL. Thus, an empty uterus at these levels of β-hCG strongly supports ectopic pregnancy. CT scan or MRI may show ectopic pregnancy but are rarely used for direct investigation.

Laparoscopy/laparotomy may be used in some cases of uncertain but urgent need for diagnosis exists.

Culdocentesis involves placing a needle through the posterior cul-de-sac into the dependent portion of the peritoneal cavity and attempting aspiration of blood. This may help in priority of candidates for laparoscopy/laparotomy.

During assessment, evaluation should be made to determine if rupture has occurred acutely which may lead to acute worsening of symptoms or hemodynamic instability.

Treatment

Stabilize the patient as needed.

Expectant management may be appropriate in patients who are asymptomatic or have only minimal symptoms.

Medication includes methotrexate which is a folinic acid antagonist that destroys proliferating trophoblast. Leucovorin may be added for increased efficacy. Exclusion criteria include: ruptured ectopic, adnexal mass ≥ 3.5 cm, noncompliance, peptic ulcer disease, immunodeficiency, pulmonary disease, liver/renal disease, blood dyscrasia, free abdominal fluid with pelvic pain, or sensitivity to methotrexate. The most effective use is in conjunction with an ectopic which shows no heartbeat on U/S, tubal location, and ≤ 2 cm diameter in size.

Surgical treatment may be used in other cases although specific indications depend on location and potential damage the growing fetus poses to those structures. Tubal ectopics may undergo **salpingostomy**.

Laparotomy is indicated in ovarian, abdominal, or intraligamentary ectopic pregnancies.

Take Home Points

- Always think of ectopic pregnancy in the female patient who presents with lower abdominal pain.
- Diagnosis is best done with transvaginal ultrasound.
- Methotrexate with or without leucovorin may be used for a medical treatment. Otherwise, surgery is indicated.

Gestational Diabetes Mellitus

Diabetes mellitus onset during the time of pregnancy. Pathophysiologically, gestational diabetes mellitus (GDM) is similar to type II DM in that it consists mainly of a lack of peripheral insulin sensitivity. In the majority of cases, glucose regulation will return to normal after delivery. GDM is commonly controlled by diet or insulin but untreated disease has profound implications for the fetus and mother.

Complications:

Maternal

- Polyhydramnios
- Preeclampsia
- Miscarriage
- Infection
- Postpartum hemorrhage
- Diabetic emergencies such as hypoglycemia, ketoacidosis, diabetic coma

Fetal

- Macrosomia
- Shoulder dystocia
- Erb palsy
- Delayed organ maturation
- Reflexive postpartum hypoglycemia
- Congenital malformations including cardiovascular defects, neural tube defects, caudal regression syndrome, situs inversus
- Intrauterine growth restriction (IUGR)

Symptoms

Generally asymptomatic, but may present with classic symptoms of DM including fatigue, weight loss, polyuria, and polydipsia.

Diagnosis

GDM is found most often with the 1 hour GTT screening test at 26–28 weeks' gestation. After screening is positive, confirmation must be made with a 3 hour GTT. See tables below.

TABLE 9.13 One Hour Glucose Tolerance Test*

Test	Normal Range
Fasting	< 105 mg/dL
1 hour	< 140 mg/dL

*After 50 g glucose load

TABLE 9.14 Three Hour Glucose Tolerance Test*

Test	Normal Range
Fasting	< 105 mg/dL
1 hour	< 190 mg/dL
2 hour	< 165 mg/dL
3 hour	< 145 mg/dL

* After 100 g glucose load. Two or more of these levels must be abnormal to diagnose GDM.

TABLE 9.15 Partial White Classification System of GDM

Type	Description
Class A$_1$	GDM; Diet controlled
Class A$_2$	GDM; Insulin controlled

Treatment

Tight glycemic control is required during pregnancy to reduce complications and birth defects. With class A$_1$, diet can be used to regulate glucose but frequent monitoring must be maintained. In class A$_2$, regular and NPH insulin are used to keep levels in control. Most oral hypoglycemics are contraindicated because of potential teratogenic effects.

Prenatal care changes: After 30 weeks, monitor fetal well-being q4–6 weeks by nonstress tests or biophysical profiles. Consider induction and delivery at 38–40 weeks to avoid complications of larger babies. The patient should be referred to a dietician for diabetic education and diet plan.

After delivery, GDM patients usually do not require insulin. However, since 25–35% will go on to have non-gestational DM in the subsequent 5 years, a 6 week postpartum glucose tolerance test is usually done. Of those with GDM, approximately 50% will develop the disease in future pregnancies.

Take Home Points

- GDM may first be screened for with a 1 hour GTT at 26–28 weeks, then confirmed with two abnormal values on a 3 hour GTT.
- GDM is commonly classified using the White classification system.
- Most GDM can be controlled with diet and exercise alone.

Preeclampsia/Eclampsia

A pregnancy-related hypertensive disorder of unknown etiology. Current theories of pathogenesis are many and varied, of which endothelial injury is a common theme. Central features of this disease include the presence of hypertension and proteinuria during pregnancy. Risk factors include: primigravida, maternal extremes of age, lower socioeconomic class, collagen disorders, African American, history of renal disease, chronic hypertension, multiple gestation, and family history of 1st degree female relative with preeclampsia/eclampsia.

Symptoms

Distinction is made between degrees of preeclampsia, mild and severe. Symptoms are few for mild disease, but may include increased edema (not required for diagnosis) often occurring in the hands and face or rapid weight gain. Severe preeclampsia may include oliguria, new onset headache, change of consciousness, visual disturbances (scotomata), pulmonary edema, cyanosis, right upper-quadrant (RUQ) pain, or fetal growth restriction.

Eclampsia: Presence of grand mal seizure activity not attributable to other cause. Most often associated with preeclampsia but sometimes occurs de novo.

HELLP syndrome: Form of severe preeclampsia that involves: **H**emolysis, **E**levated **L**iver enzymes, and **L**ow **P**latelets. Memorize this mnemonic. Often accompanied with headache, scomata, RUQ pain, and oliguria.

Diagnosis

The diagnosis relies on presence of proteinuria and high blood pressure. See table below. For strict definitions, levels in table are all that is required.

TABLE 9.16 Classifications of Preeclampsia

Preeclampsia	Blood Pressure Guidelines*	Proteinuria
Mild	> 140/90	> 300 mg/24 hour or 1–2 + urine dipstick†
Severe	> 160/110	> 5 grams/24 hours or 3–4 + urine dipstick†

*BP must be taken on two different occasions at least 6 hours apart.
†Dipstick urine measurements must be on two samples taken 4 hours apart.
Adapted from the American College of Obstetricians and Gynecologists (ACOG). Diagnosis and management of preeclampsia and eclampsia. American College of Obstetricians and Gynecologists (ACOG); 2002 Jan. 9. *ACOG Practice Bulletin,* 33.

Severe preeclampsia may also be diagnosed after fulfilling the mild criteria plus any of the following: oliguria of < 400 mL/24 hour, pulmonary edema, RUQ pain, headache, scomata, abnormal LFTs, thrombocytopenia, or IUGR (intrauterine growth restriction).

There is no one lab that will diagnose preeclampsia, but these will provide surveillance of disease:

- CBC for hemoglobin or hematocrit, and platelet count (low)
- Urine assessment of protein (24-hour is better than dipstick)

- Microscopic evaluation of urine (for RBC, renal tubular, WBC, or granular casts)
- Serum BUN and creatinine
- Serum uric acid (≥ 5.5 mg/dL)
- Alkaline phosphatase
- Liver transaminases (AST/ALT)
- Lactate dehydrogenase
- Coagulation profile (PT, aPTT, INR)
- Serum albumen
- Blood smear

Treatment

Delivery is the definitive treatment for preeclampsia/eclampsia!

Mild: Outpatient bed rest and frequent follow up may be practiced by some, others may choose to monitor with hospital admission. Blood pressure monitoring as well as strict symptom surveillance should be started. Consider atenolol to control hypertension.

Severe: Observation as inpatient. Ultrasound, nonstress test, biophysical profile, and above labs should be done. Bed rest should be in the left lateral decubitus position. Seizure prophylaxis with magnesium sulfate is indicated but start low and monitor levels closely. This may control blood pressure alone. If further lowering of BP is needed, consider hydralazine or labetalol IV. If pregnancy is after 36 weeks, consider induction and augmentation of labor.

If eclamptic or severe preeclamptic, strongly consider C-section.

Magnesium sulfate should be continued for 12–24 hours after delivery. The patient should still be monitored for symptoms of HELLP syndrome.

Take Home Points

- Preeclampsia/eclampsia is often described as a disease of endothelial injury and "leaky blood vessels."
- Proteinuria and hypertension are the cornerstones of diagnosis.
- Magnesium sulfate is used for seizure prophylaxis, not BP control.
- Delivery is the treatment!

Chromosomal Anomalies

Commonly, chromosomal anomalies are related to non-disjunction during meiosis, although translocations, deletions, and mosaicism also occur. Incidence increases with increased maternal age; after age 35 a sharp rise of occurrence is observed.

Symptoms

Abnormalities of amniotic fluid volume (poly or oligo hydramnios), decreased fetal movement, or abnormal fetal heart rate. See table on page 226 for postnatal signs/symptoms of disease.

Diagnosis

Labs: Triple test (estriol, maternal serum alpha fetoprotein (MSAFP), and β-hCG) or quadruple test (estriol, MSAFP, β-hCG, inhibin A), amniocentesis, or chorionic villous sampling. The triple/quadruple screen is part of routine labs in many practices; but remember, it gives only a probability of anomaly. A karotype and genetic testing can be done when the child is born.

TABLE 9.17 Chromosomal Abnormalities

Disorder	Associations
Down syndrome (trisomy 21)	At birth, may have hypotonia, transverse palmar crease, low set ears, absent philtrum, wide-spaced eyes. May also find congenital cardiac defects (VSD), leukemia, duodenal atresia, and early Alzheimer disease.
Edward syndrome (trisomy 18)	Females > males, mental retardation, small size, small head, hypoplastic mandible, low set ears, **clenched fist with index finger overlapping third & fourth digits**.
Patau syndrome (trisomy 13)	Mental retardation, apnea, deafness, myelomeningocele, cleft lip/palate, **rocker bottom feet**.
Turner syndrome (XO female)	Nuchal lymphedema, short stature, **webbed neck**, widely-spaced nipples, **primary amenorrhea**, lack of breast development, **coarctation of aorta**, horseshoe kidney.
Klinefelter syndrome (XXY male)	Usually silent until adulthood. Slightly decreased IQ, **infertility**, **microtestes**, gynecomastia, tall stature.
Cri-du-chat (deletion of short arm of chromosome 5)	Mental retardation and cry sounding high pitched "like a cat."

Treatment

Genetic counseling/testing of parents (relating to future pregnancies).

Follow-up should be close and with multiple specialists depending on anomaly. Heart, lungs, renal, respiratory, and GI systems should be monitored or tested for dysfunction.

Obstetric care is generally considered "high risk" but the main focus is on the fetus after birth.

Take Home Points

- Chromosomal abnormalities incidence increases as a function of maternal age.
- Screening may be done with the triple/quadruple test in normal pregnancies at 16–20 weeks.
- If high risk, amniocentesis can be done at 15–17 weeks or chorionic villous sampling at 9–12 weeks.

Multiple Fetuses

Incidence of multiple-fetus pregnancies has increased over the last 20 years, assumedly due to increased use of fertility-assistance techniques. Twins may be monozygotic, occurring from the same zygote; or dizygotic, from different fertilized ova. Dizygotic twins account for about 70% of twins and show hereditary predilection while monozygotic twins are less common and more random.

Symptoms

Women at advanced ages or using ovulation induction have increased rates of multiple-fetus gestations. Symptoms may include increased symphysis-fundal height for gestational age, rapid enlargement of uterus, excessive weight gain, etc. There are also more maternal complications during pregnancy, such as preeclampsia/eclampsia, GDM, cervical incompetence, placenta previa, anemia, postpartum hemorrhage, and preterm labor. Risks to the fetus include twin–twin transfusions, small for gestational age, and malpresentation.

Diagnosis

Physical exam: Doppler fetal heart rate and physical exam may suggest multiple fetuses.
Imaging: Ultrasound is the best way to diagnose.
Labs: Increased β-hCG and MSAFP are commonly present.

Treatment

Referral to specialist is mandatory. Close monitoring of pregnancy is indicated. Preterm labor is very common. Currently, twin pregnancies are usually delivered by C-section. Perinatologists should be available and on hand.

Vaginal delivery may be attempted, but perform C-section if either fetus is breech.

Take Home Points

- Twinning incidence increases with age and use of fertility techniques.
- Look for early signs and symptoms of accelerated uterine size and obtain an ultrasound.
- Referral to a high risk obstetrician is necessary with early C-section common.

10   Renal, Urinary, and Male Reproductive Systems

Malignant Neoplasm of the Bladder

Bladder cancer in the U.S. is most commonly of the histologic type, transitional cell carcinoma (TCC). However, other cancers exist and are most commonly epithelial in origin such as squamous cell carcinomas (SCC), adenocarcinomas, and small cell (neuroendocrine) tumors. In other areas of the world where the organism *Schistosoma haematobium* is prevalent, histologic types differ significantly, with SCC the most common. In some areas, bladder cancer is so prevalent that it is divided into schistosomal and non-schistosomal, indicating the significant role of this organism in the development of disease.

Symptoms

Bladder cancer often presents as asymptomatic hematuria. Urinary symptoms such as urgency, urge incontinence, frequency, nocturia, and dysuria may exist. Abdominal pain is a late finding that may accompany local invasion and metastasis. History often reveals the patient to be a **smoker** or working in an occupation with exposure to **aniline dyes**.

Diagnosis

Labs: Urinalysis for gross and microscopic blood is the first step. Cytology should also find malignant cells in the urine. Several bladder cancer specific biomarkers exist but do not play a role in screening and are currently not recommended for diagnosis alone.

Imaging: Cystoscopy with biopsy combined with imaging of the upper urinary tract is the standard workup. Imaging is most commonly done with spiral CT scan.

Intravenous pyelogram (IVP) combined with ultrasound may also be used.

Obtain extra renal CT scan, chest x-ray, and abdominal films for staging if necessary.

Treatment

Transurethral resection of superficial local cancers is effective. Some superficial cancers may also be amenable to instillation of intravesical chemotherapy (mitomycin C, doxorubicin, or bacille Calmette-Guerin (BCG)).

Deep tumors that invade into the bladder musculature may require partial or total cystectomy with diversion and pelvic lymph node dissection. Diversion will involve several options of new bladder creation often outside the body.

Systemic chemotherapy and radiation therapy have been used in patients with deep tumor spread although are rarely curative for metastatic disease.

Take Home Points

- In the U.S., transitional cell cancer is the most common form; worldwide, schistosomiasis is a major cause of squamous cell bladder cancer.

- Workup commonly involves cystoscopy and CT scan.

Neurogenic Bladder

A neurologic disorder of the bladder involving increased or decreased tone resulting in lack of muscular control. This occurs in patients with significant peripheral or central nervous system damage.

Symptoms

Two types:

Hypotonic (flaccid) bladder: Symptoms include painless, flaccid, distended bladder with nearly constant leaking of urine. UTIs are very common. History usually involves congenital or local injury to nerves supplying detrusor muscle.

Spastic (contractile) bladder: Unpredictable emptying and urge incontinence. History may include upper spinal cord damage or lesion.

Diagnosis

Labs: Check UA and urine culture for UTI.

Imaging: Serial intravenous urography (IVU), ultrasound, cystography, and urethrography may be useful.

Voiding cystometrogram can check for obstruction and give some prognostic information.

Treatment

Behavioral changes such as scheduled bathroom breaks may help in mild cases or during recovery from injury. Otherwise, it is important to distinguish between different types in order to treat.

For hypotonic bladder: Indwelling or self catheterization are treatment options. Females tend to do better with indwelling catheters, as males with indwelling catheters experience higher rates of urethritis. The cholinergic medication bethanechol (Urecholine) may also increase detrusor muscle tone.

For spastic bladder: Condom catheters may be used with men, or external sphincterotomy in advanced cases to reduce outflow resistance.

Medications for either type: **Ditropan (oxybutynin)** and **Detrol (tolterodine)** are very effective but best for spastic bladder. *Watch for anticholingeric side effects in the elderly.* Several other medications including imipramine (Tofranil) and propantheline are also effective.

Certain α-sympathetic blockers such as doxazosin (Cardura), prazosin (Minipress), and terazosin (Hytrin) are effective as well.

Surgery: Exteriorization of the bladder or suprapubic catheterization may be needed in severe spinal cord injury or medicine refractory, extreme cases.

Take Home Points

- Neurogenic bladder comes in two types; hypotonic and spastic.
- Culture urine for possible UTI.
- Treat with both behavioral modification and medications such as oxbutynin and tolterodine.

Uncomplicated Cystitis

Inflammation of the bladder or lower urinary tract is commonly caused by infection with *E coli, S saprophyticus,* or *Enterococcus.* Incidence is directly correlated to sexual contact in women. In men, cystitis is fairly rare so an alternate etiology should be sought if suspected, such as STD or prostatitis in the elderly.

Symptoms

Dysuria, bladder tenderness, urgency, and frequency. Fever and costovertebral angle tenderness are not part of uncomplicated cystitis.

Diagnosis

Urinalysis and urine culture-clean catch is acceptable but catheterization is best (but impractical in many situations). Bagging in children is usually not useful because of contamination. In children suprapubic tap may provide the best sample.

UA may show increased specific gravity, bacteria, leukocyte esterase, and/or nitrite. Pyuria (WBCs in urine) is widely regarded as the most sensitive and specific test in the panel. Always order sensitivities with culture to guide treatment.

Treatment

Trimethoprim/sulfamethoxazole (TMP/SMX) or ciprofloxacin are still currently first line, although resistance is emerging. Course should be for 3 days for uncomplicated nondiabetics; 7–10 days for elderly, diabetics, or mildly immunocompromised.

Prophylactic treatment may be given to women with recurrent and diagnosable UTIs linked to sexual intercourse before times of increased sexual activity (honeymoon).

Asymptomatic bacturia in pregnancy may be treated with amoxicillin or nitrofurantoin.

Consider use of phenazopyridine (Pyridium) for treatment of dysuria.

Take Home Points

- Urine culture should always be done along with urinalysis when infection is suspected.
- Rely on the presence or absence of pyuria more than other findings in the UA.
- Consider supplying the female patient a prophylactic course of appropriate treatment before periods of increased sexual activity.

Acute Pyelonephritis

Infection of the kidney by bacteria also commonly found in cystitis. Namely, *E coli, Enterococcus, S saprophyticus*, etc. In children, frequent, recurrent, or early kidney infection may herald abnormal urinary anatomy; therefore, consider investigation of urinary architecture in pediatric kidney infection patients.

Symptoms

Fever, chills, back pain, nausea/vomiting, malaise, anorexia, or headache, accompanied by urinary symptoms such as frequency, urgency, incomplete voiding, and dysuria. History may reveal frequent UTIs, diabetes, or Foley catheter.

Diagnosis

Physical exam: Increased temperature, costovertebral angle tenderness on percussion, and bladder pain. **Labs:** CBC for leukocytosis, UA may show WBCs, bacteria, casts, leukocyte esterase, or nitrite. Urine culture and sensitivities should be sent at the time of UA. Send blood cultures as well.

Treatment

Evaluate for urosepsis and make sure patient is stable.

Mild to moderate cases should be placed on oral fluoroquinolones such as ciprofloxacin, moxifloxacin (Avelox), levofloxacin (Levaquin).

Close follow up is indicated if treated as an outpatient.

For severe cases, consider admission and IV antibiotics including ampicillin plus gentamycin or a fluoroquinolone such as ciprofloxacin (Cipro) or levofloxacin (Levaquin).

All pregnant women with pyelonephritis should be admitted!

Take Home Points

- Consider the cause of ascension of bacteria in the kidneys, such as, prolonged cystitis, abnormal anatomy, immunocompromise, etc.
- Essentially, renal infection is a clinical diagnosis with signs of bacterial infection in the urinary tract.
- Treat with broad spectrum antibiotics before a focused regimen can be given per the urine culture. Fluoroquinolones are the usual class.

Nocturnal Enuresis

Loss of bladder control at night. Approximately 80% of children attain nighttime bladder control by 5 years old with a significant portion progressing to control by age 7 years.

Monosymptomatic primary nocturnal enuresis occurs in children who have never achieved consistent nocturnal dryness.

Secondary enuresis occurs in children who have achieved consistent dryness, usually for approximately 6 months, then relapsed into bedwetting.

Symptoms

Look for symptoms of UTI such as dysuria, frequency, and urinary urgency although these are often not present.

Diagnosis

Have caregivers/patient keep a urinary diary. This should highlight times of increased urination, periods between urination, or connection to sleep.

Labs: Urinalysis and urine culture to evaluate for UTI.

Imaging: In children older than age 5–6 with a history of frequent UTIs, investigate whether a structural abnormality is present. This may be done with VCUG (voiding cystourethrogram) or sonogram.

Treatment

Reassure families of children ≤ 7 years of age, spontaneous resolution occurs in the vast majority of cases.

Behavioral modification is very important in the first step. Motivational therapy, bladder training, fluid restriction before bed, late night alarms, and **enuresis alarms** are all very effective.

Pharmacologic treatment should only be considered after age 7 and attempt at non pharmacologic methods have failed. Options include desmopressin (DDAVP) or imipramine (Tofranil) (as well as other TCAs). DDAVP should be considered first and may also work as a short term (e.g. summer camp, etc.) treatment if needed.

Take Home Points

- There is generally no cause for concern under the age of 7 years although history and investigation should be considered starting at 5 years.
- Consider pharmacologic therapy only if other techniques have failed and the child is ≥ 7 years old.
- Enuresis alarms have proved very effective in most children.
- DDAVP is the first line medication.

Malignant Neoplasm of the Kidney

Renal cell carcinoma is the most common primary tumor occurring in 80–85% of primary renal malignancies. Others include transitional cell carcinomas of the renal pelvis, oncocytomas, and renal sarcomas. Nephroblastoma (Wilms tumor) is common in children and renal medullary carcinoma may be seen in sickle cell patients.

Symptoms

Hematuria or microhematuria is most common although advanced cases may involve flank pain, palpable mass, and fever of unknown origin.

Diagnosis

Physical exam: New scrotal, left-sided varicocele is sometimes the presenting finding. Abdominal mass may be felt or weight loss may be evident. Vital signs may show hypertension or fever.

Labs: Urinalysis or hematuria and renal function testing are the first labs to get. CBC may also show erythrocytosis or anemia. Hypercalcemia may be found on an electrolyte panel.

Imaging: CT scan is the best test if suspected. US or intravenous pyelogram (IVP) will demonstrate a mass but suggest little about local extension. MRI shows local extension to adjacent tissue and gives further information on density but is not the first test to order. Selective renal angiography may be done before surgery to determine local vessel involvement but does not play a role in initial diagnosis.

Don't forget to investigate possible metastatic sites such as the lungs, liver, and brain!

Treatment

Surgery for **nephrectomy** (with/without lymph node dissection) for tumors > 3 cm or partial wedge nephrectomy if the tumor is ≤ 3 cm.

Medications include interleukin-2 (IL-2) and other chemotherapeutic agents but response appears erratic.

Most tumors are fairly resistant to radiation therapy although this may be palliative in advanced cases.

Take Home Points

- Renal cell carcinoma is the most common primary renal malignancy.
- Hematuria is the most common sign (in the UA) and symptom of renal carcinoma.
- CT scan is the imaging test of choice.
- Surgery is the mainstay of treatment.

Nephrotic Syndrome

A syndrome of **glomerular proteinuria, hyperlipidemia, and hypoalbuminemia** secondary to renal disease. Primary renal diseases predominate in children while secondary causes such as diabetes mellitus, hepatitis B or C, carcinoma, amyloidosis, lupus, preeclampsia/eclampsia, and medication effect (gold, penicillamine, mercury, NSAIDs) predominate in adults.

Symptoms

Frothy urine may be the first symptom, followed by **edema**, anorexia, malaise, puffy eyelids, abdominal pain, anasarca, ascites, and breathing difficulty due to pleural effusion.

Diagnosis

Presence of > 3.5 g/24 hours, albumin < 3.0 g/dL, and generalized edema.

Labs: Urinalysis for the presence of protein is the first test. Urinary protein/creatinine ratio (> 0.2 being concerning and ≥ 3.5 indicating nephrotic syndrome) should be checked. Analyze urine sediment for casts including hyaline, granular, fatty, waxy and epithelial cells which are typical. Test urine for lipiduria.

Twenty-four hour urine protein collection is the gold standard for determining amount of proteinuria and gives information on the source of renal damage. > 3.5 g/24 hours is considered nephrotic range.

TABLE 10.1 Likely Location of Dysfunction by Level of Urinary Protein

Urinary Protein (gm/day)	Likely Source
0.15–2	Mild glomerulonephropathies, tubular proteinuria overflow proteinuria
2.0–4.0	Usually glomerular
> 4.0	Always glomerular

Adapted from McConnell KR, Bia MJ. Evaluation of proteinuria: an approach for the internist. *Resident Staff Phys* 1994;40:41–8.

Assess CBC for platelet levels, coagulation profile which may show prolongation of clotting time, lipids for hyperlipidemia, albumin which may be low, BMP for renal function (although impairment is rarely seen), and sodium level for hyponatremia.

Screen for common systemic diseases such as diabetes, SLE, amyloidosis, and multiple myeloma.

TABLE 10.2 Specific Nephrotic Diseases

Disease	Associations	Clinical Features	Diagnosis	Treatment
Minimal change disease	Most common cause of nephrotic syndrome in **children**.	Nephrotic syndrome, increased BP, renal impairment, renal NSAID damage.	Renal biopsy shows fusion of the epithelial cell foot processes on electron microscopy.	**Steroids** are very effective.
Focal and segmental glomerulosclerosis	Primary type often has greater proteinuria than secondary types. Secondary disease commonly caused by HIV, excess NSAID use, and previous renal injury.	Hematuria, hypertension, and decreased renal function are common.	Renal biopsy shows focal mesangial collapse and sclerosis.	Treat primary disease with steroids and immunosuppressive agents (tacrolimus, cyclosporine) and secondary disease with ACE-I, ARB, and lipid-lowering agents. However, treatments do overlap.
Membranous glomerulonephritis	Commonly idiopathic but associations include hepatitis B, lupus, thyroiditis, carcinoma, and drugs such as gold, penicillamine, captopril, and NSAIDs.	Nephrotic syndrome is usually the primary presentation.	Renal biopsy shows basement membrane thickening with little or no cellular proliferation or infiltration, and the presence of electron dense deposits across the glomerular basement membrane.	Spontaneous total or partial remission is common. Consider steroids and immunosuppressive drugs. Start ACE-I or ARB, and lipid-lowering agents.

Treatment

Restrict dietary protein to less than 1 g/kg/day with low-fat meals.

Start an ACE inhibitor to protect the kidneys.

Consider starting a statin for hyperlipidemia.

Steroids are usually the mainstay.

Treat hypercoagulable state with anticoagulation therapy.

Treat edema with low salt diet and loop diuretics such as Lasix. Add metolazone for synergism if needed.

Diagnosis of the underlying cause and/or referral to nephrology is the best course of action.

Take Home Points

- Look for the triad of nephrotic range proteinuria, hyperlipidemia, and hypoalbuminemia.
- Renal biopsy is the test of choice and delineates subclassification of disease.
- Steroids are commonly part of the treatment.

Glomerulonephritis (Nephritic Syndrome)

A syndrome of clinical disease caused by glomerular inflammation. Commonly involves the triad of hematuria, non-nephrotic range proteinuria, and decreased renal function.

Clinical Features

Common presentation is of "smoky-brown" urine (macroscopic hematuria), edema, oliguria, proteinuria, renal failure, and possibly hypertension. RBCs or **RBC casts** in the urine are a hallmark but may not always be present.

TABLE 10.3 Specific Glomerulonephritis Diseases

Disease	Associations	Clinical Features	Diagnosis	Treatment
Anti-GBM including Goodpasture syndrome	Lung and kidney involvement. Young adults.	Hemoptysis, dyspnea, renal failure.	Renal biopsy shows linear anti-GBM deposits. CXR shows diffuse infiltrates.	Steroids, cyclophosphamide. Plasma exchange therapy may be needed.
IgA nephropathy (Berger disease)	**Most common cause** of GN worldwide. Often young males.	Gross hematuria common. Attacks commonly precipitated by infection.	Renal biopsy and IF shows IgA and C3 deposits.	ACE inhibitors for mild disease, corticosteroids for moderate-severe disease. 20% progress to end-stage renal disease.
Post-streptococcal glomerulonephritis	Strep throat infection often proceeds by weeks.	Edema, hypertension, hematuria, oligouria, RBC casts on U/A.	Hematuria (casts present), proteinuria. Renal biopsy shows immune deposits and "lumpy-bumpy" appearance on IF.	**Supportive care**. Full recovery common.
Wegener granulomatosis	Lung and kidney involvement. Commonly sinus symptoms also present.	Hemoptysis, dyspnea, fever, wt loss.	**c-ANCA** positive.	Steroids and cyclophosphamide combination. Consider further immunosuppressants if needed. Poor prognosis.

IF = Immunofluorescence.

Take Home Points

- Look for the triad: hematuria, non-nephrotic range proteinuria, and decreased renal function.
- Look for RBC casts in the urine as a clue between glomerulonephritis and nephrotic syndrome.

Acute Renal Failure (ARF)

TABLE 10.4 Causes of Derangement by Location of Renal Failure

Etiology	Derangement
Pre-renal	Most commonly, dehydration. Renal artery occlusion. Shock.
Intrinsically renal	Intrinsic renal disease or toxin. Includes NSAIDs, Wegener, Goodpasture, SLE, DM, polyarteritis, and acute tubular (ATN) or glomerular injury.
Post-renal	Bladder outlet obstruction such as oversized prostate, renal caliculi, bladder cancer, etc.

Symptoms

Rarely symptomatic, especially in the hospital. Generally, urine excretion is preserved but oliguria or anuria may be seen especially with pre-renal/post-renal causes. Cola-colored urine may precede decrease in urine volume. Symptoms may progress to mental status change and metabolic derangement if extreme.

Diagnosis

Order urine electrolytes and plasma electrolytes, specifically sodium and creatinine. Calculate the FENa (fractional excretion of sodium).

$$FENa = \frac{UNa(PCr)}{PNa(UCr)}$$

U = urine, P = plasma, Na = sodium, Cr = creatinine.

< 1% pre-renal, > 2% intrinsically renal.

Urinalysis for proteinuria, hematuria, and osmolarity. Urinary sediment for brown granular, coarse granular, red cell or hemoglobin casts. Cellular exam for RBCs, WBCs, epithelial cells, or eosinophils.

Consider a 24-hour urine collection for creatinine clearance to estimate the glomerular filtration rate (GFR).

Labs: Creatinine, CO_2, K, Na, Ca, ionized Ca, phosphate, BUN, uric acid, and CK. Antistreptolysin-O and complement titers, ANA and antinuclear cytoplasmic antibodies may be useful if the cause is not clear. BUN/creatinine ratio > 15–20 supports ARF.

ABG for possible modest acidosis.

Insert a Foley catheter to evaluate for post-renal obstruction.

Ultrasound or CT of kidneys to look for possible hydronephrosis, sclerosis, nephrolithiasis, or mass.

Abdominal x-rays may be useful to find radio-opaque stones.

Renal biopsy if cause is still unclear.

Treatment

Treat the underlying cause, especially if reversible.

Start low sodium/fat/protein diet.

Stop all NSAIDs, aminoglycosides, or other offending agents.

Correct metabolic and electrolyte abnormalities.

Copious fluid replacement in severe dehydration or rhabdomyolysis may be kidney saving.

Dialysis with biocompatible membrane is the definitive treatment, although debate exists on when to start, how often, and for how long it should be continued.

Consider Mannitol or other diuretics for increased filtration.

Don't forget to renally dose all meds!

Take Home Points

- Determine the zone of dysfunction; pre-renal, intrinsically renal, or post-renal. Use the FENa and clinical impression for this.

- Stop all offending medications such as NSAIDs, aminoglycosides, etc. Consider aggressive fluid administration.

Chronic Renal Failure/Insufficiency

The substantial, irreversible and long term loss of renal function. Degrees of disease severity range from insufficiency to end stage.

Symptoms

Insufficiency is asymptomatic but may progress to failure. Failure also is often asymptomatic but may begin with nocturia, fatigue, and decreased mental acuity with onset of uremia. If this progresses, the patient may experience muscular twitches, peripheral neuropathies, sensory phenomena, muscle cramps, convulsions, anorexia, stomatitis, and unpleasant taste. This progresses to malnutrition and wasting, GI ulceration, bleeding, dehydration, yellow-brown skin color change, "uremic frost" (uremic crystals precipitating on the skin from sweat), pruritus, osteomalacia, and further symptoms of systemic disease such as hypertensive CHF, pericarditis, and other end-organ damage.

Diagnosis

History usually reveals a cause such as hypertension or DM.

Labs: BMP for creatinine (often > 1.5–2.0 mg/dL) and BUN. Na is often normal or only slightly abnormal. CBC will reveal normochromic/normocytic anemia and possibly thrombocytopenia. Look for increased ammonia, K, PTH, and phosphorus. Decreased vit D, and Ca.

Estimation of glomerular filtration rate (GFR) should be done by direct measurement of 24 hour creatinine or by use of the following formula:

Cockcroft-Gault equation:

$$\text{Creatinine clearance (estimated)} = \frac{140 - age\ (yr) \times lean\ body\ mass(kg)}{serum\ creatinine\ \left(mg/ml\right) \times 72}$$

This equation is for males; multiply by 0.85 for females.

TABLE 10.5 Range of Dysfunction by GFR

GFR (Estimated by creatinine clearance)	Range of Dysfunction
30–50 mL/min	Mild
10–29 mL/min	Moderate
< 10 mL/min	Severe
< 5 mL/min	End stage

Use of this equation should only be done on those with *stable* renal function and must only be relied on after consideration of the patient's applicability (less accurate for the morbidly obese, elderly, pregnant, etc.)

ABG may show metabolic acidosis.

UA may reveal osmolarity close to that of serum (300–320 mOsm/kg) due to inability to concentrate urine. Waxy casts are common in advanced disease.

Renal biopsy is the best test for determining etiology. May not be possible in advanced disease with small, sclerotic kidneys.

Imaging: Ultrasound early on to evaluate possible cause and extent of sclerosis.

Treatment

Correct metabolic disorder, correct vitamin deficiency, restrict protein in the diet.

Importantly, control glucose levels in DM patients and hypertension in hypertensive patients. These often occur together.

Consider treating anemia with erythropoietin (epoetin alfa (Epogen)) although weigh the risks/benefits for adverse cardiovascular events.

Dialysis in advanced cases.

Add an **ACE-I** to protect kidneys in early stages. Debate exists for later stages and is contraindicated if patient has bilateral renal artery stenosis or only one kidney.

Surgery: Parathyroidectomy may be indicated.

Renal transplant is definitive.

Don't forget to renally dose all meds!

Take Home Points

- Diabetes mellitus and hypertension are the most common causes of CRF/I in the U.S.

- Calculation or measurement of the creatinine clearance may be done to estimate the GFR.

- Dialysis or renal transplant are treatments for end-stage disease.

Polycystic Kidney Disease

An autosomal dominant disease with the main manifestation of multiple fluid-filled cysts on the kidneys. Rarely, an acquired form may develop in those on long-term dialysis. This is a progressive disease which is linked to other abnormalities including cerebral "berry" aneurysms, colonic diverticulae, liver cysts, ovarian cysts, or mitral valve prolapse.

Symptoms

Largely asymptomatic unless in advanced stage. When kidneys become polycystic or cysts become > 10 cm diameter, they may contribute to lumbar back pain, abdominal pain, hematuria, recurrent UTIs, or colic due to kidney stones. In late disease, symptoms of uremia may dominate, including mental status change.

Diagnosis

Labs: Urinalysis may show mild proteinuria and hematuria. Consider urine culture for symptoms of UTI.

CBC may show elevated hematocrit.

Imaging: Intravenous pyelography findings are typical. Ultrasound and CT show a characteristic "moth-eaten" appearance of bilateral kidneys.

Obtain MRI or cerebral angiography of the brain to evaluate for berry aneurysms.

Genetic testing of family members is indicated.

Treatment

Early detection (by age 25) is possible and may afford extra time to monitor new symptoms.

Otherwise, treatment of hypertension and supportive care is the mainstay.

Monitor for UTIs.

Dialysis may be used to prolong life in later stages.

Surgery: Hopeful alternative but genetic component of disease often limits possible donors.

Take Home Points

- PKD is autosomal dominant and may be associated by cerebral "berry" aneurysms.

- CT and renal US shows a characteristic "moth-eaten" appearance.

- Detect early and treat hypertension.

Urolithiasis

The existence of calculi in the urinary drainage system. Calcium oxalate/phosphate make up the majority of stones, struvite are the next most common, followed in order by uric acid and cystine stones.

Symptoms

Excruciating colicky abdominal pain. Pain is described as sharp, 10 on a 0–10 scale, and "worse than having a baby." Pain may also be referred, classically to the genitals. Hematuria may be observed along with dark urine. Fever is sometimes present, as is UTI. Symptoms of uremia or urosepsis may be present in advanced disease.

Diagnosis

Labs: UA shows micro or gross hematuria or may be typical of UTI.

Basic chemistry with serum calcium, ionized calcium, PTH, phosphorus, magnesium, uric acid, and creatinine.

Imaging: Non-contrast helical CT scan has replaced IVP as first line for finding all kinds of stones. It should be ordered using a "urolithiasis protocol" so CT slices are taken 3–5 mm apart instead of the usual 8 mm. IVP is, however, still used in some centers as first line. KUB (kidney/ureters/bladder) plain film may be used although can miss very small stones and those that are radiolucent (uric acid). Ultrasound may be useful but only with an experienced tech.

If the stone has passed and was captured, send it for analysis.

Treatment

Hydration is key and most often indicated IV.

Pain control is absolutely necessary. Use opiates including meperidine (Demerol) and morphine liberally.

Strain urine until stone passes or 72 hours after cessation of pain.

If stone ≤ 5 mm it will likely pass in < 48 hours.

If stone > 5 mm see table below.

TABLE 10.6 Treatment of Urolithiasis > 5 mm

Treatment	Indications/Associations
Extracorporeal shockwave lithotripsy (ESWL)	Criteria: Stone in renal pelvis or upper ⅔ ureter, < 2 cm, noninfected
Intracorporeal fragmentation lithotripsy (laser, electrohydraulic, pneumatic)	Used to fragment stones which are then removed with graspers or allowed to pass
Urethroscopy with/without lithotripsy	Criteria: Lower ⅓ of ureter, normal anatomy
Percutaneous nephrolithotomy	Criteria: Renal collecting system or upper ⅔ ureter, > 2 cm, ureter stricture, non-calcium stone, infection
Stenting	Upper or lower ⅓ of ureter
Open surgery	Complex anatomy, obstruction

Recurrent calcium stones may respond to hydrochlorothiazide (HCTZ), uric acid stones to allopurinol (Zyloprim), and cystine stones to penicillamine (Cuprimine).

Treat underlying UTIs with TMP/SMX or levofloxacin.

Consider further metabolic and urinary workup and referral to urologist if recurrent.

Take Home Points

- Always consider urolithiasis in abdominal pain patients.
- The most common type is the calcium oxalate/phosphate stone, however, if UTI is present, consider the "septic" stone.
- Imaging is best done with "urolithiasis protocol" helical CT scan.
- HCTZ is a common medication for the prophylaxis against calcium stones.

Urinary Incontinence

Involuntary loss of urine. Most common in older females, varieties include stress, obstructive, mixed, urge, or overflow.

Symptoms

Involuntary loss of urine associated usually with certain situations. Stress incontinence happens with coughing, laughing, rising from seated position, or straining. Urge incontinence is associated with quick onset uncontrollable urges to urinate. Overflow and obstructive types may happen after much time has passed between voids.

Diagnosis

Voiding diary is useful but generally diagnosis made by clinical history.

Physical exam: In women, pelvic exam may reveal rectocele, cystocele, or pelvic prolapse. In men, prostate exam may suggest prostatic hypertrophy.

Labs: UA and urine culture for possible UTI.

Urodynamic testing may be useful such as uroflowmetry, pressure flow, post-void residual, and urethroscopy.

Cystometrogram is most useful and may show abnormal sphincter pressure or bladder dysfunction.

Treatment

Treat underlying cause if found.

Avoid drugs that may aggravate symptoms such as caffeine, diuretics, anticholinergics, narcotics, Ca channel blockers, prostaglandin analogs, ACE-Is, and α-adrenergic blockers.

Maintain good perineal hygiene.

Behavioral modification such as biofeedback and bladder training.

Urinary pads.

For women

Intermittent or indwelling catheter may be indicated in extreme cases.

For females, pelvic floor (Kegel) exercises may help to strengthen urinary control musculature.

Vaginal cones or pessary devices may be useful in older women. These come in multiple sizes and need individual fitting.

Medications: Topical estrogen to increase urethral tone, pseudoephedrine (Sudafed) 3×/day, and imipramine (Tofranil) commonly help.

Periurethral injection of collagen may be useful but often requires more than one injection. Benefits are usually immediate and this technique requires only local anesthetic.

Surgery: Various bladder neck suspension and pubovaginal sling procedures exist. Refer to specialist if refractory to above treatments.

For men

Condom catheters may be used to avoid urinary tract infections sometimes found with indwelling catheters.

Surgery: Prostate-reducing surgery such as transurethral radical prostatectomy (TURP) is effective, but consider the common side effect of impotence.

Take Home Points

- Make sure the patient does not have a chronic UTI responsible for symptoms of urine loss.
- Types of incontinence include: stress, obstructive, mixed, urge, and overflow.
- Always do a thorough pelvic exam in females.
- Treatment consists of a combination of surgical procedures and injections and medication use.
- Since this can be a socially crippling disorder, effective treatment is very important.

Acid/Base Disorders

Principles

CO_2 is an acidic gas.

HCO_3 is alkaline.

Primary changes in CO_2 are termed respiratory, primary changes in HCO_3 are termed metabolic.

Steps to Classification of Acid/Base Disorders

1. Look at the pH: Is there acidosis or alkalosis?

2. Look at the pCO$_2$: is it consistent with the pH (i.e. low pCO$_2$ indicates alkalosis, high indicates acidosis)?

3. Look at the HCO$_3$: is it consistent with the pH (i.e. high HCO$_3$ indicates alkalosis, low indicates acidosis)?

4. If pCO$_2$ or HCO$_3$ are inconsistent with the pH and do not completely correct the pH, the change denotes an appropriate compensatory response.

TABLE 10.7 Acid/Base Disorders

	Respiratory Acidosis	Respiratory Alkalosis	Metabolic Acidosis		Metabolic Alkalosis
pH	< 7.36	> 7.45	< 7.36		> 7.45
pCO$_2$	↑	↓	↓*		↑*
HCO$_3$	↑*	↓*	↓		↑
Common causes	Acute lung disease, chronic lung disease, drugs (opiates, sedatives), respiratory failure	Hyperventilation, asthma, PE, CHF, pregnancy, thyrotoxicosis, high altitude	Anion gap: (**MUDPILES**) **M**ethanol **U**remia **D**KA **P**araldehyde **I**NH, Iron **L**actate **E**thylene glycol/ethanol **S**alicylates	Non-anion gap: Diarrhea, RTA, TPN, hyperchloremia, Addison disease, ammonium chloride ingestion	Vomiting, K depleting diuretics, burns, base ingestion

*Denotes appropriate compensation response.

Consider the possibility of a mixed disorder in the situation of no obvious compensatory response.

Diseases of the Male Reproductive System

Malignant Neoplasm of the Prostate

Cancer of the prostate is most commonly adenocarcinoma of the acinar cells and is the second most common cancer in adult men. Risk factors include family history, exposure to carcinogens, and age > 60 years, although it remains unclear how many patients die "with" prostate cancer as opposed to "of" prostate cancer.

Symptoms

Commonly, this cancer is asymptomatic, but it may present with symptoms of enlarged prostate including hesitancy, urgency, incomplete voiding, nocturia, frequency, and anuria. Ask the patient to identify lower back pain, rib pain, or other new, persistent discomfort that may potentially lead to discovery of metastasis.

Diagnosis

Physical exam: Digital rectal exam may reveal an asymmetrically hard, lumpy, or firm prostate as opposed to BPH, which is large and boggy.

Screening: Screening is a controversial subject in the general population. The United States Preventive Services Task Force (USPSTF), American Academy of Family Physicians (AAFP), American College of Preventive Medicine (ACPM), and American College of Physicians (ACP) recommendations state that there is, to date, no evidence strong enough to recommend routine population screening for prostate cancer. The American Cancer Society (ACS), however, states that since PSA and DRE have proven useful in cancer detection, yearly screening should start at age 50 (or age 45 in high-risk individuals). Thus, there is apparent disagreement amongst authoritative groups with the consensus siding to not routinely screen for prostate cancer (although providing the patient with information is highly encouraged).

The table below illustrates accepted action when PSA is used for screening.

TABLE 10.8 Recommended Action by PSA Level

Total PSA(ng/mL)	Action
< 4.0	Normal, do nothing
4.0–10.0	Consider prostate biopsy
> 10.0	Biopsy and investigate metastatic spread

PSA is also commonly used to follow prostate cancer after treatment.

When elevated PSA is found and biopsy confirms cancer, grading is with the **Gleason score**. This scale grades the histologic appearance 1 thru 5, the lower being the most differentiated and higher the least differentiated. The score is done on the most prominent *and* the second most prominent appearance of abnormal cells in the biopsy. Thus, there are two scores of 1–5 added together. The total end Gleason score will then be between 2 and 10.

Imaging: After diagnosis, obtain imaging for staging and to look for metastasis. This includes radionucleotide bone scan, abdominal/pelvic CT, and intravenous pyelogram. Other less used modalities include ProstaScint scan and endorectal MRI.

Treatment

Transurethral radical prostatectomy (TURP) is the most common treatment, although beware the many complications including neurovascular impotence and incontinence. Surgery has better long-term efficacy but patient life expectancy should be taken into account.

External beam radiation as well as brachytherapy (radioactive implants) are also used although are less effective than surgery for the long term. Radical prostatectomy is an alternative to TURP in select patients.

Radiation and chemotherapy can be used for metastasis and advanced disease although overall cure rates are very low. Keep in mind the rectal consequences of radiation.

Anti-androgen therapy is often used in advanced disease. Castrate therapy may prolong survival.

Take Home Points

- Prostate cancer is one of the slowest growing carcinomas in men.
- PSA use in screening is controversial and has limitations such as frequent false positives. These may be due to prostatitis, BPH, etc.
- Surgery including TURP is the mainstay of therapy, although other modalities may be used.

Testicular Cancer

Most common solid tumor in young males (age 20–40 years). Varieties include, in order of frequency, seminoma, teratoma, Sertoli or Leydig cell tumors. Spread is often lymphatic and, since this drainage ascends along the aorta, may present in abdominal, mediastinal, or lung lymph nodes.

Symptoms

A mass on the testicle often found by the patient self-palpating and is sometimes noticed after trauma leads to greater attention to the area. History may reveal cryptorchidism, which increases the chances of malignancy > 20 fold and is *unaffected by surgical correction.*

Diagnosis

Physical exam: Hard, solid mass. Negative for transillumination.
Labs: Tumor markers **β-hCG** (choriocarcinoma) and **α-fetoprotein** (yolk sac tumors) should be measured and may be useful in post treatment follow up.
Imaging: Initially, ultrasound to evaluate. CT of chest, abdomen, pelvis, and CXR are used in staging. Standard staging is with TNM system.

Treatment

Radical orchiectomy is the mainstay. Depending on the type of cancer, radiation with/without lymph node dissection may be done. Chemotherapy has shown good results in some types of cancer. Prognosis is generally very good.

Take Home Points

- Testicular cancer spreads via lymph drainage, thus may metastasize to abdominal, mediastinal, or lung lymph nodes.
- Cryptorchidism dramatically increases the chances of malignancy in the affected testis.
- Radical orchiectomy is the mainstay of treatment.

Prostatitis

The syndrome of inflamed prostate tissue which may be chronic or acute. Risk factors include age > 50 years, urinary tract infection, dehydration, trauma, chronic indwelling catheter, HIV positivity, and urethral stricture.

Symptoms

Urinary frequency, urgency, hesitancy, dysuria, nocturia, hematuria, fevers, chills, and myalgias.

Diagnosis

Physical exam: Exquisitely tender prostate which may be enlarged.
Labs: Urinalysis and culture are indicative of UTI. Prostate massage and culture of secretions may be done although should only be after adequate blood levels of antibiotics are achieved to avoid bacteremia. Practically, prostate massage is rarely done. CBC, CRP, ESR may be indicative of infection.
Causes:

Age < 35 years → *N gonnorhea* and *Chlamydia*
Age > 35 years or chronic disease → *Enterobacteria*

Treatment

Age < 35 years → ofloxacin or ceftriaxone (Rocephin) + doxycycline
Age > 35 years → ciprofloxacin or TMP-sulpha

Take Home Points

- Prostatitis is most commonly a disease of older men. If found in the young, suspect STDs.
- Digital rectal exam characteristically reveals an exquisitely tender prostate.
- Therapy should be directed toward the cultured or most likely organism, duration ranges from 10–28 days depending on clinical presentation.

Benign Prostatic Hypertrophy

A benign adenomatous enlargement of the prostate. It's still controversial if this disease represents a normal part of aging, but it is rare before the age of 40 years.

Symptoms

Symptoms of bladder outlet obstruction such as difficulty starting a stream, weak stream, hesitancy, urgency, incomplete voiding, dribbling, bladder pain, stress incontinence, nocturia, and anuria. May progress to azotemia and possibly urosepsis if untreated and severe.

Diagnosis

Physical exam is the best way to clinically diagnose (although definitive diagnosis remains pathological). Symmetrically boggy prostate on digital rectal exam.
Imaging: Ultrasound may be used to estimate gland size or investigate other prostate disease.
Biopsy is not useful for diagnosis although may eliminate cancer as a possibility.

Treatment

Acutely decompress the bladder with a Foley or suprapubic catheter if needed.

Long term, use the α-blockers doxazosin (Cardura), terazosin (Hytrin), tamsulsin (Flomax), prazosin (Minipress) and 5α-reductase inhibitors finastride (Proscar) and dutasteride (Avodart).

Avoid anticholinergics, antihistamines, and narcotics.

Surgical treatment with TURP is definitive.

Other approaches include stents, microwave thermotherapy, high-intensity focused ultrasound thermotherapy, laser, electrovaporization, and radiofrequency vaporization, although these are rarely used.

Alternative therapies include the use of saw palmetto (serena repens) and South African stargrass, although supporting evidence is inconsistent.

Take Home Points

- BPH shows a very common association with aging, prompting some to believe it's a normal consequence of hormonal effect on prostate tissue.
- Symptoms include those of bladder outlet obstruction.
- Medication treatment consists of α-blocking agents and 5α-reductase inhibitors.

Masses Referable to the Testes

TABLE 10.9 Testicular Masses

Mass	Associations/Diagnosis	Treatment
Hydrocele	Painless. No signs of inflammation. **Transilluminates**. May obtain ultrasound for definitive diagnosis if needed.	Observation unless growing or very large. Aspiration may provide relief but often recurs. Surgery has several options including ligation, tying procedures, or removal of tunica vaginalis.
Varicocele	Dilation of the pampiniform plexus (10× more likely on the left). Does not transilluminate. Usually benign but may affect fertility. Varies in size with standing/sitting position. Exam classic for **"bag of worms"** feel.	Surgical.
Inguinal Hernia	May be direct or indirect in relation to the inguinal canal. In extension into the scrotum, exam will reveal no cord superior to bulge (thus differentiating from other masses). Often reducible when change to supine position. Watch for possible strangulation or incarceration.	Surgical (either open or laproscopic); immediate surgery if complicated.

Urethritis

Inflammation of the urethra commonly due to a sexually transmitted disease (STD). In males, the most common complication of untreated disease is urinary stricture, which is fairly uncommon overall.

Symptoms

May be asymptomatic, but dysuria is common in men. Purulent or milky, non-bloody discharge. History may suggest other STDs or multiple sexual partners.

Diagnosis

Physical exam: Purulent discharge may be obvious on exam or evident upon "milking" the penis forward. Pain from this procedure is uncommon.

Labs: Urinalysis and culture are indicated. Urine PCR is diagnostic but of limited availability. Culture or Gram stain of discharge may reveal *N gonorrhoeae*.

Urethral DNA probe for *N gonorrhoeae* and *Chlamydia trachomatis* may also be useful as a screening test.

Treatment

Treat with ceftriaxone (Rocephin) or cefixime (Suprax) for gonorrhea and give doxycycline or azithromycin to treat chlamydia. Give metronidazole (Flagyl) for trichomonas, although this is almost always asymptomatic in men.

Always treat both sexual partners.

Screen for other STDs as indicated.

Take Home Points

- Urethritis is most commonly a disease of younger males with an STD.
- Diagnose with a urethral DNA probe, or culture and Gram stain.
- Treat for gonorrhea and chlamydia as indicated.

Orchitis/Epididymitis

Infection and inflammation of the testis and epididymis, respectively. Adjacent structures such as the scrotal wall may show edema and erythema from extension of inflammatory response.

Symptoms

Pain of the testis, which may be localized to the testicle itself or worse on palpation of the epididymis. Erythema, dysuria, pain with ejaculation, and symptoms of bladder outlet obstruction may be present (from accompanying prostatitis). History may reveal recent urologic surgery, prostatitis, UTI, or recent STD.

Diagnosis

Physical exam: Erythematous, tender epididymis may be evident. Epididymitis pain is classically relieved somewhat by elevation although this is not as obvious as in testicular torsion, which must be ruled out.
Labs: Urinalysis and culture. Urethral swab for *N Gonorrhoeae* and *Chlamydia*. CBC, CRP, ESR show signs of infection.
Imaging: Ultrasound may show inflammation and localized infection. Importantly, Doppler US shows normal blood flow.
Causes:

Age < 35 years → *N Gonorrhoeae* and *Chlamydia*
Age > 35 years → Enterobacteria

Treatment

Treat for both gonorrhea and chlamydia if under age 35 or STD suspected:
Age < 35 years ceftriaxone (Rocephin) or cefixime (Suprax) and doxycycline or azithromycin.
Age > 35 years ciprofloxacin or levofloxacin.
Treatment should be for 10–14 days.

Take Home Points

- Orchitis and epididymitis commonly go hand-in-hand.
- Physical exam may reveal tender testicle or epididymis, although this is not as pronounced as in testicular torsion.
- Treat for STDs.

Testicular Torsion

Twisting of the testicle and spermatic cord leading to distal ischemia. Torsion may happen in two ways: Intravaginal torsion occurs with spermatic cord twisting within the tunica vaginalis; extravaginal torsion occurs with the twisting of the testis, spermatic cord, and processus vaginalis.

Symptoms

Acute severe testicular pain. May be referred to the abdomen and cause nausea/vomiting. Typical patients are infants, toddlers, and children. Risk factors may include trauma but most commonly is idiopathic.

Diagnosis

Physical exam: Affected testicle may be high riding and is exquisitely tender. Elevating testis may relieve some pain. Opposite testis may lie horizontally instead of vertically (Angell's sign).

Imaging: Doppler ultrasound may reveal diagnosis by demonstrating absent or decreased blood flow to the effected testis.

Treatment

Immediate referral to urologist for emergency surgical correction.

While waiting, manual reduction may be attempted (although adequate analgesia is needed). Classically, turn the affected testis laterally "like opening a book." Depending on time to correction, the affected testis may be completely salvaged, completely lost, or salvaged but with future low sperm count.

Take Home Points

- Testicular torsion usually occurs in the prepubescent boy.
- Physical exam may reveal an exquisitely tender, high riding testicle.
- Doppler ultrasound is the imaging test of choice.
- Emergently, while awaiting surgical evaluation, manual reduction may be attempted by turning the testis laterally—"like opening a book."

Male Infertility

Inability to conceive a child after 12 months of unprotected intercourse, due to male factors. An estimated 10–15% of couples are said to be infertile by this definition, 20–40% may be due to a male factor. Intrinsic factors include Klinefelter syndrome, hypogonadism, erectile dysfunction, and others.

Diagnosis

Labs: Semen analysis. This should be done twice to confirm if the first test is abnormal. Factors in a semen analysis include:

Measurement of semen volume and pH

Microscopy for debris and agglutination

Assessment of sperm concentration, motility, and morphology

Sperm leukocyte count

Search for immature germ cells

Microscopic exam

Three factors are important, including concentration, motility, and morphology. Concentration is normal with at least 20 million/ml, with 48 million/ml considered fertile (between these values the patient is considered subfertile). Motility is normal if at least 50% are motile and 25% are considered rapidly progressively motile. Morphology is normal if at least 15% are seen as normal.

If the above does not elicit the diagnosis, specialized semen tests may be done and include: Sperm autoantibodies, biochemistry, semen culture, sperm cervical mucus interaction, and a battery of sperm function tests (computer-aided sperm analysis, acrosome reaction, zona-free hamster oocyte penetration test, human zona pellucida binding test, sperm chromatin and DNA assays).

Genetic analysis may be considered and includes sex chromosome and somatic mutations testing.

Evaluate with hormonal testing to include testosterone, LH, FSH to evaluate gonadal and pituitary function.

Treatment

Treatment largely depends on production of some amount of sperm. Otherwise, correction of underlying abnormality must be attempted. In reversible hormone-related dysfunction, treatment may include dopamine agonists for hypoprolactinemia, pulsatile GnRH analogs for pituitary dysfunction, or steroids for autoantibodies. Testosterone injections may be used in hypogonadism.

Surgery may be a viable option to treat varicocele, retrograde ejaculation, and other structural defects.

Assistive reproductive techniques are gaining popularity and effectiveness, including intracytoplasmic sperm injection (ICSI), intrauterine insemination, artificial insemination with donor semen, and in vitro fertilization.

Take Home Points

- By definition, the inability to conceive after 12 months of normal, unprotected intercourse.

- On microscopy, look for concentration, motility, and morphology.

- Treatment depends on abnormality, but strategies may include hormonal manipulation, surgical correction, or assistive reproductive techniques.

Infections and Parasitic Diseases

Scabies

Scabies is an infestation of the skin by the mite *Sarcoptes scabiei* that results in an intensely pruritic eruption occurring commonly in the intertriginous areas, waistline, and interdigital web spaces. This contagious mite transmits easily, especially under crowded conditions where epidemic outbreaks may occur.

Symptoms

Itching and soreness between fingers and toes. Vesicles or papules may be seen, crusting may occur in extensive disease. Often, burrows appear as excoriated areas due to scratching from the intense pruritis.

Diagnosis

Physical exam: Look for burrow tracks between fingers or toes. The "ink trick" is performed by placing a dot of ink from a felt tipped marker over the suspected burrow. After washing the ink from the skin surface, ink absorbed into the burrow track will appear as a dot leading into the skin surface.

Labs: Scrape tracks and look under microscope. Classic picture is of microscopic parasite.

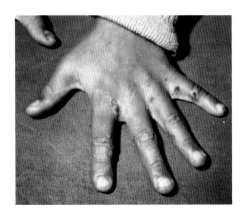

FIGURE 11.1 Scabies papules seen in the typical distribution of hands and finger web spaces. Reprinted with permission from Saxe N, Jessop S, Todd G. *Handbook of Dermatology for Primary Care.* 2007, Oxford University Press.

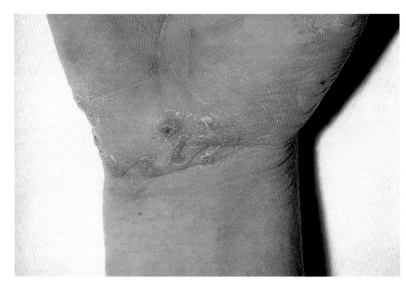

FIGURE 11.2 Scabies involving the flexor aspect of the wrist. Reprinted with permission from MacKie, RM. *Clinical Dermatology*, 5th edition. 2003, Oxford University Press.

Treatment

Permethrin (Elimite, Nix) or crotamiton (Eurax) topical cream applied from the neck to the soles of the feet. This is left on then washed off 12 hours later. Reapplication in one week may be needed. Lindane (Kwell, Scabene) may also be used in this manner but is somewhat more toxic and should not be used in the very young, pregnant, or old. Use precipitated sulfur in pregnant patients and ivermectin (Stromectol) in the immunocompromised.

Diphenhydramine (Benadryl), hydroxyzine, or other antihistamine for itching.

Take Home Points

- Scabies is highly contagious and causes intense pruritis.
- Diagnose with scrapings or the "ink trick."
- The prototypic drug is permethrin topical (Elimite, Nix).

Candidiasis

Candida albicans and related species cause a variety of infections, which manifest as a mucocutaneous or cutaneous rash. These include: candida intertrigo, folliculitis, balanitis, onychomycosis, diaper rash, perianal rash, "yeast infection" vaginal involvement, oral mucous membrane (thrush) involvement, and disseminated disease. Disseminated disease is the most life-threatening form and occurs in the immunocompromised and patients with heme or solid malignancies.

Symptoms

Erythematous, painful, itchy, well-demarcated patches often in the intertriginous areas. Lesions are often moist and malodorous and often reveal classic "satellite lesions."

History may reveal immunocompromised state (or risk factors) or diabetes.

Diagnosis

Usually a clinical diagnosis that can be made by exam. Rash is erythematous which may or may not show classic satellite lesions.

Labs: Skin scrapings may be examined on potassium hydroxide slide. Branching pseudohyphae are pathopneumonic.

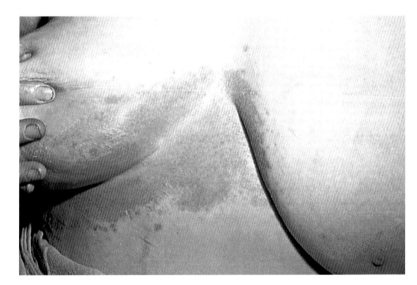

FIGURE 11.3 Infra-mammary candidiasis in a female diabetic patient. Reprinted with permission from MacKie, RM. *Clinical Dermatology,* 5th edition. 2003, Oxford University Press.

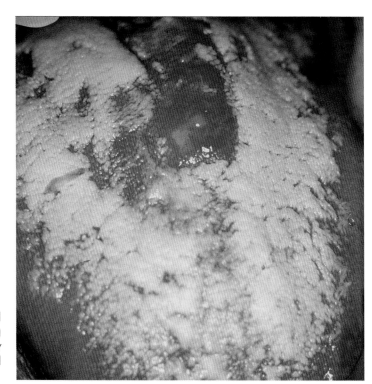

FIGURE 11.4 Oral candidiasis. Reprinted with permission from Humphreys H, Irving WL. *Problem-Oriented Clinical Microbiology and Infection*, 2nd edition. 2004, Oxford University Press.

Treatment

Topical therapy is often effective and includes nystatin (Mycostatin) cream, powder, or in combination with a topical steroid (or may be mixed) to add itch relief. Clotrimazole cream (Lotrimin, Mycelex) or miconazole (Micatin) are second line.

Systemic antifungals for disseminated disease include caspofungin (Cancidas), fluconazole, itraconazole, variconazole, or amphotericin B. At a minimum, liver function tests should be carefully monitored on these medications.

Take Home Points

- Candida is most commonly a superficial mucocutaneous infection, but in the immunocompromised may be disseminated and life threatening.
- Diagnose with scrapings from the rash and examination after prep with KOH.
- Treat with topical nystatin or azoles. Systemic antifungals are reserved for refractory or disseminated disease.

Acne Vulgaris

Acne is caused by the development of four main characteristics within the pilosebaceous follicle, including keratin plug formation, increased sebum production, infection of the follicle complex by *Propionibacterium acnes*, and resulting inflammation.

Symptoms

Open or closed comedones, nodules, papules, or pustules. Scarring may or may not be present.

Diagnosis

Characteristic appearance and history.

Physical exam: Lesions usually on face, forehead, neck, superior back, and anterior chest. Comedones and cystic lesions usually have an erythematous base.

TABLE 11.1 Types of Acne

Type 1	Mainly comedones with occasional small inflamed papules or pustules; common in early adolescence or early teenage years; no scarring is present.
Type 2	Comedones, papules, and pustules (mainly facial) are present; mild scarring may be seen.
Type 3	Numerous comedones, papules, and pustules, which have spread to the back, chest, and shoulders, with occasional cysts or nodules; scarring may be moderate.
Type 4	Numerous large cysts and/or nodules on the face, neck, and upper trunk. Scarring has progressed to severe.

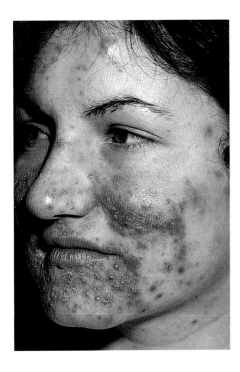

FIGURE 11.5 Moderately severe (type 2) acne vulgaris of the face. Reprinted with permission from MacKie, RM. *Clinical Dermatology*, 5th edition. 2003, Oxford University Press.

Treatment

Treatment should be stepwise. Anecdotal evidence exists that decreasing fat intake and basic daily hygiene shows improvement. Wash face with non oil-based soap at least twice per day.

Topicals

Start with benzoyl peroxide in the morning or at night. Increase to twice per day.

Tretinoin (Retin-A) may be added, starting with cream of lowest concentration and titrating up. Highly effective but has several side effects such as sun sensitivity, reddening, severe drying, and interaction with benzoyl peroxide. These lessen with time so counsel the patient on compliance.

Adaplaene (Differin) cream or gel, tazarotene (Tazorac), or azelaic acid (Azelex) may be tried but have similar side effects as tretinoin.

Antibiotic topicals such as erythromycin (Emgel, EryDerm), clindamycin (Cleocin-T), or metronidazole (Metrogel) may be effective.

Systemic Antibiotics

Systemic antibiotics such as tetracycline, minocycline, doxycycline, erythromycin, or TMP-SMX (Bactrim or Septra) are the next step. Avoid tetracyclines in young children/pregnant patients and counsel that photosensitivity is most common side effect.

Hormonal Treatment

Consider systemic birth control pills for their favorable side effect of reducing acne in women.

Spironolactone may be effective because of anti-androgen properties but watch for side effect of gynocomastia in men.

Flutamide (Eulexin) is an anti-androgen used in prostatic pathology and has been shown somewhat effective for acne, although its hepatotoxicity limits its use.

Oral steroids (prednisone) may decrease moderate inflammatory acne.

Isotretinoin (Accutane)

As a last resort, referral may be considered to dermatology for isotretinoin (Accutane). This medication is very effective, especially against severe, nodulocystic form, but is very teratogenic and has a grave side effect profile. Patients must use at least two methods of birth control and be fully informed about increased rates of cancer and psychiatric disturbances.

All treatments take at least 4 weeks (commonly 6–8 weeks) to show improvement and should not be expected to be immediate.

Take Home Points

- Acne is very common in the peripubertal period and is produced by a combination of mechanical obstruction, hormonal influences, and inflammation/infection with typical bacteria.

- On exam, it's important to classify the type of acne to aid treatment decisions.

- Treatment often starts with topical medications and may progress to systemic drugs if needed. Isotretinoin may be used but careful management is needed.

Onychomycosis

Infection of the nail (commonly toenails) caused by a variety of dermatophytes, but other organisms such as *Candida* and molds also occur. Risk factors include nonbreathable shoes, wool socks, excess moisture, diabetes, immunocompromise, or hyperhidrosis.

Symptoms

Yellow, brittle, thickened nails, usually of the toenails. This is generally a non painful condition and it may spread between nails and to opposite foot or hands.

Diagnosis

Labs: KOH preparation for branching hyphae is sensitive and specific. If negative, yeast culture is available but takes 4–6 weeks and sensitivity only mildly improved.

Biopsy is also characteristic of yeast infection and may be most the sensitive technique but is often unnecessary.

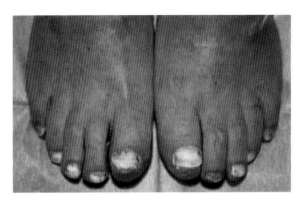

FIGURE 11.6 Thickened, yellowish, irregular toenails in *tinea unguium*. Reprinted with permission from Saxe N, Jessop S, Todd G. *Handbook of Dermatology for Primary Care.* 2007, Oxford University Press.

Treatment

Various topical regimens exist but are widely regarded as ineffective against the vast majority of infections. If used, occlusive dressing and/or keratinolytic preparations may improve outcomes. Topicals include the lacquer ciclopirox (Penlac), or clotrimazole (Lotrimin, Mycelex), terbinafine (Lamisil), tolnaftate (Tinactin), among others.

Long term oral therapies have been the classic treatments and include terbinafine (Lamisil), itraconazole (Sporanox), and fluconazole (Diflucan). Effectiveness varies, with terbinafine (Lamisil) being the best but also most expensive. Drawbacks include treatment duration, which should be 12 weeks or longer. Obtain transaminases and CBC (for platelet count) at baseline and for routine monitoring while on terbinafine or transaminases while on itraconazole. Intervals of monitoring are approximately 4–6 weeks. These medications are contraindicated with pre-existing significant hepatic or renal disease. Have patient abstain from EtOH during therapy.

Surgical excision of nail is an option if infection is isolated to only that nail and this is acceptable to patient.

Take Home Points

- Onychomycosis is usually an infection of the toenails but can spread to fingers.
- Generally, this infection is resistant to topical therapy, necessitating long systemic therapy.

Cellulitis/Erysipelas

Both these infections are caused preferentially by gram positive skin bacteria; the difference being erysipelas is a superficial infection of the superficial dermis/epidermis and lymphatics, while cellulitis also involves the deep dermis and subcutaneous fat layer. Methicillin-resistant *Staphylococcus aureus* (MRSA) is a growing concern and is commonly seen with cellulitis.

Symptoms

Red, erythematous, painful skin area which may contain a central abscess or pustule. Erysipelas tends to appear less focal with a greater surface area involved and well-demarcated borders. A break in the skin is commonly identifiable but is not necessary for diagnosis. Often on extremities, although erysipelas is more common on face.

Diagnosis

Physical exam: Commonly a macular skin area with a reasonably well-demarcated border in both infections, although erysipelas has more defined borders. Area will be tender and warm, although should not significantly constrict movement of the underlying joint. If fluctuance under the skin is apparent, abscess is present. Lymphadenopathy or lymphangitis may be especially in erysipelas.

Labs: WBC may be increased. Culture any expressible fluid from skin breaks. Consider blood cultures as warranted.

Imaging: Unnecessary unless exclusion of septic joint or osteomyelitis is indicated. Ultrasound may reveal underlying fluid collection if abscess is present.

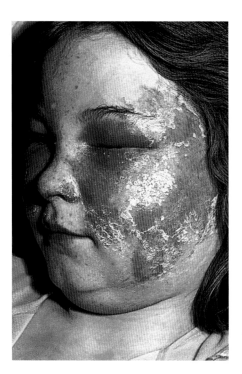

FIGURE 11.7 Erysipelas demonstrating well defined borders and facial location. Reprinted with permission from MacKie, RM. *Clinical Dermatology*, 5th edition. 2003, Oxford University Press.

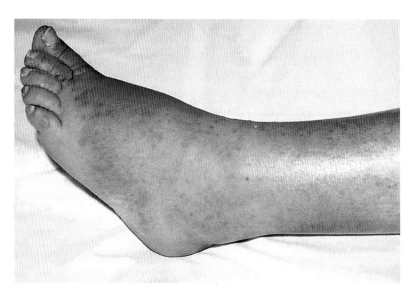

FIGURE 11.8 Cellulitis of lower extremity demonstrating swelling and erythema. Reprinted with permission from MacKie, RM. *Clinical Dermatology*, 5th edition. 2003, Oxford University Press.

Treatment

Clean area and de-roof any scab or skin break to evaluate for underlying abscess.

Oral antibiotics active against Gram-positive bacteria are highly effective and may be used on an outpatient basis as first line. Use dicloxacillin, cephalexin (Keflex), TMP-SMX (Bactrim DS, Septra DS), erythromycin, or clindamycin.

Admission should be considered for toxic-appearing children, presence of sepsis, facial cellulitis, poor follow up is likely, or suspicion of osteomyelitis is present.

Inpatient management should include an IV regimen of penicillin G, nafcillin, clindamycin, cefozolin, or vancomycin for empiric therapy. If MRSA prevalence is high in the local area, consider more than one antibiotic such as IV or PO clindamycin and PO TMP-SMX (Bactrim DS, Septra DS). Vancomycin is also effective against MRSA but requires good kidney function and has its own resistance patterns. New medications illustrate the ongoing problem of bacterial resistance development to antibiotics.

Take Home Points

- MRSA is now a common cause of cellulitis and erysipelas.
- Give antibiotics with good Gram-positive activity.

Skin Abscess

Formation of local fluctuant mass which occurs due to a point inoculation, commonly with Gram-positive skin bacteria such as *Strep* and *Staph* sp. This infection is then recognized and "walled off" by the body which acts to contain the infection as well as starving it from a blood supply. For this reason, antibiotics are ineffective.

Symptoms

Usually focally and exquisitely tender area of the skin which may be surrounded by cellulitis or erysipelas. This area also demonstrates erythema, nonpitting edema, warmth, and possibly drainage. De-roofing of the scab or opening of the skin break may demonstrate pus or fluid drainage. Gentle pressure may be needed. History may reveal use of IV street drugs, prior skin break, or superficial injury.

Diagnosis

Usually a clinical diagnosis by physical exam findings such as fluctuance, erythema, focal tenderness, and/or drainage. If no obvious skin break is detected, needle aspiration may be used and can distinguish an abscess from other cystic structures.

Lab: Culture all fluids from the abscess. Blood cultures are warranted as well but are often negative unless sepsis is present.

Imaging: Ultrasound may be useful in demonstrating fluid-filled pocket under the skin.

If IV drug user, consider HIV or drug screen.

Treatment

"The only way to treat an abscess is to cut an abscess." Incision and drainage is the standard of care, although antibiotics are warranted for any accompanying skin infection (see cellulitis/erysipelas). Once drained, break up cavitary loculations with a sterile instrument and pack with sterile packing (Iodoform gauze). Change/repack daily or 2x/day until healed. Packing ensures further fluid won't accumulate and healing will occur from the inside wall of the abscess.

Take Home Points

- Abscess is commonly caused by the same skin organisms causing cellulitis/erysipelas.
- The only way to treat an abscess is to cut an abscess.

Folliculitis

Folliculitis is a superficial infection of hair follicles. In contrast, carbuncles are collections of multiple infected hair follicles in close proximity. Further, a furuncle is an infection of the hair follicle that extends into the deeper dermis where a small, punctate abscess forms. The most common bacteria involved are *Staph aureus*, although fungal infections may occur comorbidly and *Pseudomonas* is involved in the clinical syndrome of "hot tub folliculitis."

Symptoms

Often occurring in groups, lesions may generally be < 5 mm diameter, pruritic, erythematous, tender, and with the central protrusion of the hair shaft. Lesions may occur in bathing suit distribution in "hot tub folliculitis."

Diagnosis

Culture of expressible fluid is usually not necessary but may reveal group A *Strep*, *S aureus*, or *Pseudomonas*.

Treatment

Warm compresses improve healing and help resolution.

Topical mupirocin (Bactroban) may be used and is usually sufficient therapy.

In more severe cases, give cephalexin (Keflex), erythromycin, or dicloxicillin.

Recurrent folliculitis often indicates carrier state which is most commonly in the anterior nares. Treat with mupirocin (Bactroban) topical, 3x/day for five days, every month for two months, to reduce outbreaks.

Hot tub folliculitis is usually self limited and systemic antibiotics do not shorten course.

Take Home Points

- Folliculitis is an infection of the superficial hair follicle.
- Gram-positive bacteria are the causative agent except in "hot tub folliculitis" caused by *Pseudomonas*.
- Topical mupirocin is usually effective.

Impetigo

A superficial skin infection caused mainly by *S aureus* or *Strep* species. This infection spreads readily and may be worse in young children or those with preexisting skin conditions (e.g. psoriasis). Variants include a bullous form in which large fluid-filled bullae form and often rupture, leaving extensive crusting.

Symptoms

Classic "honey crusted" appearance of grouped lesions with mild surrounding erythema. Brief history of a tender, vesicular stage before rupture and crusting is usual. Often lesions are tender but generally nonpurulent. Distribution, especially in the young, is often around mouth, lower face, and on fingers/hands.

Diagnosis

Clinical diagnosis by typical appearance.

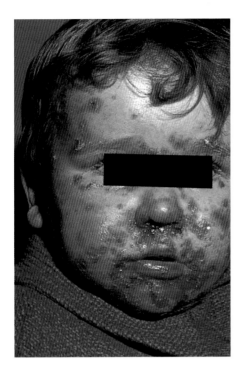

FIGURE 11.9 Classic impetigo. Reprinted with permission from MacKie, RM. *Clinical Dermatology*, 5th edition. 2003, Oxford University Press.

Treatment

Topical treatment with mupirocin (Bactroban) is often adequate for mild to moderate disease. Consider systemic antibiotics for the very young, severe cases, or bullous form. PO regimens include dicloxacillin, erythromycin, and cephalexin (Keflex).

Cover or dress affected areas to keep children from scratching and autoinfecting other body parts.

Take Home Points

- Impetigo is commonly caused by *S aureus* and *Strep* species.
- Impetigo is not an infection of the hair follicle as in folliculitis and is not as deep as erysipelas or cellulitis.

Viral Warts (Human Papilloma Virus)

Warts are a localized viral infection caused by the HPV virus, of which over 100 different serotypes exist. A common infectious site is on the hands and fingers during childhood, during which time most will develop immunity toward the virus. However, that immunity does not extend to other serotypes, thus, further infection may occur. Once the virus is present, treatment methods ultimately succeed only if there is an immune response against the virus and the immune identification of the particular viral serotype occurs.

Symptoms

Nonerythematous skin-colored or slightly hyperpigmented nodules. Often occur on hands, plantar surface of feet, genitals, or practically anywhere on the body. Caused by various serotypes of HPV.

Diagnosis

Physical exam: Verrucous appearance. Plantar warts have characteristic "black dots" in the lesion itself which consist of capillaries induced by the virus.

Labs: Biopsy often not needed.

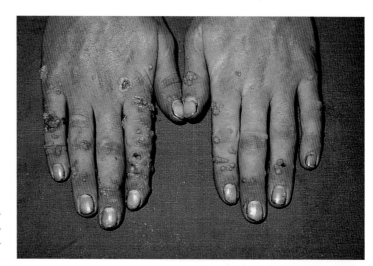

FIGURE 11.10 Multiple warts on hands. Reprinted with permission from MacKie, RM. *Clinical Dermatology*, 5th edition. 2003, Oxford University Press.

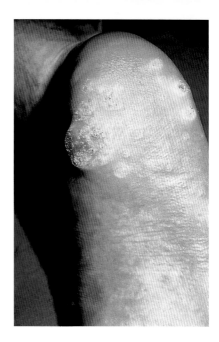

FIGURE 11.11 Extensive plantar warts. Reprinted with permission from MacKie, RM. *Clinical Dermatology*, 5th edition. 2003, Oxford University Press.

Treatment

Various treatments and topicals exist. Vaccination is recommended to avoid certain subtypes that cause warts.

In-office procedures include paring the lesion down with a scalpel or razor, then applying electrocautery, laser desiccation, or cryotherapy. Have the patient return every week until lesion is cured. Some laser treatments also exist for stubborn plantar warts.

Cryotherapy technique: Particularly on plantar warts, paring down of the lesion should be done before application. Application of liquid nitrogen with a mist-forming device is the most effective method to cause a sharp temperature drop. Focus the mist to avoid a large freeze diameter with the use of an otoscope cover or small spurts of mist. Application of nitrogen should be for 5–10 seconds. Allow to thaw completely. Repeat freeze/thaw cycles 3–4 times. Each cycle should be less painful for the patient as superficial cutaneous nerves are destroyed.

Medications include salicylic acid 40% topical, trichloroacetic acid (Tri-Chlor), imiquimod (Aldara). In severe cases, poldophyllin topical or bleomycin injection may be used. Topicals take on the order of months so don't expect quick results!

Take Home Points

- Viral warts occur due to one of the over 100 serotypes of the HPV virus although serotype tropisms do occur.

- Treatments with local cyrotherapy, laser, or electrocautery are all effective with cryotherapy most widely used. Topical medications may be better tolerated for venereal form.

Cutaneous Squamous Cell Carcinoma

This common cutaneous tumor originates from epithelial cells arising from keratinocytes preferentially in a sun-exposed distribution. Risk factors include older age, male gender, sunlight exposure, fair skinned ancestry, and tendency to sunburn rather than tan. Metastasis is rare.

Symptoms

Small, usually isolated lesions occur in sun-exposed areas and consist of exophytic nodules which are commonly scaly, red, crusting, and occasionally bleed and become tender. Patient may have previously been treated or diagnosed with **actinic keratosis**.

Diagnosis

Characteristic appearance: Biopsy shows abnormal, cancerous cells all the way to the dermis.

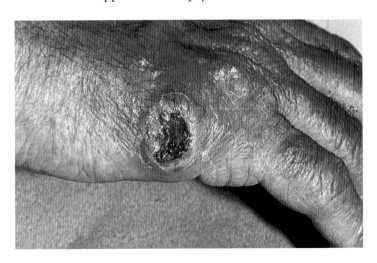

FIGURE 11.12 Invasive squamous carcinoma. Reprinted with permission from MacKie, RM. *Clinical Dermatology*, 5th edition. 2003, Oxford University Press.

Treatment

Prevention is the key. Use high SPF rated sunscreens with UVA and UVB light protection.

In treating this carcinoma, assessment of risk of malignancy for suspicious lesions can be taken into account.

Surgery is the best treatment for most lesions or those that occur in sensitive sites such as around the mouth, ear, or genitals. Surgical excision may be done in conjunction with biopsy of lesions with high initial malignancy suspicion but care must be taken to include the whole lesion within the margins of the biopsy.

Mohs micrographic surgery is another option for skin cancer and involves specialty surgery referral. Indications include recurrent lesion, ill-defined borders, underlying tissue involvement, multiple clumped lesions, or lesion in prior radiation-exposed areas.

Other techniques such as cryosurgery, electrodessication, topical 5-FU, and other topicals exist but should only be used for low-risk lesions.

Radiation therapy may be used for those lesions that involve cosmetically sensitive areas *and* are low risk. Side effects, however, do exist which may be intolerable to the patient.

Take Home Points

- Cutaneous SCC is common in sun-exposed areas of the elderly and suspicious lesions should always be biopsied.
- Actinic keratosis is a premalignant lesion associated with SCC.

Basal Cell Carcinoma

This most common form of skin cancer originates in the basal cells and their appendages. Risk factors are similar to SCC and include: chronic sun exposure, outdoor occupation, advanced age, light complexion, tendency to sunburn instead of tan, male gender, and family history of skin cancer. Metastasis is rare.

Symptoms

Often occurs in sun exposed areas and on the face, it appears like a small nodule or papule with translucent covering or ulceration, commonly with overlying telangiectasias. May have pearly white areas and bleed without healing. Central ulceration may occur in larger lesions contributing to the nickname of "rodent ulcers."

Diagnosis

Characteristic appearance on exam.
Biopsy is mandatory.

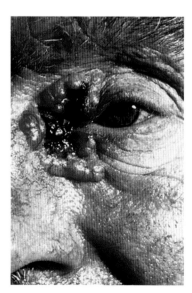

FIGURE 11.13 Basal cell carcinoma of left peri-nasal region. Reprinted with permission from MacKie, RM. *Clinical Dermatology*, 5th edition. 2003, Oxford University Press.

Treatment

Biopsy results, location, age, and cosmetic outcome must be taken into account when choosing treatment.
  Options include electrodessication, cryotherapy, local radiation, and surgical excision.
  Mohs micrographic surgery is an option but involves specialty surgery referral.

Take Home Points

- Characteristics including causes, risk factors, treatment, and metastatic potential are similar to SCC (although appearance is not).

- These lesions commonly occur on the head and neck.

Malignant Melanoma

Melanoma is the most aggressive skin cancer and may occur anywhere on the body, although sun-exposed areas are at higher risk. Growth generally occurs in nondiscrete stages, including a superficial or radial growth phase in which the lesion grows horizontally on the skin followed by the vertical or invasive growth phase that leads to invasion of the underlying skin and structures. Types of disease include superficial spreading, nodular, lentigo maligna, and acral lentiginous melanoma. Metastasis usually occurs by lymphatic spread.

Symptoms

May be asymptomatic for years, hence the opportunity for lethal metastasis. Otherwise lesions are usually discrete and occur in sun-exposed areas.

Diagnosis

Physical exam: Look for border irregularity, asymmetric shape, variegated color throughout the lesion, elevation above the skin surface, and large diameter (> 6 mm).

Biopsy any suspicious lesion all the way to the subcutaneous fat since grading/staging depends on depth. If this is not done, the patient is left with an incredible prognostic problem leading to the worst case scenario for treatment!

Staging is done by use of the American Joint Commission on Cancer Staging (AJCC) system to provide a pathologic stage in the TNM style of staging. This pathologic stage is based on the classification of the lesion according to one of two systems for microstaging: **Breslow's,** which classifies based on depth of invasion in millimeters; and **Clark's,** which classifies based on anatomic skin level. Prognosis is worse the higher the pathologic stage.

Evaluate for metastatic spread to other systems with appropriate imaging. Melanoma spreads almost everywhere.

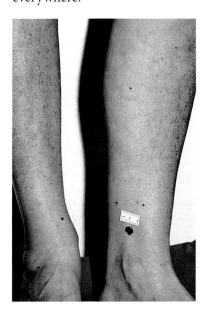

FIGURE 11.14 Superficial spreading melanoma. Reprinted with permission from MacKie, RM. *Clinical Dermatology*, 5th edition. 2003, Oxford University Press.

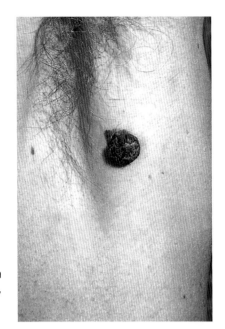

FIGURE 11.15 Nodular melanoma of left axilla. Reprinted with permission from MacKie, RM. *Clinical Dermatology*, 5th edition. 2003, Oxford University Press.

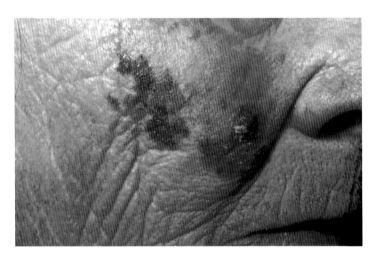

FIGURE 11.16 Lentigo maligna melanoma. Reprinted with permission from MacKie, RM. *Clinical Dermatology*, 5th edition. 2003, Oxford University Press.

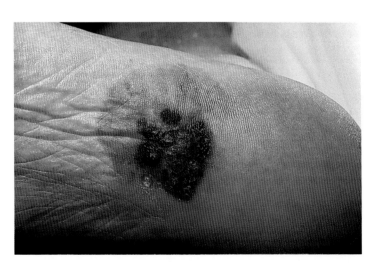

FIGURE 11.17 Acral lentiginous melanoma. Reprinted with permission from MacKie, RM. *Clinical Dermatology*, 5th edition. 2003, Oxford University Press.

Treatment

Surgical excision is the treatment in all cases. Surgery should include a wide margin to assure nondysplastic cells at the edges, horizontal and vertical amount of margin is still in debate. Sentinel lymph node biopsy is sometimes done with or without regional lymph node dissection.

For high stage or metastatic disease, radiation and chemotherapy are both effective.

After treatment, surveillance measures include weekly patient skin checks, physician-conducted skin checks every 3–6 months, and yearly chest x-rays.

Take Home Points

- Except for nodular melanoma, this malignancy starts with a superficial growth phase followed by vertical invasion.

- If melanoma is suspected before biopsy, biopsy should be carefully taken to ensure adequate depth is sampled.

- Treat and diagnose with excisional biopsy. If positive, further investigate possible metastasis.

Benign Skin Lesions

TABLE 11.2 Benign Skin Lesions

Lesion	Appearance/Associations	Treatment
Actinic keratosis	Associated with aging; appear very scaly, rough, and non painful. Conversion to squamous cell cancer uncommon but possible.	Cryotherapy, electrodesiccation, laser therapy, dermabrasion, or trichloroacetic acid topical. Biopsy if not clinically obvious to exclude malignancy.
Seborrheic keratosis	"Stuck on" appearance of elevated nodule. Brown color and rough feel. Clinically appears similar to basal cell cancers.	Cryotherapy, electrodesiccation, shave biopsy, or topical trichloroacetic acid.
Hypertrophic scar formation (keloid)	More common in dark-skinned individuals. Complication of late healing phase in susceptible persons.	Steroid injection, radiation therapy, dermabrasion, pressure dressings, or surgical removal and debulking. Recurrence is common.
Acrochordons (skin tags)	Small, often pedunculated, skin-colored lesions usually on opposing surfaces of skin such as under breasts, between legs, and axilla. Often also occur on lateral neck.	Cryotherapy, shave biopsy, electrodessication.
Keratocanthoma	Usually rapid onset, flesh-colored lesion with eventual central depression exhibiting plug of kertatinous material. Clinical appearance is similar to squamous cell cancer but this lesion has no malignant potential.	Excisional biopsy is most common but 5-FU or steroid injection may also be effective with better cosmesis. Eventual involution often occurs.
Lipoma	Subcutaneous rubbery mass that feels unattached to the overlying skin. Literally a benign fat cell tumor often occurring in the subcutaneous layer.	Surgical removal. Recurrence is common so repeat surgery may be needed.
Pyogenic granuloma	Usually rapidly growing, often pedunculated mass which is characteristically friable with frequent bleeding. May occur on extremities after minor skin trauma. Often occur in pregnancy.	Surgical excision, electrocautery, or cryotherapy are the usual treatments.

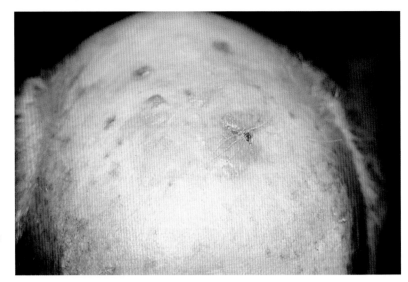

FIGURE 11.18 Actinic keratoses on scalp. Reprinted with permission from MacKie, RM. *Clinical Dermatology*, 5th edition. 2003, Oxford University Press.

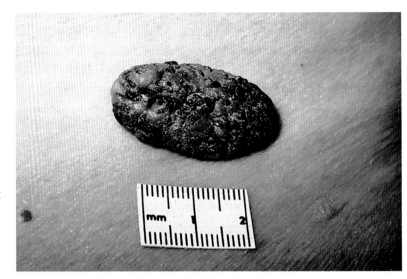

FIGURE 11.19 Classic seborrheic keratosis with "stuck on" appearance. Reprinted with permission from MacKie, RM. *Clinical Dermatology*, 5th edition. 2003, Oxford University Press.

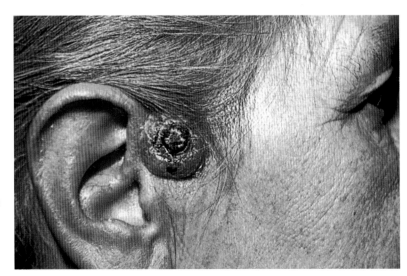

FIGURE 11.20 Keratocanthoma of the right peri-aural skin. Reprinted with permission from MacKie, RM. *Clinical Dermatology*, 5th edition. 2003, Oxford University Press.

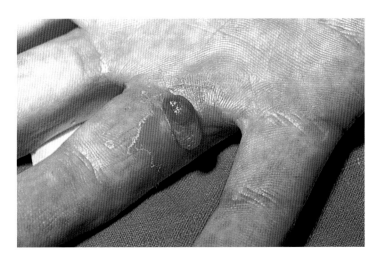

FIGURE 11.21 Pyogenic granuloma of finger. Reprinted with permission from MacKie, RM. *Clinical Dermatology*, 5th edition. 2003, Oxford University Press.

DERMATOLOGY

Atopic Dermatitis (Eczema)

A chronic and extremely itchy dermatitis with a strong genetic component, this disease commonly begins in infancy or early childhood and is frequently associated with asthma and rhinitis (atopic triad = eczema, asthma, rhinitis).

Symptoms

Pruritis is the most common and recognizable symptom. Lesions commonly appear as reddened, scaly, dry plaques which are first reported as extremely itchy. Lichenification of lesions commonly follows outbreaks, especially in the older child or adults.

Diagnosis

Physical exam: Distribution of dry, itchy plaques is a major clue to etiology. Infants are often affected by plaques on the cheeks, scalp, extensor aspects of extremities, and face (sparing the nasolabial folds) although lesions may appear crusted, exudative, or involve blisters. In older children and adults, less exudation is seen and lesions often demonstrate lichenified plaques in a **flexural** distribution, such as of the antecubital and popliteal fossae, volar aspect of the wrists, ankles, and neck. In adults or especially severe cases, any aspect of the skin may be affected.

The most validated clinical definition for atopic dermatitis is from The United Kingdom Working Party Diagnostic Criteria:

TABLE 11.3 The U.K. Working Party Criteria for Atopic Dermatitis

Presence of:	An itchy skin condition within the past year
PLUS three of the following	History of flexural involvement
	History of asthma/hay fever (or a history of atopic disease in first degree relatives if child < 4 years old)
	History of generalized dry skin within the past year
	Onset of rash under the age of 2 years (this criterion not used for children < 4 years old)
	Visible flexural dermatitis at the time of presentation

Adapted from Williams, HC, Burney, PGJ, Pembroke, AC, Hay, RJ, on Behalf of the U.K. Diagnostic Criteria for Atopic Dermatitis Working Party: Validation of the U.K. diagnostic criteria for atopic dermatitis in a population setting. *Br J Dermatol* 1996, 135:12-17.

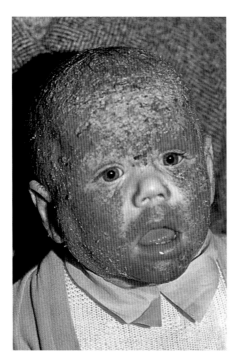

FIGURE 11.22 Atopic dermatitis in infancy. The face and scalp are often affected in young children, and relative sparing of the perioral and nasal region is common as seen here. Reprinted with permission from MacKie, RM. *Clinical Dermatology*, 5th edition. 2003, Oxford University Press.

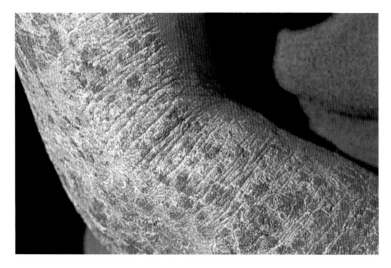

FIGURE 11.23 Severe atopic dermatitis in an adult. Note gross lichenification and superimposed excoriations. Reprinted with permission from MacKie, RM. *Clinical Dermatology*, 5th edition. 2003, Oxford University Press.

Treatment

General measures for treatment can help with maintenance of disease and include: Treating bacterial colonization with antibiotics if infection is present, reduce stress and anxiety, use antihistamines for sedation and control of itch while sleeping, and avoiding trigger factors such as heat, perspiration, and low humidity.

Topical prevention with emollients after bathing is a mainstay of prevention of outbreaks. These trap skin moisture in and avoid common recurrences.

The mainstay of treatment of active skin lesions are topical steroids. Potency level should be matched to the clinical severity of disease.

Examples are shown in Table 11.4.

TABLE 11.4 Topical Steroid Examples and Classification

Topical Steroid Potency	Examples	Group Classification
Low potency	Hydrocortisone 1%, 2.5% cream; fluocinolone 0.01% cream	IV
Medium potency	Fluocinolone 0.025 % cream/ointment; hydrocortisone (Westcort) 0.2% cream/ointment; triamcinolone 0.1 % cream/ointment	III
High potency	Amcinonide 0.1% cream/ointment; fluocinonide 0.05% cream/ointment/gel; triamcinolone 0.5% cream/ointment	II
Very high potency	Clobetasol 0.05% cream/ointment; halobetasol 0.05% cream/ointment	I

Limit use of corticosteroids for extended periods of time (due to striae, telangiectasias, and skin atrophy), use on the face, or high potency on those patients < 2 years old.

Other topical agents include tacrolimus (Protopic) and pimecrolimus (Elidel) which provide a good alternative to topical steroids. However, these agents have been linked to rare malignancies.

Oral steroids have shown good effect for short term, abortive use in acute outbreaks.

Other oral immunomodulatory medications such as cyclosporine and interferon gamma have shown good effect but only for severe cases. Use of these agents should be limited in duration and to select cases.

Other therapies, including UVA/UVB light therapy, have shown positive results but rebound flare ups after cessation may be limiting.

Take Home Points

- An itchy, dry skin rash on the flexoral surfaces of a child is most commonly eczema.
- Children comprise the majority of cases and patients commonly "outgrow" the disease.
- Corticosteroids are the mainstay for acute flairs although other topical are also effective.

Psoriasis

An inherited, autoimmune disorder caused by shortening of the keratinocyte cell cycle resulting in hyperproliferation of keratinocytes in epidermal skin. Ongoing research points toward a derangement of T lymphocyte function although exact etiology remains unclear. This disease tends to manifest as silvery, scaly, erythematous plaques occurring in preferential sites on the body according to type. Types include: discoid or plaque form, guttate, pustular, inverse-flexural, erythroderma, and ostraceous. Involvement of joints causing arthritis or the presence of other autoimmune disorders is not uncommon.

Symptoms

Patients present with intermittent **silvery, scaly**, erythematous, well-demarcated, ovoid or circinate patches or plaques. Sometimes these are pruritic and may occur on the scalp, knees, nails, extensor surfaces of extremities, elbows, eyebrows, sacral area, buttocks, penis, axillae, umbilicus, or more rarely, may be generalized. Family history may be positive for psoriasis or other immunologic abnormality. Flares may occur after direct skin injury (Koebner phenomenon), use of antimalarial agents, β-blockers, and lithium. Other medications may make existing disease worse including ACE-Is, NSAIDs, tetracycline, amiodarone, salicylates, and penicillins.

Diagnosis

Physical exam: Scaly, silvery, flaking patch or plaques as described above. Nails may show stippling, pitting, and onycholysis which resembles onychomycosis.

Clinical diagnosis is usually adequate.

Biopsy is rarely indicated and exhibits immune involvement and characteristic appearance.

Labs: Fungal studies may or may not reveal overlying fungal infection, rheumatoid factor should be negative, leukocytosis and increased ESR may be present in acute flair, rarely anemia with vitamin B12/folate or iron deficiency is present.

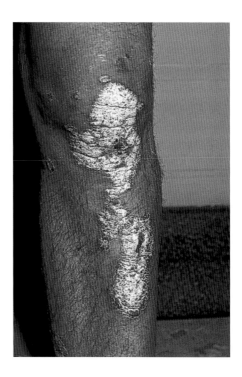

FIGURE 11.24 Typical appearance of psoriasis vulgaris occurring on the leg. Reprinted with permission from MacKie, RM. *Clinical Dermatology*, 5th edition. 2003, Oxford University Press.

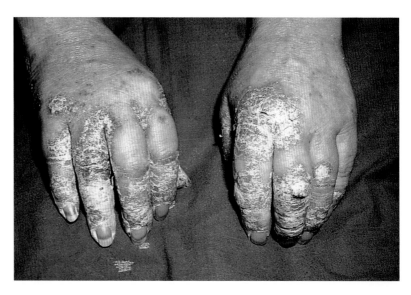

FIGURE 11.25 Severe psoriasis of the hands with associated nail involvement. Reprinted with permission from MacKie, RM. *Clinical Dermatology*, 5th edition. 2003, Oxford University Press.

Treatment

Sun exposure and UVA/UVB phototherapy is commonly used with good results mainly in generalized disease. Add Psoralen plus ultraviolet A (PUVA) for additional efficacy.

Topical moisturizers and occlusive dressings that are aimed at decreasing dryness are effective.

Topicals such as corticosteroids, coal tar solutions, retinoids such as tazarotene (Tazorac) and calcipotriene (Dovonex), or topical immunomodulators such as tacrolimus (Protopic), anthralin, or pimecrolimus (Elidel) may be used for mild-moderate disease.

For generalized or severe disease, methotrexate (classic), cyclosporine, or newer systemic immune modulating therapies such as alefacept (Amevive), efalizumab (Raptiva), or etanercept (Enbrel).

Refer to dermatology as needed.

Take Home Points

- Psoriasis is an inherited, autoimmune, hyperproliferation of the skin cells in which T lymphocytes likely play a central role.
- Treat with light therapy (as opposed to other autoimmune rashes which may be made worse by sun exposure).
- Corticosteroids are the mainstay for acute flairs although other topicals are also effective.

Neurofibromatosis

The disorder of neurofibromatosis is the most common of the neurocutaneous syndromes and has two types. These types are both autosomal dominantly inherited, although the causative gene loci have been shown to occur on two separate chromosomes.

Type I: Von Recklinghausen disease
Type II: Bilateral acoustic neurofibromatosis

Symptoms/Diagnosis

Symptoms vary depending on type. Family history is often positive for autosomal dominant inheritance in either type.

Type I:

- **Café-au-lait macules** (≥ 6 if prepubertal, ≥ 15 if adult) measuring 5 mm or more
- Two or more **neurofibromas**
- Axillary or inguinal freckling
- Two or more Lisch nodules of the eye (hamartomas of the iris)
- Optic glioma
- Characteristic osseous lesions: (long bone cortical thinning, mild scoliosis)
- First degree relative with NF1

Also may be associated with learning disabilities or ADHD.

Imaging: Obtain screening plain films of spine, long bones, skull. Obtain MRI of brain including optic nerves and spine.

Examine retina with slit lamp.

Type II:

- Bilateral acoustic/vestibular schwannomas
- Family history of NF 2
- Family history of neurofibroma, meningioma, glioma, or unilateral schwannoma

Imaging: MRI of the brain.

Consider brainstem auditory evoked response (BAER) with audiologic evaluation.

Treatment

Type I:

- General outpatient follow up with symptomatic control as needed.
- Referral to neurosurgeon for complications of CNS tumor or glioma.
- Consider psychological referral for learning disability if present.
- Referral to neurosurgery/orthopedic surgery for scoliosis as needed.

Type II:

- Annual exams including neurologic, ophthalmologic, and audiologic.
- Hearing aids as needed.
- Speech therapy as needed.
- Neurosurgery evaluation for any CNS tumors.

Families with either type will benefit from genetic counseling.

Take Home Points

- Although named similarly, these two disorders are distinct in genetics and presentation.

12 Orthopedics and Rheumatology

Paget Disease of the Bone (Osteitis Deformans)

A local or generalized inflammatory bone disorder characterized by a high rate of bone turnover with resultant weakened structure which is, characteristically, highly vascularized. Etiology remains unclear although a viral cause is the most accepted theory. Comorbid conditions include high output heart failure, osteosarcoma, and mechanical hearing loss/deafness.

Symptoms

This disease is most commonly asymptomatic but patients characteristically complain of bone pain and deformity in certain areas such as the spine, skull, pelvis, and femur (classically, they complain of hat size increasing). Because of disordered bone structure, fractures may be frequent and disfiguring, leading to bowing of the legs or kyphosis. Neurologic (including cranial nerve) symptoms may arise from compression of nerve roots.

Diagnosis

Physical exam: Long bone bowing, kyphosis, or focal bone enlargement may be evident on exam. Classically, this is seen as "frontal bossing" of the skull.
Labs: Alkaline phosphatase is characteristically increased. N and C telepeptide and urinary pyridinoline are special labs that are increased in Paget disease. Serum calcium and phosphate are normal.
Imaging: Bone scan shows increased uptake in focal patterns and is the single best imaging test.
Plain x-ray: Characteristic skull pattern of disease "osteoporosis circumscripta" shows scattered areas of hyperlucency in a "moth-eaten" type pattern. Otherwise, focal areas of callus and hyperlucency may be evident. Osteosarcoma may rarely be seen.

Treatment

Treatment is aimed at suppressing osteoclastic activity.

Bisphosphonates such as etidronate (Didronel), alendronate (Fosamax), zoledronic acid (Reclast), risedronate (Actonel), and pamidronate (Aredia) are effective and may be given in several forms in many different regimens.

Salmon or human calcitonin is also commonly used.

Treat bone pain preferentially with NSAIDs and acetaminophen.

Refer to orthopedic surgery for fractures, tumors, or nerve compression as needed.

Take Home Points

- Most Paget disease is asymptomatic, but look for bone bowing, fractures, and pain.
- Alkaline phosphatase combined with normal calcium should raise suspicion for Paget disease.
- Look for the characteristic "moth-eaten" skull on x-ray.

Systemic Lupus Erythematosus

A multi-system autoimmune disease with a fluctuating and chronic course. Etiology is due to multiple autoantibodies being produced against various native antigens which either may have a direct effect or deposit bound complexes within tissues. This disease may be seen in any race but occurs more often in women and those of African descent.

TABLE 12.1 Symptoms of Lupus

System	Symptoms
Constitutional	Fatigue, fever, weight loss
Skin	Malar (Butterfly) rash, photosensitive rash, alopecia, mucous membrane lesions, Raynaud phenomenon, purpura, urtcaria
Musculoskeletal	Arthritis (multiple joints), arthralgia, myositis
Renal	Hematuria, proteinuria, cellular casts
Hematologic	Anemia, thrombocytopenia, leucopenia
Lymph	Lymphadenopathy, splenomegaly
Neurological	Seizures, transverse myelitis, cranial neuropathies, peripheral neuropathies
Psychiatric	Psychosis, depression, anxiety
Gastrointestinal	Nausea, vomiting, abdominal pain, peritonitis
Cardiac	Pericarditis, endocarditis, myocarditis, pericardial effusion

Symptoms

Diagnosis

Diagnosis is based on a combination of signs/symptoms and laboratory testing. The following are the criteria from the American College of Rheumatology. SLE diagnosis needs **4 of the 11** criteria during any period of observation.

TABLE 12.2 Criteria for Lupus

Criteria	Description
1. Malar rash	Rash on face in "butterfly" pattern, sparring the nasolabial folds.
2. Discoid rash	Erythematous, raised patches with scaling and follicular plugging. Scarring possibly present.
3. Photosensitivity	Skin rash made worse by sun exposure.
4. Oral ulcers	Painless oral or pharyngeal ulcers.
5. Arthritis	Nonerosive, swollen, tender joints. Two or more in peripheral areas.
6. Serositis	Pleuritic chest pain, pleural rub, or pleural effusion. Pericarditis, pericardial effusion, EKG changes, or cardiac rub.
7. Renal disorder	Proteinuria > 500 mg per 24 hours or > 3+ on dipstick. Cellular casts in urine.
8. Neurologic disorder	Seizures or psychosis in the absence of other reason for either.
9. Hematologic disorder	Hemolytic anemia, reticulocytosis, or leukopenia, lymphopenia, or thrombocytopenia on two or more occasions.
10. Immunologic disorder	Anti-dsDNA, anti-SM, anti phospholipids antibody as measured by anti-cardiolipin antibody IgG and IgM. Presence of lupus anticoagulant. False-positive testing for syphilis (VDRL).
11. ANA	Anti-nuclear antibody titer positive.

Summarized from Hochberg, MC. Arthritis Rheum 1997; 40(9):1725.

In addition, ESR will likely be elevated.

Treatment

Sunscreen and UV light avoidance for those who are photosensitive.

Skin manifestations respond well to topical (intermediate-high strength) glucocorticoids.

Mild disease, arthralgias, mild fevers, etc, may respond well to NSAIDs. A short course of glucocorticoids is commonly clinically indicated although no specific evidence has shown benefit.

Antimalarials, classically hydroxychloroquine (Plaquenil), are the next step for mild-moderate disease. In practice, several antimalarial regimens have shown good response.

Systemic corticosteroids are indicated for more serious, multiorgan disease. Prompt initiation may prevent irreversible damage to the kidneys and liver. Admission and high dose IV corticosteroids may be indicated.

Other immunomodulating medications may be added if disease is thought to be severe or progressive. These include cyclophosphamide (Cytoxan), methotrexate (Trexall), chlorambucil (Leukeran), cyclosporine (Gengraf), or nitrogen mustard. Use of these medications should only be attempted with guidance of a rheumatologist.

IVIG may be helpful in those with severe thrombocytopenia.

If steroids are used, minimize dose and length of therapy to avoid steroid-associated side effects.

Some medications such as hydralazine and procainamide may produce a secondary SLE syndrome that resolves on their discontinuation.

Remember to vaccinate and refer for routine ophthalmologic exams.

Take Home Points

- Any organ system may be affected by SLE.
- Four of 11 criteria must be present to diagnosis SLE.
- Management consists of antimalarials, immunomodulators, and steroids.

Rheumatoid Arthritis (RA)

A chronic systemic inflammatory disease that most commonly involves joints but may affect any system of the body. The arthritis is symmetrical and may be remitting, but uncontrolled disease leads to destruction of joints from focal erosion of cartilage and bone, leading to deformity. HLA-DR4 antigen is highly correlated with RA.

Symptoms

Pain, morning stiffness, deformity, heat, and resistance to motion occurs in multiple joints including shoulders, wrists, knees, elbows, ankles, feet, and subtalar joints. Deformity of especially the hands is often noticed in later stages. Systemic symptoms may be present as well and include fatigue, depression, malaise, anorexia, rheumatoid nodules, and entrapment neuropathies.

Comorbid conditions include **atlantoaxial joint subluxation**, carpal tunnel syndrome, Baker's cyst rupture, episcleritis, Sjögren syndrome, pulmonary fibrosis, hepatosplenomegaly, Hashimoto thyroiditis, pleuritis, lung nodules, pericarditis, and myocarditis.

Diagnosis

Physical exam: Inflamed, stiff joints especially in the hands. In later stages, classic hand deformities show MCP (metacarpophalangeal) and PIP (proximal interphalangeal) joint involvement, producing **"swan-neck"** finger deformity, "Boutonnière's deformity," ulnar deviation of the fingers, and **sparing of the DIP joints**.

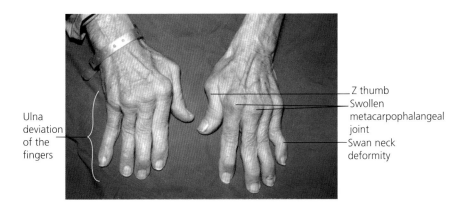

Ulna
deviation
of the
fingers

Z thumb
Swollen
metacarpophalangeal
joint
Swan neck
deformity

FIGURE 12.1 Rheumatoid arthritis of the hands. Note relative sparring of the DIP joints. Reprinted with permission from Cox NLT, Roper TA. *Clinical Skills.* 2005, Oxford University Press.

Diagnosis is made by combination of history, physical exam, x-ray, and laboratory results.

The following are the criteria from the American College of Rheumatology.

TABLE 12.3 Criteria for Diagnosis of RA

Criteria	Description
Morning stiffness	Lasting > 1 hour
Arthritis in 3 or more joints	Soft tissue swelling or effusion in the wrist, PIP, MCP, elbow, knee, ankle, or MTP
Hand joint involvement	Involvement of the wrist, MCP, or PIP joints
Symmetric arthritis	Both right and left joints involved
Rheumatoid nodules	Subcutaneous nodules in areas surrounding affected joints
Serum rheumatoid factor positive	Positive RF
Radiological changes	Typical erosions or loss of density in affected joints

Diagnosis should include 4 or more criteria which are required to be present for ≥ 6 weeks.
Adapted from Saraux A, et al. Ability of the American College of Rheumatology 1987 criteria to predict rheumatoid arthritis in patients with early arthritis and classification of these patients two years later. *Arthritis Rheum* 2001; 44: 2485–91. And Arnett FC, Edworthy SM, Bloch DA, McShane DJ, Fries JF, Cooper NS, et al. The American Rheumatism Association 1987 revised criteria for the classification of rheumatoid arthritis. *Arthritis Rheum* 1988;31:315–24.

Labs: CBC for mild anemia, ESR/CRP usually elevated, ANA positive in 20–30% patients, RF as above, CMP for electrolytes, renal and liver involvement.

Joint aspiration and fluid analysis.

Imaging: Obtain plain radiographs of chest, cervical spine, and affected joints as needed.

Treatment

NSAIDs should be used for first line therapy but should not be used alone.

Glucocorticoids are very effective in RA treatment but have long-term side effects. Thus, they may be useful in shorter courses for acute flares or as "bridging" therapy when DMARDs are started. Intra-articular injections may also be used for acute flares of joint symptoms.

Disease-modifying anti-rheumatic drugs (DMARDs) are the mainstay of therapy and include: methotrexate (Trexall), cyclosporine (Gengraf), hydroxychloroquine (Plaquenil), sulfasalazine (Azulfidine), infliximab (Remicade), gold (Myochrysine), and etanercept (Enbrel).

Sulfasalazine or hydroxychloroquine often are started first, but in more severe cases, methotrexate or combination therapy may be first-line treatment.

Newer DMARDs that show very promising effects include TNF-α antagonists leflunomide (Arava) and anakinra (Kineret) as well as monoclonal antibodies such as rituximab (Rituxan).

Monitoring is common for each DMARD and often done with periodic CBCs and surveillance for infection.

Non-medicinal treatments such as therapeutic fasting, dietary supplementation of essential fatty acids, journaling, spa therapies, and exercise have shown benefit. Evidence for acupuncture, herbal medications, and splinting is inconclusive.

Take Home Points

- RA is a systemic autoimmune disease.
- Proximal joint involvement with nodule formation characterizes RA.
- Management consists of DMARDs and steroids.

Osteoarthritis

A degenerative disease of the joints involving narrowing of joint space due to loss of articular cartilage, osteophyte formation, and subarticular bone sclerosis. This is the most common form of arthritis and may be due to a myriad of disorders.

Symptoms

Classically, pain that worsens during the day. Arthritis is noninflammatory but often limits range of motion and is characterized by a dull ache in or around the joints. In advanced disease, erosion may produce inflammatory picture, including swelling and erythema of joints. Risk factors include obesity, advanced age, female sex, previous joint injury, and family history.

Diagnosis

Physical exam: Tenderness on passive range of motion may be seen. Crepitus is a sign of advanced disease. Bony enlargement called **Heberden nodes,** in the DIP joints, or **Bouchard nodes**, in the PIP joints, may be seen in the hands. This disease is generally asymmetric although often occurs in multiple joints.

Labs: No specific lab tests exist for OA although exclusion of other arthropathies may be indicated with screening labs. ESR is not reliable for diagnosis.

Imaging: Plain x-rays of joint in question often show narrowing of joint space and osteophyte formation. Joint space narrowing, formation of subchondral cysts, and sclerotic walls may develop later. MRI may show greater detail of these changes but is commonly not needed due to reliability of plain x-rays.

Aspiration of joint is often not needed and shows noninflammatory processes with normal WBCs. Crystal disorders and inflammatory arthritis may be excluded.

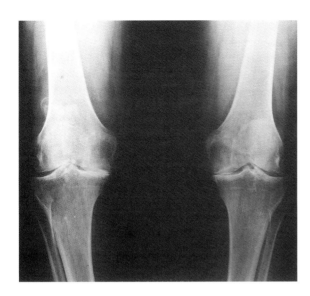

FIGURE 12.2 Bilateral knee osteoarthritis. Note the asymmetric joint space narrowing, bony sclerosis, and presence of osteophytes. Reprinted with permission from Warrell DA, Cox TM, et al. *Oxford Textbook of Medicine*, 4th edition. 2003, Oxford University Press.

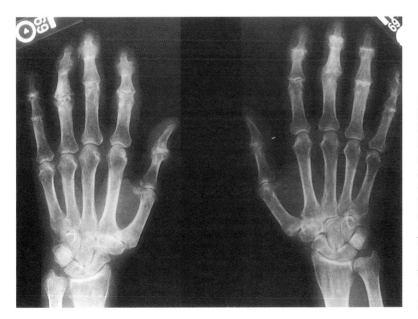

FIGURE 12.3 Osteoarthritis of the hands. Note changes in the distal interphalangeal joints and proximal interphalangeal joints as well as the base of the thumb. These changes are typical for OA and show loss of joint space, bony sclerosis, and presence of osteophytes. The bony changes seen in the DIP and PIP joints correspond to Bouchard's and Heberden's nodes on physical exam. Reprinted with permission from Warrell DA, Cox TM, et al. *Oxford Textbook of Medicine*, 4th edition. 2003, Oxford University Press.

Treatment

Weight reduction, heat to affected joint, and occupational modification or assistance is the first step in treatment.

NSAIDs and acetaminophen are the pharmacologic mainstays of treatment. In the elderly, monitor for GI bleeding or renal failure.

COX-2 inhibitors (NSAIDs) have been an acceptable alternative to regular NSAIDs in the past although recent concerns have been raised about safety, regarding cardiovascular risks. Benefits include fewer GI symptoms and less risk of bleeding. Monitor closely if these are used.

Topical capsaicin cream is often helpful.

Opioid analgesics are rarely indicated for OA.

Intra-articular corticosteroid injections often improve symptoms although repeated injection commonly needed. Limit to 3–4 injections per year, never exceeding 12 injections per any one joint.

Intra-articular injection of hyaluronic acid has been shown to provide some relief but further investigation is needed to define benefit.

Surgery, including total joint arthroplasty, is acceptable and effective when disease has proven refractory to medical therapy. Symptom reduction and joint mobility are often significantly improved.

Take Home Points

- Osteoarthritis involves cartilage degeneration, osteophyte formation, and subarticular sclerosis.
- Obesity is a risk factor for weight-bearing joints.
- Monitor for side effects of long term NSAID therapy if this is used.

Gout

Acute or chronic arthritis caused by inflammatory urate crystals deposited in joint synovial fluid. The primary form is associated with overproduction or underexcretion of uric acid. Acute attacks are associated with some medications including: hydrochlorothiazide, aspirin, and allopurinol.

Symptoms

"Podagra," an inflammatory presentation of the great toe MTP joint, which is, classically, the first place of presentation. Otherwise, it is seen as mono or pauciarticular arthritis. Gout is associated with obesity, excess EtOH use, and purine (protein) rich diet.

Diagnosis

Gold standard is **aspiration and exam of synovial fluid** in polarized light. Gout has negative birefringent crystals, Pseudogout (a related crystalline arthritis) has positive birefringent crystals.

Imaging: Classically shows "punched out" lesions with preserved joint space. May also show tophi presence.

Check blood urate levels to support the diagnosis but this test is not specific enough to rule it out.

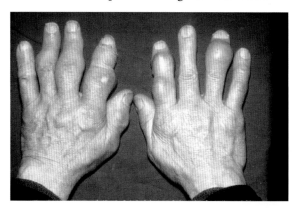

FIGURE 12.4 Chronic gouty arthritis with tophaceous formation. Reprinted with permission from Cox NLT, Roper TA. *Clinical Skills*. 2005, Oxford University Press.

Uric acid excretion test: 24-hour urine collection. If gout confirmed by joint aspiration and uric acid secretion is:

< 800 mg/day on unrestricted diet or < 600 mg/day on purine free diet → patient is **underexcreter**.

> 800 mg/day on unrestricted diet or > 600 mg/day on purine free diet → patient is **overproducer**.

Treatment

General measures: Patients need to increase fluid intake dramatically, abstain from EtOH use, reduce protein in their diet, and lose weight.

Acute attack: Colchicine in acute attacks is classic but also controversial secondary to side effects, including severe abdominal pain, N/V, and diarrhea. If used, colchicine must be given in first 24 hours of onset of attack to abort it. NSAIDs (not ASA) are also used with great efficacy. Indomethacin (Indocin) is a favorite. Oral or intra-articular steroids have been shown to relieve symptoms. In severe cases use narcotics for pain relief.

Chronic prophylaxis: Colchicine can be given to ward off attacks but side effects generally prevent this.

Classic prophylactic medications are:

Allopurinol for overproducers
Probenecid for underexcreters

Take Home Points

- Gout has negatively birefringent crystals under polarized light exam.
- Aspiration of joint synovium is the gold standard test.
- Colchicine has significant GI side effects and is an abortive medication.
- Prophylaxis includes allopurinol or probenecid. Don't give allopurinol acutely.

Internal Derangement of the Knee

TABLE 12.4 Knee Derangements

Derangement	Typical Injury	Physical Exam
Anterior cruciate ligament tear (ACL)	Twisting or rotary motion of the knee. Often in planting-then-turning motions.	*Lachman test*—Best overall test. Flex knee to 30°, stabilize the femur, and apply anterior/posterior force to proximal tibia. Positive test is "soft" or "boggy" endpoint. *Anterior drawer sign*—In 90° flexion, lower leg is stabilized and anterior force applied to tibia, anterior laxity with "boggy" endpoint indicates positive.
Posterior cruciate ligament tear (PCL)	Fall while foot is plantar flexed with knee in flexion or as a dashboard injury in motor vehicle accident.	*Posterior drawer sign*—In 90° flexion, stabilize the lower leg and apply posterior force to anterior tibia, posterior laxity with "boggy" endpoint indicates positive.
Medial collateral ligament (MCL)	Stress or blow to knee on the lateral side. Often occurs in football tackling injuries.	*Valgus stress test*—Place knee in 30° flexion and apply valgus stress to lower leg, medial laxity or pain indicates positive.
Lateral collateral ligament (MCL)	Skiing, football, or soccer injuries.	*Varus stress test*—Place knee in 30° flexion and apply varus stress to lower leg, lateral laxity or pain indicates positive.
Meniscal tear	Running, basketball, football, or unknown injury.	*Apley compression test*—In prone position with knee in 90° flexion, place downward force on heal to load knee, pain or click on rotation of foot indicates positive. *McMurray test*—While supine, begin with 90° flexion and simultaneously apply varus and valgus stress while extending and flexing knee. Pain or clicking indicates positive.

Imaging: MRI is the best modality for all above since it allows visualization of ligaments. Plain x-rays may assess fracture.

Treatment

NSAIDs acutely and subacutely. Further pain control may be necessary at the time of injury. Rest, ice, elevation may help with initial swelling.

Definitive treatment is surgery and repair. PCL injuries are often deferred without surgery.

Physical therapy and rehab are often useful.

Knee brace may symptomatically help in the phase of acute symptoms but has not been shown to improve outcomes.

Afflictions of the Shoulder

TABLE 12.5 Shoulder Derangements

Derangement	Injury	Physical Exam
Rotator cuff tear	Fall on outstretched arm, fall on shoulder, excessive pulling (lawn mower engine starting), etc. SITS muscles of rotator cuff: Supraspinatus Infraspinatus Teres minor Subscapularis	Test range of motion, strength of motion, and isolate muscles as needed. Specific tests are as follows: *Drop arm test*—Fully abduct the shoulder and have patient actively, slowly lower extended arm to side. Pain on attempt or "dropping" of the arm indicates supraspinatus weakness/tear. *Isometric supraspinatus test*—With elbow flexed 90°, abduct the shoulder 45° and have the patient attempt abduction against isometric resistance, pain indicates positive. *Isometric infraspinatus/teres minor test*—With shoulder hanging to side and elbow flexed 90°, have patient externally rotate against isometric resistance, pain indicates positive. *Subscapularis (lift off) test*—Place dorsum of hand against surface of back with elbow at 90° flexion. Pain or inability to externally rotate arm such that the hand lifts off the back is positive for subscapularis tendon injury.
Impingement	Rotator cuff tendon inflammation	*Hawkins test*—Stabilize the shoulder with one hand, 90° flex the shoulder and 90° flex the elbow. Pain on internal rotation indicates impingement. *Neer test*—Stabilize the scapula, place shoulder in 90° flexion and forearm in full pronation with the elbow extended. Flex shoulder to 180°, pain indicates subacromial impingement. *Passive painful arc maneuver*—With arm at side, in full internal rotation, and elbow flexed at 90°, stabilize the shoulder with one hand and passively flex the shoulder. Pain or shrugging indicates impingement. *Empty can test*—With shoulder flexed at 90° with extended elbow and hand in pronation (as if pouring out a can); pain with attempting full flexion against resistance indicates impingement.

TABLE 12.5 Continued

Derangement	Injury	Physical Exam
Biceps tendonopathy	Repetitive motion or weight bearing on flexed arm. May occur with occupation of repetitive lifting.	*Speed's test*—With extended elbow and shoulder flexed to 30°, have patient flex shoulder against resistance. Pain indicates positive. *Yergason test*—With shoulder hanging at side and elbow flexed to 90° and forearm in full pronation, grasp patient's hand (as if to shake) and have patient supinate against resistance; pain indicates positive.
Dislocation	Anterior dislocation occurs with blow to lateral or posterior shoulder, often repetitive. Posterior dislocation is associated with seizures, electrocutions, and motor vehicle accidents.	Look for deformity and prominent humoral head. Often acutely painful. *Apprehension test*—With abduction of the shoulder to 90° and flexion of elbow 90°, fear of dislocation or pain on external rotation and anterior pressure to shoulder indicates positive.

Imaging: Shoulder x-ray (three views!) is indicated if acute injury is suspected. Rotator cuff tear or pathology is sometimes visible by narrowing of joint space. Shoulder arthrography has historically been useful but is now being replaced by MRI/MR arthrography. Ultrasound may demonstrate large tears but is limited with tears < 1 cm.

MRI is indicated if a tear is suspected.

Treatment

NSAIDs are effective for anti-inflammation and pain control. Rotator cuff and impingement: Injection of painful area with mix of local anesthetic and steroid is often useful. This reduces inflammation and provides acute relief. Be certain not to inject tendons. Relative rest and referral to physical therapy is often helpful. Consider surgery after conservative treatment failure.

Anterior dislocation: Common reduction techniques include hanging weights, scapular manipulation, external rotation, and the use of towels and pulling for traction/countertraction. The humeral head often relocates after a matter of minutes. A short duration in a sling is usually adequate for full recovery. If recurrent, consider referral to orthopedist for possible surgery to tighten ligaments.

Surgery is indicated for posterior shoulder dislocation and repair of rotator cuff tears.

Physical therapy and rehab are often useful.

Take Home Points

- NSAIDs acutely, consideration of steroid injection, and relative rest comprise conservative treatment and is effective for the majority of cases.

Bursitis

Inflammation of a bursal sac which may involve effusion or local cellulitis. Cause may be traumatic, infectious, inflammatory, or gout associated.

Symptoms

Pain, tenderness, and mildly limited range of motion of affected joint. Effusion inside bursa may form, which may become secondarily infected. History is often positive for overuse or repeated direct trauma when not otherwise seen, such as in the "weekend warrior."

Diagnosis

Physical exam: Tender area to direct palpation over bursal area. Pain is generally superficial and easily evoked. If infection is present, erythema, effusion, swelling, and fluctuance may be appreciated. Common sites are olecranon, prepatellar, infrapatellar, subdeltoid, trochanteric, and radiohumeral.

Labs: CBC shows leukocytosis with infection. Obtain aspiration and fluid analysis including crystal presence, leukocytes, Gram stain, differential, and culture/sensitivities of effusion fluid. This distinguishes between inflammatory, crystalloid, and infectious bursitis.

Treatment

NSAIDs are helpful for pain.

Rest, **i**ce, **c**ompression, **e**levation (RICE) therapy may be helpful acutely.

Treat infection (if present) with broad spectrum oral antibiotics, cover for skin bacteria.

Injection with steroid/lidocaine mix may help pain and speed healing, although should not be done if infectious etiology is present.

Take Home Points

- Distinguish between bursitis and other conditions such as infectious arthritis and cellulitis.
- NSAIDs and RICE therapy will successfully treat bursitis in the majority of cases, injection of steroid/lidocaine mixture is appropriate for non-infectious bursitis.

Tendonopathy

A group of inflammatory states of various areas of the tendon. These may include tendonosis (microtearing or stretching of tendon fibers), tenosynovitis (inflammation of the tendon sheath), epicondylitis (tendonitis near the forearm epicondyles), chronic paratendonitis (inflammation around the tendon, i.e. Achilles' tendon), and enthesiopathy (inflammation at the point of tendon insertion into bone).

Symptoms

Pain and tenderness commonly at the tendon origin of muscle or insertion into bone. Often after exertion and made worse by flexion of nearby joints. History may be positive for overuse in a sporting event or vigorous repetitive exercise.

Diagnosis

Physical exam: Tenderness on isolated contraction of the affected muscle and tendon. Weakness is elicited by the same maneuver but tendon integrity should be preserved.

Imaging: If in doubt, MRI is the best visualization modality if tear of any degree is suspected; however, is often not needed. Plain x-ray may show calcific deposits in repeated or chronic tendonitis.

Treatment

Limit affected muscle use and exertion. This may be done with sling or counseling.

NSAIDs are often helpful for pain and decreasing inflammation.

Advance to physical therapy after the area is pain free.

For epicondylitis, forearm bands may be helpful in long term recovery and work by limiting range of motion.

Injection of steroid/lidocaine mix to surrounding tendon sheath provides acute relief, however, should be limited to no more than 3 injections per year.

Complete healing generally takes 4–6 weeks.

Take Home Points

- Tendonitis is a group of related inflammatory disorders causing symptoms involving the muscular tendon.
- Treatment is commonly NSAIDs and relative rest.

Infectious Tenosynovitis of the Hand

This condition consists of bacterial infection of the tendon sheaths of the flexor or extensor tendons controlling the fingers. Mode of entry into the tendon sheaths may be minor ("fight bite" or cat bite) and start with simple cellulitis. The infection quickly takes hold of the inner sheath compartment and commonly travels proximally.

Symptoms

Pain, limited range of motion, swelling, and red streaking (lymphangitis) from the infected finger.

Diagnosis

Physical exam:
Kanavel's signs

1. Symmetric swelling along tendon sheath
2. Tenderness and erythema along tendon sheath
3. Semiflexed posture of the involved finger
4. Severe pain on passive extension.

Labs: CBC shows leukocytosis. Obtain cultures before antibiotics. Cultures often positive for *Staph* and *Strep* spp.
Imaging: Plain x-rays of hand depending on mode of injury.

Treatment

Surgical incision and drainage of tendon sheath should be done as soon as possible.
IV antibiotics initiated after surgery may include IV penicillin, nafcillin, or cephalosporin.
Place hand in Murphy's splint during recovery (hand kept above level of the heart).
NSAIDs or opiate pain control as needed.
Refer to orthopedics or plastic surgery.

Take Home Points

- Tenosynovitis of the hand is basically an abscess tracking along finger tendon sheaths.
- Kanavel's signs are important to diagnosis.
- Incision and drainage with subsequent antibiotics is the treatment (not antibiotics alone).

Ganglion Cyst

A cystic extension of the joint capsule or tendon sheath, often forming a palpable mass under the skin. The capsule or sheath herniates from the main compartment and fills the cyst with synovial fluid.

Symptoms

Painful or non-painful rubbery mass over joint, commonly of wrist or hand.

Diagnosis

Physical exam: Rubbery, discrete subcutaneous mass over the joint or tendon sheath. These commonly occur in the hand, volar and dorsum aspects of the wrist, and ankles.

Transillumination is useful and demonstrates fluid-filled cyst.

Treatment

Reassurance that the mass is benign and common.

Aspiration and steroid injection may be effective acutely but counsel the patient it is not curative; the mass will likely recur.

Surgical excision is the only definitive method of removal. Recurrence is, however, common. Recovery is usually fast without complication.

Take Home Points

- Ganglion cysts are outpouchings of the joint capsule or tendon sheaths.
- Aspiration commonly leads to recurrence. Many resolve on their own, but some require excision.

Rhabdomyolysis

A syndrome of skeletal muscle breakdown and release of breakdown products (mostly myoglobin) into the systemic circulation. Myoglobin may consequently rise to toxic levels, harming organs such as the kidneys and liver. Etiologies include heat injury, crush injury, compartment syndrome, sepsis, shock, statin medications, etc.

Symptoms

Severe muscle aches, tenderness and dark urine. A classic scenario is of alcoholics who fall and remain in the same position for long periods of time, effectively creating a crush injury. If severe, the condition may be accompanied by mental status change or evidence of other organ damage.

Diagnosis

Physical exam: Tender muscles. Muscular injury may be obvious. Evaluate for compartment syndrome even if this is not the inciting event.

Labs: CBC may show hemoconcentration; CK is significantly elevated; urine positive for myoglobin (may be followed); CMP may show electrolyte abnormalities of Na, K, Ph, Ca. Abnormalities in Ph and Ca may be followed, LDH elevated (may be followed), AST/ALT, often > 3 times normal (may be followed), PT/aPTT/INR may show liver injury or early DIC, ABG shows metabolic acidosis.

Note that a urine dipstick commonly turns positive for blood but microscopic exam reveals only a few RBCs. Blood reaction is due to myoglobin.

Treatment

Most important initial step is to start IV fluids. Generous bolus at first then at least 2 times maintenance. Follow urine myoglobin which should turn positive, indicating when to normalize rate of fluid administration.

Monitor for pulmonary edema or ARDS in severe cases. Give furosimide (Lasix) as needed.

Treat seizures with benzodiazepines as needed.

Manage concurrent organ damage and its effects.

DIC may be an indication of eminent crash, be vigilant.

Alkalinization of the urine with sodium bicarbonate is controversial but may help clear myoglobin more effectively; consider in severe cases.

Take Home Points

- Rhabdomyolisis occurs as a result of severe skeletal muscle breakdown.
- Treat with high rate parenteral fluid and close monitoring.

Myositis

TABLE 12.6 Types of Myositis

Disease	Associations	Diagnosis	Treatment
Polymyositis/ dermatomyositis	Proximal muscle **weakness and pain;** difficulty raising arms, ascending stairs, brushing teeth. Characteristic skin rash may accompany.	Based on history, physical exam, and labs showing **increased CK,** LDH, AST/ALT, creatinine, ESR, aldolase. EMG and muscle biopsy clinch the diagnosis.	**Prednisone** is the classic choice and may require long term use. Refractory cases may benefit from methotrexate, azathioprine, cyclophosphamide, chlorambucil, or cyclosporine. Use lowest effective dose for the shortest interval.
Polymalgia rheumatica	Proximal muscle **pain without weakness;** soreness in pelvic or pectoral girdle. AM stiffness or after inactivity. **Temporal arteritis** may be comorbid.	ESR and CRP often very elevated. Normocytic anemia. CK normal. EMG normal. Arterial biopsy for temporal arteritis.	Prednisone is very effective and dramatic response can be diagnostic. Long term maintenance is usually required, use lowest effective dose.

Collagen Vascular Diseases

TABLE 12.7 Types of Collagen Vascular Diseases

	Associations	Diagnosis	Treatment
Marfan syndrome	Tall, gangly limbs, long/thin fingers, pectus deformity, high arched palate, **scoliosis.** Associated with heart abnormalities such as aortic dissection, aortic regurg/insufficiency, mitral regurg/prolapse. Eye manifestations include subluxation of lens, myopia, or retinal detachment.	Plain x-rays of spine for scoliosis during childhood years. Annual echocardiograms for premorbid aortic root dilatation.	Multidisciplinary surveillance for aortic or vascular dilatation, ophthalmologic disorders, and spinal malformations. Treat individual abnormalities with surgery. β-blockers and calcium channel blockers along with avoidance of strenuous exercise may be advised. Consider exogenous estrogen to induce premature puberty in girls to avoid excess height.

(continued)

TABLE 12.7 Continued

	Associations	Diagnosis	Treatment
Ehlers-Danlos syndrome	Several different types with variable genetic genotypes/phenotypes. Hyperflexibility of joints (often hands), hyperextensible skin, poor wound healing, easy bruising, and, rarely, subcutaneous spheroids. Vascular involvement may be present but is less common.	Most often clinical unless genetic analysis is done. Pedigree with affected relatives should be analyzed. Many different inheritances and mutations may produce variations of disease.	Reassurance that for mild disease, there will likely never be disability. For more severe disease, treat individual conditions.

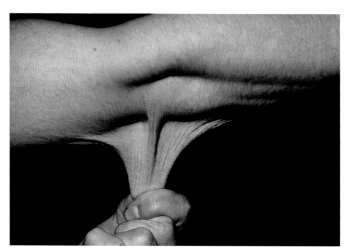

FIGURE 12.5 Ehlers-Danlos syndrome. The skin is elastic and distensible. Reprinted with permission from MacKie, RM. *Clinical Dermatology,* 5th edition. 2003, Oxford University Press.

Osteoporosis

A disorder of the skeletal bone structure involving low bone mass and change in bone microarchitecture. Risk factors include: personal history of fragility fracture, low body weight, current smoking, use of oral corticosteroid therapy for more than 3 months, estrogen deficiency at an early age (< 45 years), poor health/frailty, northern areas, low calcium intake (lifelong), low physical activity, and alcohol in amounts > 2 drinks per day.

Symptoms

Often an asymptomatic disease until the complication of fracture. Fractures may commonly be seen in hip or vertebrae. Spine may develop many "micro-fractures," developing into severe kyphoscoliosis, which may progress to respiratory compromise in late stages.

Diagnosis

TABLE 12.8 World Health Organization (WHO) Criteria for Diagnosis of Osteoporosis

Normal	BMD not more than 1 standard deviation below PABM. T-score > –1.
Osteopenia	BMD between 1 and 2.5 standard deviations below PABM. T-score between –1 and –2.5
Osteoporosis	BMD value more than 2.5 standard deviations below PABM. **T-score ≤ –2.5.**
Severe Osteoporosis	Osteoporosis with T-score ≤ –2.5 plus one or more fragility fracture.

PABM = Peak adult bone mass

Dual-energy x-ray absorptiometry (DEXA) scanning at the hip or spine and elucidation of the T-score is commonly used for classification of bone mineral density (BMD).

Plain bone or spine x-rays should be sought on any suspected fracture.

Recommendations on screening show little variations amongst expert groups. The United States Preventive Services Task Force (USPSTF) and the National Osteoporosis Foundation (NOF) recommend universal screening of all women over the age of 65 and screening of postmenopausal women under age 65 with one or more risk factors (not including being female, white, and postmenopausal). The NOF further recommends screening of postmenopausal women that present with fragility fractures. Recommendations for follow-up exam and interval testing is inconsistent amongst groups at this time, but a repeat DEXA scan is usually performed every 2 years for those on medication.

Treatment

Oral calcium/vitamin D intake throughout life but especially after menopause is highly recommended. Calcium dose is generally 1200 mg/day with vitamin D 400–800 IU/day.

Recommend regular strength training exercise.

Bisphosphonates such as alendronate (Fosamax), zoledronic acid (Reclast), risedronate (Actonel), pamidronate (Actonel) are effective at both prevention and treatment. These drugs should be taken while upright (sitting/standing) for at least 30 minutes and on an empty stomach to avoid common GI side effects.

Calcitonin (Miacalcin) has shown good effectiveness with little side effects.

Raloxifene (Evista) is a selective estrogen receptor modulator (SERM) that is approved for postmenopausal osteoporosis, although common side effects include hot flashes and possible DVT.

Progesterone and estrogen hormone replacement therapy (HRT) has shown positive effects on BMD in postmenopausal women but has recently been shown to cause disproportionate cardiovascular and breast cancer risks by the Women's Health Initiative study. However, it is commonly still used for short term relief of menopausal symptoms and if all other options for osteoporosis have been exhausted.

Take Home Points

- Osteoporosis involves low bone density and change to bone microarchitecture.
- Osteoporosis is defined as BMD T-score of ≤ -2.5.
- Treatment consists of prevention, bisphosphonates, SERMs, calcitonin, and HRT in select patients.

Developmental Musculoskeletal Deformities

TABLE 12.9 Developmental Hip Deformities

	Diagnosis	Treatment
Hip dysplasia	Often at birth with positive Barlow/Ortolani test. Unequal number of thigh folds and uneven height of knees. For neonates obtain **hip U/S**; for older infants, plain x-rays in AP and frog lateral leg positions. CT, MRI may be beneficial.	Positioning in "frog leg" position with hip flexed and abducted. Double or triple diapers effective in neonates, older infants may require **Pavlik harness**. In infants > 6 months, closed reduction and hip spica cast is indicated. Duration usually 1–3 months.
Legg-Calvé-Perthes disease (avascular necrosis of femoral head)	Presents as "painless limp" around 7 years old. Plain x-rays in AP and frog lateral positions are usually adequate to diagnose. MRI may catch early disease but not adequate to follow course.	Abduction brace for most. Surgical correction for severe cases.

(continued)

TABLE 12.9 Continued

	Diagnosis	Treatment
Slipped capital femoral epiphysis (SCFE)	Classically, overweight male adolescent. Pain in thigh or knee (referred) with external rotation of hip. Plain x-rays in AP and frog lateral positions show abnormality.	Surgery including internal fixation and pinning, osteotomy, and hip spica cast immobilization.

Spondylosis

Degeneration of the intervertebral disc spaces (osteoarthritis) leading to increased weight-bearing on alternate intervertebral joints and osteophyte formation. Osteophyte formation or narrowing of the joint space may place pressure on exiting nerve bundles from the neural foramina, causing symptoms.

Symptoms

Localized back pain commonly in lumbar and cervical regions. If advanced, may produce radicular pain including sciatica or following a dermatomal distribution. Progression may lead to neurogenic claudication and signs of spinal stenosis.

Diagnosis

Physical exam: Tenderness at the level of defect, increased pain on back extension. Pain is exacerbated by ipsilateral bending to the side of the affected joints.
Labs: CBC and ESR are usually normal.
Imaging: Plain spinal x-rays reveal intervertebral disc degeneration and osteophyte formation. MRI and CT are not indicated unless spinal stenosis is suspected.

Treatment

NSAIDs and acetaminophen are the mainstays of treatment.

Physical therapy, such as core muscle strengthening, TENS, and ultrasound therapy, has shown benefit in the short term.

Surgery (spinal fusion) is indicated for significant neurologic symptoms although long term benefit is controversial.

Decompression laminectomy may be used if stenosis is suspected.

Take Home Points

- Spondylosis may cause local or radiating back pain.
- Treatment consists of initial trial of medical therapy then consideration of surgery.

Ankylosing Spondylitis

A chronic and systemic inflammatory disease involving the point of tendon and ligament attachment to bone (enthesis), causing new bone formation (osteophyte). Commonly, this disease occurs in the relatively young (20–40 years) male and involves the sacroiliac joint. Genetic analysis shows a strong correlation with HLA-B27.

Symptoms

Insidious onset lower back pain and stiffness are the hallmarks of disease. Morning stiffness which is relieved by activity. Pleuritic chest pain and constricted chest expansion may be reported. Constitutional symptoms such as fever, weight loss, and fatigue may be present and correlate with back pain flares. Rarely, anterior uveitis and cardiovascular abnormalities are present in history.

Diagnosis

Physical exam: Tenderness on palpation of sacroiliac (SI) joint, limited range of motion of the SI joint, and relative loss of lumbar lordosis (leading to "question mark" posture). Decreased chest expansion may be present. Heart exam should be focused on presence of murmur, indicating aortic valve sclerosis.

Labs: Antigen testing for HLA-B27 (common), ESR/CRP often elevated. CBC may show a mild normocytic anemia.

Imaging: Plain x-rays (including oblique view) of lumbar spine may show "bamboo" spine with squaring of vertebrae. Early disease is seen by sclerosis of the SI joint with late disease seen by ankylosis and osteopenia. Peripheral joints showing symptoms should be imaged as well. MRI may be used if plain radiography is inconclusive. Increased signal in the area of the SI joint indicating surrounding edema may be present.

EKG is recommended but may be inadequate if valvular disease is present. Consider echocardiography if murmur exists.

DEXA scan is indicated for possible osteoporosis (an associated condition).

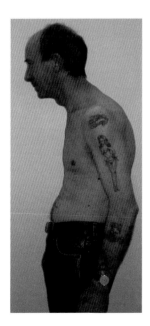

FIGURE 12.6 Ankylosing spondylitis. Note the typical question-mark posture of AS. Reprinted with permission from Cox NLT, Roper TA. *Clinical Skills*. 2005, Oxford University Press.

Treatment

Physical therapy with focus on strengthening back extensors is effective.

NSAIDs are the mainstay of initial therapy and indomethacin (Indocin) is most common. Good response supports diagnosis.

Interarticular corticosteroid injection provides temporary relief.

Other anti-rheumatic drugs such as etanercept (Enbrel), sulfasalazine (Azulfidine), and methotrexate (Trexall, Rheumatrex) have shown excellent benefit in recent studies.

Surgery may include total hip replacement, fusion, or vertebral wedge osteotomy.

Take Home Points

- Ankylosing spondylitis is associated with HLA-B27.
- AS may be associated with other comorbidities such as valvular malformation or osteoporosis.
- X-ray characteristically shows a "bamboo" spine.
- DMARDs may help treat AS.

Intervertebral Disc Herniation

The condition of herniation of the nucleus pulposus of the intervertebral disc leading to nerve compression and possibly, spinal stenosis. The herniation can occur due to bone degeneration, disc degeneration, trauma, overuse, or idiopathically. Herniation may or may not lead to symptoms and its presence in a patient with back pain does not necessarily imply causation, thus making direct diagnosis difficult.

Symptoms

Localized back pain and radiating neurological pain. While the vast majority of cases are mild to moderate, severe herniation accompanied by nerve impingement may result in sensory or motor symptoms. History may reveal heavy lifting or traumatic event.

"Red Flag" Symptoms

Bowel/bladder incontinence

Fever

Weight loss

Bilateral sensory or motor dysfunction

Saddle anesthesia

Diagnosis

Physical exam: Tenderness at herniation site. Flexion or extension at the site may produce radicular symptoms. Straight leg raise or crossed straight leg raise reproduces radicular symptoms (not back pain). Sensory or motor dysfunction may be seen in spinal nerve root distribution.

Imaging: Plain x-rays are rarely indicated in acute workup unless red flag symptoms are present. After 4–8 weeks of continued symptoms despite therapy, AP and lateral views may be obtained. MRI is the best technique for evaluation and may show disc herniation or nerve compression.

EMG may reveal nerve root compression and slowed conduction after acute phase.

Treatment

NSAIDs and physical therapy are the mainstays of therapy. Corticosteroid injection may also reduce local inflammation and treat acutely.

Surgery (laminotomy, microdiscectomy, spinal fusion, or laminectomy) is needed in only a small proportion of individuals with progressive, acute neurologic dysfunction, chronic progressive pain, or refractory chronic symptoms.

Cauda equina syndrome is an emergent condition that is characterized by a patchy loss of sensory and motor function of the lower extremities. Classic signs are saddle anesthesia, loss of bowel/bladder function, and leg weakness. It requires prompt neurosurgical consultation and constitutes an emergency.

Take Home Points

- "Red flag" symptoms should always be kept in mind if disc herniation is possible.
- Presence of herniation does not necessarily imply causation.

Spinal Stenosis

The condition of narrowing of the spinal canal with resultant compression of the spinal cord or nerve roots. Etiologies include: spondylosis, spondylolisthesis, trauma, skeletal disease (RA, ankylosing spondylitis, Paget disease), neoplasm, spina bifida, and myelomeningocoele.

Symptoms

Nonspecific lower back pain is usually the inciting complaint; followed by lower extremity complaints such as fatigue, pain, numbness, or weakness. Often occurring upon walking or running, these symptoms are loosely referred to as "neurogenic claudication."

Diagnosis

Physical exam: Symptoms are classically reproduced by back extension and relieved by flexion. Neurologic exam may be normal if patient is seated during exam, thus a repeat exam should be done after patient has been walked.

Imaging: Plain x-rays are not adequate for diagnosis but may show disc space narrowing and general degeneration of the joints. Spondylolisthesis (anterior slippage of one vertebra upon another) may be evident if present. MRI is the much preferred modality of imaging and most clearly demonstrates narrowing of the spinal canal. CT with injection myelography is also useful but is invasive.

EMG may demonstrate nerve root compression but is often not needed.

Treatment

Conservative therapy with NSAIDs, weight loss, and back strengthening may be tried initially.

Injection therapy including epidural and/or soft tissue injection with a mix of local anesthetic and corticosteroid have provided some relief, although is rarely long lasting.

Decompressive surgery, commonly with laminectomy, is the definitive treatment which has shown good outcomes. Recent meta-analysis, however, has not proven long term benefits as compared with non-surgical treatments.

Take Home Points

- "Neurogenic claudication" is associated with spinal stenosis.
- Classic presentation includes partial relief of symptoms with back flexion.

Osteosarcoma

The most common primary bone tumor (although rare overall) and occurs with predilection toward children and adolescents. The tumor itself commonly occurs in the femur, proximal tibia, and proximal humerus.

Symptoms

Most patients present with insidious bone pain in one of the characteristic locations. Pathologic fracture may be a presenting situation. Constitutional symptoms including fever, malaise, and weight loss are atypical.

Diagnosis

Physical exam: Palpable mass may be present in a characteristic location which should raise suspicion.

Labs: Alkaline phosphatase, lactate dehydrogenase (LDH), and ESR may be elevated but do not correspond to extent of disease.

Imaging: Plain radiographs often show an abnormal osseous focus with a characteristic "sunburst" pattern. Codman's triangle is a spicule of bone formed at the diaphyseal end of the lesion.

Biopsy of the lesion reveals final diagnosis.

Treatment

Surgical removal is the mainstay. Limb sparing surgery or amputation is the decision to be made. Chemotherapy is commonly given due to the high rate of metastasis of osteosarcoma (preferentially to the lung) and a high susceptibility to current regimens.

Take Home Points

- Osteosarcoma is the most common primary bone cancer and occurs primarily in the young.
- Osteosarcoma has a characteristic presence of a "sunburst" pattern and Codman's triangle on x-ray.
- Treatment is surgical coupled with chemotherapy.

Malignant Metastases

Metastatic spread of distant primary cancers. Common cancers that spread to the bone are prostate, breast, and lung.

Symptoms

Bone pain, commonly in spine, may be presenting symptom (may be associated with fracture). Pain may be in other areas including the hip, femur, ribs, sternum, or humerus. Rarely in smaller bones. History may show prior treatment for cancer or risk factors for cancer.

Diagnosis

Physical exam: Tenderness to palpation over bone in effected area. Swelling, erythema, warmth, or deformity may accompany a pathologic fracture.

Labs: CBC to evaluate for signs of infection. Serum and ionized calcium increased. Alkaline phosphatase increased.

Imaging: Plain x-ray is useful in evaluating for fracture but **nuclear medicine bone scan** (skeletal survey) is most important. Bone scan will show lytic lesions.

Biopsy the lesion as well as the suspected sight to evaluate grade of carcinoma.

Treatment

Treat according to best treatment guidelines for primary sight. This often includes local radiation therapy and chemotherapy. By the time bone metastases are seen, advanced stage is usually present. Therapy is often palliative.

Give pain control with narcotics as needed. Do not limit regimen for fear of dependence.

Take Home Points

- Look for possible distant primary cancers if malignancy is found in the spine.
- Obtain a bone scan (skeletal survey) if metastasis is suspected.

Skull Fracture

Fractures of the skull may come in several types: basilar skull fractures where the fracture line falls in the area of the skull base and foramen magnum, linear skull fracture with a discrete fracture line, depressed skull fracture involves fracture and involution of the area of injury, and Le Fort fractures which are classified on their location in the face.

Symptoms

Usually, these cases present in a trauma format. Pain and bruising are cardinal symptoms. May be accompanied by change in vision, double vision, alteration of consciousness, paralyzed extraocular muscles, eye pathology, clear otorrhea or rhinorrhea, or movable fracture regions of face.

Diagnosis

Physical exam: Basilar: bruising "battle sign" (postauricular ecchymosis) "raccoon eyes" (periorbital ecchymosis), hemotympanum, CSF otorrhea, CSF rhinorrhea, Depressed: area of obvious "dent" in the skull, area of softness in the skull, Le Fort: facial bone crepitis and facial tenderness.

Imaging: Plain x-rays of head and cervical spine. Multiple views may be needed to visualize fractures. CT may also reveal fractures and is inevitably done for evaluation of intercranial bleeding. MRI will also show fractures but is less commonly done acutely.

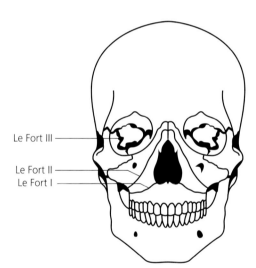

FIGURE 12.7 Le Fort classification of facial fractures. Reprinted with permission from Brown J. *Oxford American Handbook of Emergency Medicine.* 2008, Oxford University Press.

Treatment

Surgical correction with neurosurgeon, ENT, or plastic surgeon ASAP if indicated, although patients with a normal neurologic exam, nondepressed fracture, and no intracranial injury may be managed outpatient.

Monitor carefully for rise in intracranial pressure (ICP) if significant injury has occurred.

Give IV broad spectrum antibiotics if there has been any possible mechanism of entry.

Wires and stabilization bars may be placed temporarily for stabilization.

Give adequate pain control.

Take Home Points

- Skull fractures are commonly basilar, linear, depressed, or Le Fort.

Fractures

TABLE 12.10 Fracture Features by Type

Fracture	Description	Common Context	Management
Boxer's fracture	Fracture of 5th metacarpal neck.	Closed fist punch of hard surface or object.	Closed reduction and ulnar gutter splint. If good opposition of ends is not accomplished, consider ORIF.
Scaphoid fracture	Fracture of the carpal scaphoid bone. Most commonly in the central portion (waist) but also occurs at either pole.	Fall on outstretched hand. Look for tenderness in the **anatomical snuff box**. Major complication is avascular necrosis.	Use a thumb spica splint even if initial radiographs are neg. Obtain bone scan, CT, or MRI of wrist if needed acutely 3–4 days after injury. Otherwise, plain radiographs 7–14 days after injury to confirm. Refer to orthopedics if severe.
Colles fracture	Fracture of distal radius. Often dorsally displaced and dorsally angulated.	Fall on outstretched hand.	Closed reduction with eventual long arm cast.
Greenstick fracture	Incomplete fracture of children's immature bones.	Fall or direct trauma often to forearm.	If angulation is insignificant, casting not needed. Otherwise, long arm cast.
Salter-Harris fracture	Pediatric fracture with break affecting the physis. Five types exist.	Multiple.	Closed reduction in types I and II, higher types require ORIF.
Clavicle fracture	Majority occur in middle ⅓, next most common in distal ⅓, and rarely in medial ⅓.	Multiple. Common football injury.	Ipsilateral sling often adequate. Figure of eight cast or surgery only needed if significant misalignment seen.
Rib fracture	Often hairline or complete. Evaluate for pneumothorax.	Blunt trauma to ribcage such as in car accident. If in pediatric patient, posterior/lateral location, consider child abuse.	Pain control is commonly all that is needed. Treat complications.
Vertebral body fracture	Compression fracture involving body of vertebrae. May be in "burst" or "wedge" pattern.	Osteoporosis in the elderly is common. Car accident in the young.	Pain control and bedrest acutely. Evaluate need for steroids secondary to spinal compression. Closed management common if uncomplicated. Vertebroplasty/kyphoplasty if not.
Hip fracture	Several types exist but most involve femoral neck and danger to vascular supply.	"Step off" mechanism common in the elderly. Seated "dashboard" injuries in car accident in young.	ORIF because of delicate blood supply.
Tibia/fibula fracture	Often occur together and involve opposite proximal and distal ends.	Rotation of foreleg is the common mechanism. Common skiing fracture.	Closed management unless complicated or open.
Stress fracture	"Hairline" or incomplete fracture of bone.	Compression or stretching mechanism to bone.	Conservative therapy with immobilization and splinting except with high risk fractures or displacement.

ORIF = Open reduction, internal fixation

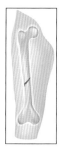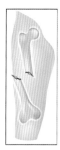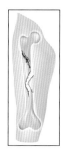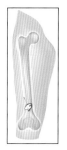

Oblique   Comminuted   Spiral   Compound   **FIGURE 12.8** Different fractures.

Infective Arthritis

Arthritic joint pain caused by primary or secondary bacterial infection. *N gonorrhoeae* is most common, *Staph* and *Strep* species are second most common although any infection may spread to joints.

Symptoms

Pain, fever, tenderness, limited range of motion, erythema, and effusion are common in septic joint. Causes are many but history may reveal recent STD, trauma, immunodeficiency state, recent joint surgery, penetrating wound (such as cat bite), or recent significant bacteremia.

Diagnosis

Physical exam: Often mono or pauciarticular. Swelling, erythema, effusion, and limited range of motion are common. Fever, myalgias, and obvious inoculation site may be seen.

Labs: Aspiration of joint fluid and Gram stain is mandatory. Fluid analysis often reveals increased WBCs and bacteria. Protein and glucose are not reliable for diagnosis. Culture the aspirate and obtain sensitivities. Evaluate fluid for crystal presence indicating gout or pseudogout. If sexually active, young patient, test for gonorrhea.

Treatment

Drainage of purulent joint fluid is most important. This may be done by aspiration but most commonly done in the OR by orthopedic surgery.

Treatment should be according to the suspected organism on Gram stain but commonly includes vancomycin. Add ceftriaxone (Rocephin) if gonorrhea is a possibility.

Narrow regimen according to sensitivities and culture results. Course of antibiotics may last 4–6 weeks and may be longer depending on host.

Surgically remove any infected artificial joints.

Take Home Points

- If infective arthritis is suspected, screen for *N gonorrhoeae*.
- Treatment may involve parenteral antibiotics or surgical "washout."

Osteomyelitis

An acute or chronic infection of the bone most commonly caused by bacteria. This disease is seeded by blood, direct inoculation, or by adjacent tissue. History may reveal source of bacteremia, comorbid vascular insufficiency, or recent operation or prosthetic device.

Symptoms

Symptoms are often localized and may include pain, overlying skin breakdown, swelling, erythema, or drainage. Constitutional symptoms such as fever, malaise, arthralgias, or headache may be present.

Diagnosis

Physical exam: Local inflammation, erythema, swelling, tenderness, ulceration, and drainage often are present in the acute form. Chronic form may be asymptomatic.

Labs: Definitive diagnosis is made by aspiration or bone biopsy and culture. Blood cultures are often positive. CBC shows leukocytosis in acute infection. ESR or CRP is often elevated.

Imaging: No single modality may be used for diagnosis or rule out. Radiographs show characteristic appearance although are often negative until weeks into the infection. Nuclear medicine bone scan is often helpful but nonspecific. CT scan may be used, MRI is the best overall modality.

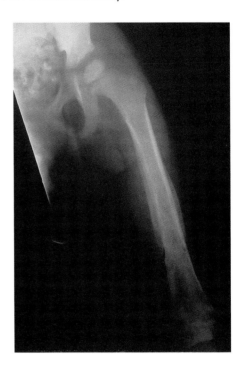

FIGURE 12.9 X-ray of femoral osteomyelitis in child. Reprinted with permission from Humphreys H, Irving WL. *Problem-Oriented Clinical Microbiology and Infection*, 2nd edition. 2004, Oxford University Press.

Treatment

Empiric therapy is warranted by most likely organism although identification and sensitivities are best. Empiric regimens include nafcillin (if non MRSA), vancomycin (if MRSA), ciprofloxacin, or levofloxacin. Start these, or combinations of these, after bone is cultured! Duration is often 4–6 weeks or longer in chronic form.

Surgical debridement and removal of necrotic tissue or hardware is essential.

Revascularization surgery is beneficial in those patients who are candidates.

Place patient on bed rest and place cast if necessary.

Amputation is a last resort.

Take Home Points

- Radiographs are not the best test to exclude osteomyelitis (especially early).

- Surgical debridement is essential to healing.

- Parenteral antibiotics are needed for acute treatment.

Ankle Sprain

Complete or partial injury to a ligament in the ankle region. History commonly reveals injury with inversion or other event. Prior ankle sprain is the main risk factor for new injury.

Ligaments commonly involved in ankle sprain:

1. Anterior talofibular ligament
2. Calcaneofibular ligament
3. Posterior talofibular ligament

Symptoms

Pain and feeling of looseness of the joint are the most common symptoms. Often acutely swollen with mild erythema. Subacutely may become ecchymotic.

Diagnosis

Physical exam: Tender to palpation over the injured ligament. May show swelling, ecchymosis, erythema, and limited range of motion. Provocative testing includes inversion, eversion, plantar/dorsiflexion, and abduction and adduction. Ankle anterior and posterior drawer signs should be tested.

Imaging: Often unnecessary unless fracture suspected. Stress x-rays and arthrography may be helpful for extent of tear but rarely used since advent of MRI. MRI may be useful in grade 2–3 sprains to evaluate extent of tear (if in question).

Treatment

TABLE 12.11 Grading of Ankle Sprain

Grade	Tear	Treatment
Grade 1	Mild sprain or stretching of ligaments	RICE, NSAIDs for pain. Stabilization wrapping followed by return to function.
Grade 2	Partial tear	RICE, pain control, and stabilization brace. Consider imaging and physical therapy.
Grade 3	Complete tear (rupture)	MRI may be helpful to confirm, brace is often indicated. Refer to orthopedic surgery for possible surgery. Surgery may or may not be of benefit.

RICE = Rest, Ice, Compression, Elevation

Adequate pain control is essential.

Physical therapy referral is helpful in rehabilitation.

Take Home Points

- The most commonly injured ligament is the anterior talofibular ligament.
- Grade the sprain clinically.
- Control pain and advise RICE therapy for Grade I and II ankle sprains.

13 Endocrinology and Metabolism

Diseases of the Thyroid Gland

Malignant Lesions of the Thyroid Gland

TABLE 13.1 Thyroid Cancer by Type

Papillary	Most common type (50–80%) but is slow growing. Usually presents after lymphatic spread and usually mixed lesion with follicular type. Histologically, has **Psammoma bodies** that are pathognomonic.
	Treatment: Surgery, either total thyroidectomy or lobectomy depending on stage. Also may use radioactive iodine for ablation but must suppress thyroid function with thyroxine afterward since these tumors are TSH responsive.
Follicular	More aggressive spread (hematogenously instead of lymphatically) and incidence increases with age. Can metastasize to bone and cause pathologic fractures. More common in females over 40 years.
	Treatment: Surgery and radioactive iodine as above. Also needs suppressive thyroxin for patients with metastases.
Anaplastic	Most aggressive type that is usually found after metastases. Death at diagnosis usually predicted in number of months. Fortunately, fairly rare (< 10%).
	Treatment: Usually palliative but radiation and chemotherapy have been tried with some success.
Medullary	Also aggressive. Tends to invade locally and can involve recurrent laryngeal nerve, causing vocal cord paralysis. May present as a patient with a hoarse voice. Associated with rapid growth. Can produce paraneoplastic syndrome and high plasma calcitonin effect from **thyrocalcitonin**. When paired with pheochromocytoma and hyperparathyroidism is called **multiple endocrine neoplasia Type II (MEN II)**.
	Treatment: Surgery and screen relatives for MEN II.

Take Home Points

- Papillary carcinoma is the most common form, anaplastic is the most aggressive.
- In thyroid scan studies, cold nodules are more suspicious for malignancy than hot ones.

Hypothyroidism

A clinical state associated with low-circulating free thyroid hormone or lack of effect of this hormone on thyroid receptors. Incidence remains 5–10/1000 in the general population but increases with age.

Myxedema is a severe hypothyroid state in which coma can develop and constitutes a true medical emergency.

Cretinism refers to a congenital untreated hypothyroid state which leads to severe mental and physical defects.

Causes

Hashimoto thyroiditis—Most common type. May have brief hyperthyroid stage then burn out. Lymphocytes infiltrate the gland and **antimicrosomal antibodies** attack it. May be associated with other autoimmune diseases and usually occurs in women.

Subacute thyroiditis (includes de Quervain)—Associated usually with viral infection/URI. Common course is initial hyperthyroid state followed by "burnout" hypothyroid phase which leads to gradual recovery. May give NSAIDs and other pain relief for often tender thyroid, but patients usually recover without need for long-term treatment.

Iodine deficiency—Historically and internationally important. Lack of iodine is the cause. Virtually eliminated in U.S. secondary to institution of iodized salt!

Euthyroid syndrome—Can be caused by any illness but usually s/p serious hospitalization. Characterized by normal TSH and low T4 and T3. Usually self limited after treatment of underlying cause.

Medications—Multiple meds can cause hypothyroidism. Classics are amiodarone, lithium, warfarin, and rifampin. Don't forget radioactive iodine from ablation of hyperthyroid state.

Symptoms

Fatigue, **hyperlipidemia**, coarse hair, weight gain, depression, slow speech, **cold intolerance**, menstrual disturbance (usually increased), constipation, carpal tunnel syndrome, decreased reflexes, anemia of chronic disease. Generally, reflective of a whole body "slow down." The severe form of hypothyroidism is **myxedema coma** characterized by altered mental status and hypothermia. The patient may or may not have a history of thyroid disturbance but often the state is precipitated by infection, myocardial ischemia, trauma, or stroke.

Diagnosis

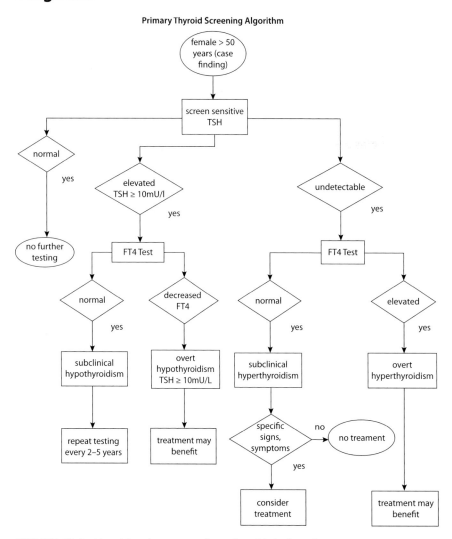

FIGURE 13.1 Algorithm for approach to thyroid dysfunction.

See figure on previous page for algorithm. Check TSH first then evaluate for T4. Look for TSH to be high and T4 to be low.

If myxedema coma is suspected, obtain labs including screening electrolytes for hypoglycemia and hyponatremia, CBC for signs of infection, and TSH, T4 levels. Cortisol levels are also indicated to assess adrenal function for possible emergent state.

Treatment

Give thyroxine (T4) as levothyroxine. The following and slow increase in dose of levothyroxine should be q6–8 weeks until patient is found to be clinically stable by repeat TSH monitoring. Some sources (and clinicians) advise to follow TSH levels, but the ultimate adjustment is still officially a clinical decision. This is due to the long time course required for TSH to actually change (up to 8 weeks).

Mortality for myxedema coma is 20–50%, so if found, remember ABCs and then give IV levothyroxine and IV hydrocortisone. Correction of hypothermia, electrolyte abnormalities, and hypoglycemia as indicated. Close monitoring is mandatory.

Take Home Points

- Myxedema is the state of severe hypothyroidism, myxedema coma is the extreme form of this.
- Replace thyroid hormone with levothyroxine and slowly adjust dosage.
- Medications such as amiodarone, lithium, warfarin, and rifampin may cause hypothyroidism.

Hyperthyroidism

A clinical state of excess circulating thyroid hormone. This state can be seen related to multiple etiologies:

Graves Disease—Most common cause of hyperthyroidism which results from production of autoactivating thyroid-stimulating immunoglobulins (TSIs), which bind to and activate thyroid TSH receptors, thus causing false overproduction of thyroxine. More common in women 20–40 years old. Causes are multiple and diverse, molecular mimicry likely plays a role. If suspected, order TFTs and thyroid-stimulating immunoglobulin for investigation.

Toxic adenoma or nodular goiter—Nodules may be multiple or singular and result in autonomous production of thyroxine. These nodules are almost always benign. Radioactive iodine scanning may reveal "hot" thyroid hormone producing nodule which reveals the diagnosis.

Thyroiditis (Hashimoto/Subacute)—Thyroid inflammation with initial hyperthyroid state followed by "burnout" hypothyroid phase which may or may not lead to gradual recovery. Associated usually with viral infection/URI. Often has low radioiodine uptake on radioactive iodine uptake (RAIU) scan. May give NSAIDs and other pain relief of often tender thyroid, but patients usually recover without need for long-term treatment.

Exogenous thyroid hormone—May be linked to mental disturbance, situation of secondary gain, or factitious disorder. Commonly tested.

Thyroid carcinoma—Medullary, follicular, or anaplastic types may produce hyperthyroid state.

Symptoms

Insomnia, palpitations, tachycardia, thinning hair, menstrual irregularities, diarrhea, hyperphagia, weight loss, anxiety, **heat intolerance, osteoporosis**, and **atrial fibrillation**. Graves disease is also associated with exophthalmos and pretibial myxedema.

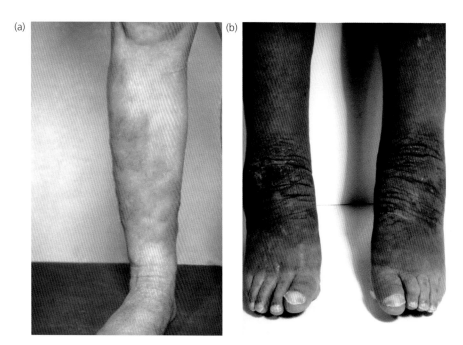

FIGURE 13.2 Pretibial myxedema. Reprinted with permission from Cox NLT, Roper TA. *Clinical Skills*. 2005, Oxford University Press.

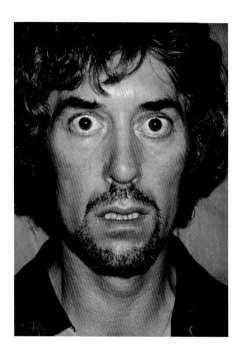

FIGURE 13.3 Exophthalmos due to Graves disease. Reprinted with permission from Cox NLT, Roper TA. *Clinical Skills*. 2005, Oxford University Press.

Diagnosis

See figure for algorithm. Check TSH first then T4. Look for TSH to be low and T4 to be high.

Treatment

Two classic drugs: Methimazole and propylthioracil (PTU). PTU is used with more severe disease while methimazole is for more moderate disease. Methimazole is also available in single daily dose and easier for compliance. Both drugs cross placental barrier and thus are ill advised in pregnancy. Use PTU preferentially if forced to make a choice but also use lowest effective dose. In all patients, use either drug for 6 months to 1 year then stop and follow T_4 for remission. Between 40% and 60% of patients relapse and need further treatment.

Propanolol—May be used to control symptoms such as tachycardia and palpitations.

Side effects of therapy: Granulocytopenia, aplastic anemia, mouth ulcers, skin rash, drug-induced lupus, PTU-induced subclinical liver injury (usually transient)

Radioactive Iodine (^{131}I) (i.e. radioactive ablation): Commonly used AFTER trying above therapy. Contraindicated in pregnancy. High incidence of induced hypothyroid state with need for levothyroxine therapy.

Surgery: Can be used with cases refractory to classic drugs and those who are not candidates for ablation (pregnancy). Side effects include both hypothyroidism and risk of hypoparathyroidism if too many parathyroids are accidentally taken.

Take Home Points

- Hyperthyroidism occurs from inflammation, infection, autoimmune derangement, or medication effect on the thyroid.

- Two medications are pathognomonic for treatment: methimazole and propylthioracil (PTU).

Diabetes Mellitus

The disease state of either lack or ineffect of insulin. Two types predominate; type I involves lack of insulin secretion by the pancreas, type II involves lack of effect of insulin upon target tissues. Both states lead to hyperglycemia, which often causes further damage to certain organ systems.

Symptoms

Classic symptoms include polyuria, polydipsia, polyphagia, and weight loss. Clues can include repeated infections (especially yeasts), blurring of vision, non-healing ulcers usually on feet, and many other varied symptoms.

Types

TABLE 13.2 Comparison of DM by Type

	Type I (Insulin Dependent)	Type II (Non-Insulin Dependent)
Mechanism	Beta cell burnout of pancreas	Peripheral insulin resistance and inadequate pancreatic compensation
Treatment	Usually insulin controlled	Usually diet or PO med controlled (may progress to insulin dependence)
Major acute complication	Diabetic ketoacidosis (DKA)	Hyperglycemic hyperosmolar nonketotic state (HHNKS)
Typical age of onset	Onset usually < 30 years old	Onset often > 30 years old
Obesity association?	Not associated with obesity	Obesity common

Diagnosis

American Diabetic Association recommendations:

One of the following categories:

1. Hemoglobin A1C (HgA1C) value of ≥ 6.5%

Or

2. A *random* plasma glucose value ≥ 200 mg/dL with classic symptoms (polyuria, polydipsia, weight loss)
    Or

3. A *fasting* plasma glucose ≥ 126 mg/dL. Fasting defined as NPO for 8 hours or more.
    Or

4. Two-hour glucose tolerance test of ≥ 200 mg/dL after a 75 g oral glucose load.

Criteria 3–4 above should be confirmed by repeat testing on a different day (in the absence of overt hyperglycemia).

HbA_1C is an average of the glucose levels over the lifespan of the red blood cell (approximately 3 months). Goal for established diabetics is generally < 7% for good diabetic glycemic control.

Treatment

Standard preventive measures are recommended, including yearly ophthalmologic exam, blood pressure control to < 130/80 mmHg, LDL level < 100 mg/dL, yearly lipid profile, periodic diabetic foot exams, and regular review of diet.

Type I diabetics are usually started directly on insulin. Use a combination of long-acting and short-acting insulin at first. Goal is to provide a somewhat constant basal insulin level with separate peaks to match meals. See Table 13.3 below. Typically, a combination of NPH and regular insulin with AM and PM dose is used. Test makers will require adjusting of these regimens, so know them.

Typical regimen involves estimated total daily insulin requirement (ETDIR) method (estimated at onset to be 0.5 U/kg). ETDIR divided into ⅔ given in AM, ⅓ given in PM. At each dosage time give ⅔ long-acting and ⅓ short-acting insulin. Typically have patient take finger stick blood glucose (FSBG) values at least 4 times per day (before breakfast, before lunch, before dinner, bedtime) and PRN. Adjust insulin regimen accordingly.

TABLE 13.3 Long-Acting Insulin

Insulin	Onset	Peak	Duration
NPH/Lente	1–4 hours	8–12 hours	12–20 hours
Ultralente	3–5 hours	10–16 hours	18–24 hours
Glargine/Lantus	1–2 hours	? Flat	24 hours

TABLE 13.4 Short-Acting Insulin

Insulin	Onset	Peak	Duration
Regular	0.5–1 hour	2–4 hours	4–8 hours
Lispro/Aspartate Humolog/Novalog	5–15 min	1–2 hours	3.5–5 hours

Somogyi effect—The theorized effect of the body's stress reaction to early morning hypoglycemia, which in turn causes hyperglycemia. The situation of too much short-acting insulin given at the evening meal producing hypoglycemia at the early hours of the morning, which starts a stress hormone release by the body, resulting in hyperglycemia upon waking. Treatment is to decrease evening insulin.

Dawn phenomenon—The effect of the body's natural early morning growth hormone release producing waking (7 am) hyperglycemia. The treatment is to increase nighttime insulin dosage, delay insulin dosage until closer to bedtime, or switch to nighttime long-acting insulin.

Type II diabetics are started on oral hypoglycemics *after* a *three month* trial of lifestyle changes including diet and exercise. Best plan is to start with monotherapy and add additional agents if not well controlling blood sugars. Goals are FPG < 126 mg/dL and HbA1C < 7. Weight reduction and increased lean body mass can sometimes lead to remission of type II DM.

TABLE 13.5 Oral Type II DM Medications

	Sulfonylureas	Meglitinides	Biguanides	Thiazolidinediones	α-Glucosidase Inhibitors
Target pop.	Recent type 2 DM diagnosis; diagnosis < 5 years	Recent Type 2 DM diagnosis	Obese, insulin resistant	Obese, insulin resistant	Elevated post prandial glucose
Advantages	Rapid FPG reduction, cost	Short acting, meal-adjusted dosing	No weight gain, decreased risk hypoglycemia	Decreased secretion of insulin, decreased risk hypoglycemia	Decreased risk hypoglycemia
Disadvantages	Weight gain, increased risk hypoglycemia	High cost, Increased risk hypoglycemia	GI side effects, high cost, metabolic (lactic) acidosis, not used with renal failure/ insufficiency	High cost, weight gain, slow onset of action, question of liver toxicity; likely negative cardiovascular effects including congestive heart failure (CHF)	High cost, GI side effects i.e. flatulence

TABLE 13.6 Oral Type II DM Medications

	Sulfonylureas	Meglitinides	Biguanides	Thiazolidinediones	α-Glucosidase Inhibitors
Prototypic drugs	Glipizide (Glucotrol), Glyburide (Micronase, DiaBeta)	Repaglinide (Prandin)	Metformin (Glucophage)	Pioglitizone (Actos) Rosiglitizone (Avandia)	Acarbose (Precose) Miglitol (Glyset)
Mechanism of action	Stimulates pancreatic insulin release	Stimulates pancreatic insulin release (non-sulphonylurea)	Decreases hepatic glucose production; increases peripheral insulin sensitivity	Increases peripheral insulin sensitivity	Inhibits intestinal enzymes, delaying glucose absorption

Take Home Points

- Classic symptoms of DM are: polyuria, polydipsia, polyphagia, and weight loss.
- Type I DM occurs mainly due to lack of secreted insulin; type II DM occurs mainly due to insulin resistance.
- Type I DM usually needs exogenous insulin for treatment; type II DM usually requires oral medications.

Diabetic Complications

Acute

TABLE 13.7 Acute DM Complications

	Diabetic Ketoacidosis (DKA)	Hyperosmolar Hyperglycemic Nonketotic State (HHNK)
Symptoms	Polyuria, polydipsia, change in mental status, "fruity" acetone breath odor, Kussmaul respirations (rapid, deep breathing presumably to blow off excess acidic ketones), abdominal pain, nausea/vomiting	Profound dehydration, mental status changes
Typical labs	Hyperglycemia, **increased anion gap**, decreased plasma pH (metabolic acidosis), serum bicarb < 15 mEq/L, serum/urine ketones, electrolyte derangement	Overt hyperglycemia (often > 600 mg/dL), plasma hyperosmosis, absence of ketones in blood or urine
Treatment	Aggressive rehydration with non-glucose containing fluid, IV insulin (often initially by drip), Potassium repletion as needed, electrolyte replacement, NPO status, (rarely bicarbonate is required when pH < 7.0)	Rehydration with non-glucose containing fluid, IV insulin, potassium repletion as needed, electrolyte replacement
Associated DM	Type I	Type II

Chronic

- Atherosclerosis—DM of either type is considered a coronary artery disease equivalent due to its proatherosclerotic effects on blood vessel walls. Significant consequences include peripheral artery disease, claudication, myocardial infarction, or stroke. "Silent MI" is seen in DM patients who have an occult MI with residual effects not initially felt due to diabetic neuropathy (see below).

- Retinopathy—Diabetic retinopathy may be proliferative, requiring laser treatment. Yearly ophthalmologic exams are required.

- Nephropathy—May lead to chronic renal failure. Check urine microalbumin periodically to detect early changes. ACE-Is or ARBs may be protective.

- Neuropathy—Commonly in the lower extremities, manifesting as numbness or pain. May lead to "Charcot foot," which is the common refracturing of the bones in the feet or joints leading to malformation.

- Gastroparesis—Due mainly to splanchnic blood vessel disease and neuropathy leading to dysfunction of the gut tract.

- Infection—DM patients are more susceptible to infection due to impaired immune system function.

Metabolic Syndrome

The clinical syndrome of increased peripheral insulin resistance in conjunction with lipid derangements, abdominal obesity, and high blood pressure. The most important of these risk factors are abdominal obesity and insulin resistance. Other associated conditions include physical inactivity, type II diabetes mellitus, older age, hormonal imbalance, and genetic or ethnic predisposition.

Symptoms

Commonly asymptomatic except for individual disease courses caused by comorbid diseases such as diabetes, etc.

Diagnosis

The Adult Treatment Panel III (ATP III), the American Heart Association (AHA) and the National Heart, Lung, and Blood Institute (NHLBI), as well as a joint committee for the international definition of metabolic syndrome define it as the presence of three of the following conditions (From Harmonizing the Metabolic Syndrome A Joint Interim Statement of the International Diabetes Federation Task Force on Epidemiology and Prevention; National Heart, Lung, and Blood Institute; American Heart Association; World Heart Federation; International Atherosclerosis Society; and International Association for the Study of Obesity, K.G.M.M. Alberti *Circulation.* 2009;120:1640–1645.).

5. Elevated waist circumference:
   - National and country specific standards.

6. Elevated triglycerides:
   - Equal to or greater than 150 mg/dL
   - Drug treatment for hypertriglyceridemia

7. Reduced HDL ("good") cholesterol:
   - Men — Less than 40 mg/dL
   - Women — Less than 50 mg/dL
   - Drug treatment for low HDL

8. Elevated blood pressure:
   - Equal to or greater than 130/85 mm Hg
   - Drug treatment for hypertension

9. Elevated fasting glucose:
   - Equal to or greater than 100 mg/dL
   - Drug treatment for hyperglycemia

Treatment

Generally, lifestyle modifications may be used to control the metabolic syndrome. These are classified into three groups: treat the overweight state, increase physical activity, and improve diet.

To address overweight state and physical activity:

Goals:

Reduce body weight by 7%–10% during the first year of therapy. Continue weight loss thereafter to the extent possible with the goal to ultimately achieve desirable weight and BMI.

Regular moderate intensity physical activity; i.e., at least 30 min of continuous/intermittent (preferably 60 min) aerobic exercise 5 days/week (preferably daily).

To address diet:

Goals:

Reduce intake of saturated fat, trans-unsaturated fat, and cholesterol.

Treat lipid and non-lipid risk factors if they persist despite these lifestyle therapies:

Treat hypertension

Use aspirin for CHD patients to reduce prothrombotic state

Treat elevated triglycerides and/or low HDL

Treat high LDL

Treat hyperglycemia

Take Home Points

- Central themes and contributing factors to the metabolic syndrome are central abdominal obesity and insulin resistance.
- The metabolic syndrome is likely on a spectrum of metabolic derangement just before type II diabetes.
- Treat with lifestyle changes focused on decreasing weight, increasing physical activity, and improving diet.

Hypoglycemia

Presence of low blood glucose levels.

Symptoms

Patient presents with sweating, tremors, tachycardia, anxiety, headache, fatigue, visual changes, and in severe cases syncope, seizure, change in mental status, hemiplegia, or coma.

One of the first things to check when any patient presents in an obtunded state, coma, or seizure is the blood glucose level!

Diagnosis

Roughly defined as FSBG < 50 mg/dL in adults. Symptoms as above. Measurement of plasma glucose and relief of these symptoms by ingestion of carbohydrates is often enough to diagnose.

The hypoglycemic state may be due to pathologic and nonpathologic issues. Most common causes in non-diabetic patients include fasting and postprandial hypoglycemia. Other causes include; alcohol use, factitious source of insulin, hypoglycemic medications (insulin, oral hypoglycemic, etc.), pituitary or adrenal insufficiency, advanced liver failure, certain non-pancreatic tumors or paraneoplastic syndromes, and insulin secreting pancreatic tumors (insulinomas).

In most cases, check C-peptide level, insulin level, and repeated FSBG.

C-peptide level is low in factitious insulin administration and is diagnostic. Look for the test question dealing with a nurse with access to insulin and a flair for the dramatic.

A supervised fast of 24–72 hours resulting in high levels of insulin despite low levels of plasma glucose is pathognomonic for insulinoma.

Treatment

Usually giving D5W in the ER is curative. One or two ampules of D50 may also be used depending on the presence of symptoms. Then, if tests for factitious insulin administration come back positive, call psychiatry. Other pathologic causes can be tested for in a controlled environment with a supervised fast. If positive, search for the cause, which may lead to surgery if a tumor is discovered.

Take Home Points

- Hypoglycemia may be a trigger for seizure or reason for obtundation.
- Exogenous insulin administration may be to blame if the patient is diabetic.
- Treat with parenteral carbohydrate solution or oral repletion.

Hyperparathyroidism

Seen in primary and secondary forms. Primary usually involves dysfunction of parathyroid glands themselves while secondary involves kidney failure. When thinking of parathyroid disease always think of PTH, phosphorus, and calcium.

Primary hyperparathyroidism: High calcium, high PTH, **low phosphorus.**

Secondary hyperparathyroidism: High calcium, high PTH, **high phosphorus.**

Symptoms

Often asymptomatic. However, may present with fractures, osteoporosis, pancreatitis, kidney stones, neurological and psychiatric disturbances. Generally, illness of bone breakdown to maintain unnaturally high blood calcium levels. Hence the mnemonic: **Stones** (renal, gall), **bones** (fractures, pain), **groans** (PUD, pancreatitis), and **psychotic overtones** (fatigue, depression, insomnia, etc.).

Diagnosis

Check electrolytes including magnesium, phosphorus, IONIZED calcium, and the main actor, PTH. Check kidney function. Expect plasma alkaline phosphatase to be elevated in bone turnover.

Expect PTH to be high in hyperparathyroidism and low in other forms of hypercalcemia. If other causes of hypercalcemia are suspected (such as ectopic secretion) check PTH-related peptide.

Treatment

Therapy is aimed at reducing the blood calcium. IV normal saline and furosemide are the mainstays of treatment. Bisphosphonates also protect bone from further resorption. Surgery is definitive treatment but hypoparathyroidism is a common side effect. After parathyroidectomy, give calcium supplements to counter the sudden decrease of plasma calcium from the bones resorbing it after withdraw of PTH.

Take Home Points

- PTH, phosphorus, and calcium derangements are heralding signs of parathyroid disease.
- Symptoms of hypercalcemia predominate: Stones, bones, groans, and psychotic overtones.
- Give IV saline and furosimide acutely.

Diabetes Insipidus

Lack of amount or effect of antidiuretic hormone (ADH).

Two types: Central DI: Often idiopathic but linked to trauma (especially chest), neoplasm, sarcoidosis, etc.

Nephrogenic DI: Medications are most common cause including **lithium**, demeclocycline, methoxyflurane, colchicines.

Symptoms

Patient presents with severe polydipsia and polyuria. Urine volumes can be amazingly high (in the tens of liters/day).

Diagnosis

High plasma osmolarity and low urine osmolarity in both central and nephrogenic forms.

Water deprivation test is gold standard and can tell the difference between the two types. The patient is restricted from water ingestion in a controlled environment until dehydration is achieved (usually judged by hypernatremia). Then, IV vasopressin (ADH) is administered. In the central DI patient, urine osmolarity increases in proper response. In the nephrogenic DI patient, urine osmolarity will not change (since the kidneys do not respond correctly).

Treatment

Central DI: Exogenous vasopressin (DDAVP) is the treatment of choice.

Nephrogenic DI: Thiazide diuretics are treatment of choice due to a paradoxical effect.

Take Home Points

- Two types exist: Primary DI and nephrogenic DI; elucidation of cause is important.
- The water deprivation test may distinguish the difference between the two types of DI.

Syndrome Inappropriate Antidiuretic Hormone (SIADH)

Excess antidiuretic hormone (ADH) in the blood produces hyponatremia, decreased serum osmolarity, and increased urine osmolarity. SIADH is a common cause of **normovolemic hyponatremia**. Excess ADH may be from malignancy, classically small cell of the lung, trauma (especially chest), postoperative status, lung infections or other causes. Medication etiologies include morphine, oxytocin, and others.

Diagnosis

Labs: Hyponatremia, decreased serum osmolarity, increased urine osmolarity. Elucidation of a cause often suggests this diagnosis but since this disorder is caused by such a wide range of problems, often the etiology is hard to find.

Treatment

Water restriction is the mainstay of treatment in most cases. Demeclocycline (Declomycin) can also be used in refractory cases. Be warned not to correct the hyponatremia too quickly, as the classic complication of central pontine myelinolysis is possible.

Take Home Points

- SIADH causes the physiologic state of water retention.
- Normovolemic hyponatremia is commonly seen with SIADH.
- Lung abnormalities such as cancer or trauma may stimulate production of excess ADH.

Cushing's Syndrome

Caused by too much **Cortisol.**

Cushing's *syndrome*

ACTH dependent causes:

Cushing's *disease* (pituitary hypersecretion of ACTH)

Paraneoplastic secretion of ACTH by distant tumor

Paraneoplastic secretion of corticotropin-releasing hormone (CRH) by distant tumors causing pituitary hypersecretion of ACTH

Iatrogenic or factitious Cushing's syndrome due to administration of exogenous ACTH

ACTH-independent causes:

Iatrogenic or factitious administration of exogenous glucocorticoids

Adrenocortical adenomas or carcinomas

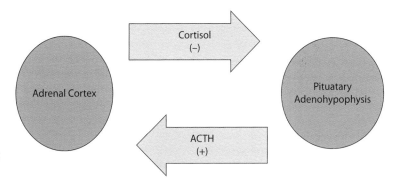

FIGURE 13.4 Normal endocrinologic feedback.

Symptoms

Classic **"moon" facies**, **buffalo hump**, central truncal obesity, striae, osteoporosis, DM. Other associations include psychiatric problems, easy bruising, poor wound healing, menstrual irregularities or viralism in women.

Diagnosis

Because of normal daily variations of cortisol in the serum, it is hard to measure these concentrations and be accurate (although AM, PM, and 24 hour totals are elevated if measured).

Urinary cortisol level is the best assay. Normal 20–100 μg/24hr; Cushing patients > **120 μg/24hr.**

Dexamethasone suppression test—Distinguishes increased cortisolism caused by pituitary abnormality vs. other forms of Cushing's syndrome. Administration of 1 mg dexamethasone PO at 11–12 pm should suppress cortisol in the normal patient in the AM the next day. In Cushing's syndrome from a nonpituitary source, cortisol will continue to have elevated levels. In Cushing's syndrome from a pituitary source (the disease), since ACTH from the pituitary is subject to feedback inhibition by cortisol (in this case, exogenous glucocorticoid), the urinary cortisol should decrease. Thus, the reaction to change proves the elevated levels are pituitary in nature.

Imaging: CT/MRI (MRI is best) to visualize pituitary or adrenal tumors. Try to visualize any other source you may suspect of being the culprit, e.g. small cell of the lung, etc.

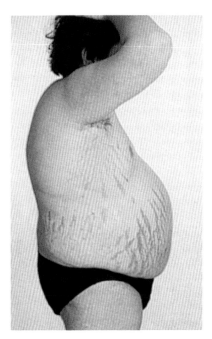

FIGURE 13.5 Classic "Cushingoid" appearance. Reprinted with permission from Flynn JA. *Oxford American Handbook of Clinical Medicine.* 2007, Oxford University Press.

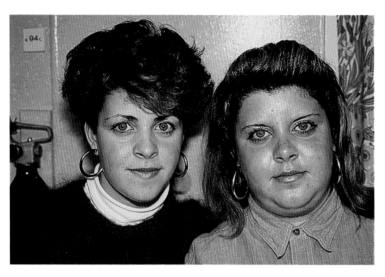

FIGURE 13.6 A young woman with Cushing's disease photographed alongside her identical twin sister. Note typical Cushing "moon" facial appearance. Reprinted with permission from Warrell DA, Cox TM, et al. *Oxford Textbook of Medicine*, 4th edition. 2003, Oxford University Press.

Treatment

Surgery wherever it may be! If the pituitary is the culprit, a transphenoidal resection; if ectopic, remove it; if adrenal, remove them (be careful of the side effects of loosing the adrenals, though).

Then **replacement** with adrenocorticoids for cortisol replacement.

If from exogenous steroids, reduce/stop them.

Take Home Points

- Cushing's syndrome is due to the effects of excess cortisol.
- Cushing's syndrome may be from ACTH dependent or independent factors.
- Find the source of excess secretion with the dexamethasone suppression test.

Addison's Disease (and Secondary Hypoadrenalism)

Technically, Addison's disease is only from hypofunctioning of the adrenals (primary hyposecretion). But symptoms and discussion can be similar in secondary adrenal insufficiency from other causes, such as pituitary hypofunction.

Etiology most commonly is due to autoimmune destruction of the adrenals, which may or may not be part of a broader "polyglandular autoimmune disorder" involving diseases such as diabetes mellitus type I, Graves disease, thyroiditis, and others. Other causes include infectious (TB, disseminated fungal infections), metastatic carcinoma or lymphoma, adrenal hemorrhage or infarction, medications (keto-conazole, rifampin, phenytoin, etc), or congenital adrenal hypoplasias.

Symptoms

Hyperpigmentation of skin (pathognomonic for Addison's disease secondary to high ACTH), postural hypotension, dehydration, anorexia, nausea/vomiting, diarrhea. Can lead to complication of Addisonian crisis which can lead to death.

Diagnosis

Cosyntropin stimulation test (aka ACTH stimulation test)—Administration of exogenous cosyntropin (Cortrosysn) will elevate levels of cortisol in the normal individual. In Addison's disease the levels will remain unchanged. This is diagnostic.

TABLE 13.8 Typical Lab Derangements in Addison's Disease

Blood chemistries	Low Na
	High K
	Low fasting glucose
	Low plasma bicarbonate
	Elevated BUN
Hematology	Elevated hematocrit
	Low WBC count
	Relative lymphocytosis
	Increased eosinophils

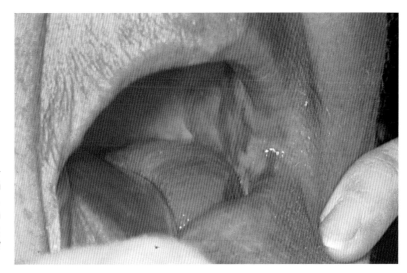

FIGURE 13.7 Intra-oral hyperpigmentation of buccal mucosa in a patient with Addison's disease. Reprinted with permission from MacKie, RM. *Clinical Dermatology*, 5th edition. 2003, Oxford University Press.

Treatment

Acute setting—Addisonian crisis needs stat administration of **hydrocortisone** to save the patient's life. Often tested as unexplained hypotension in hospitalized patient. Hydrocortisone 100 mg IV x 1. Remember your ABCs to manage the rest, such as hypotension, etc. Also monitor and manipulate electrolytes as needed.

Chronic setting—Mineralcorticoid replacement is the mainstay. **Hydrocortisone** in two divided doses. **Fludrocortisone** in one daily dose. Monitor coexisting conditions such as diabetes and thyroid problems and correct as needed.

Take Home Points

- In Addison's disease, a hypofunctioning adrenal gland leads to decreased cortisol, which leads to high ACTH levels.

- Characteristic routine laboratories should cause suspicion of Addison's disease.

- Treat Addison's disease with exogenous steroids.

Hyperaldostronism and Conn's Syndrome (Primary)

Conn's syndrome (primary) is caused by excess secretion of aldosterone most likely from an adrenal cortex adenoma. Look for low renin levels.

Secondary hyperaldostronism is more common and related to renovascular hypertension, renal artery stenosis, and edematous disorders such as heart failure, cirrhosis, and nephrotic syndrome.

Symptoms

Symptoms from electrolyte disturbances, personality disturbances, fatigue, weakness, cramps, headache, palpitations, hyperglycemia, or most commonly, **moderate hypertension.**

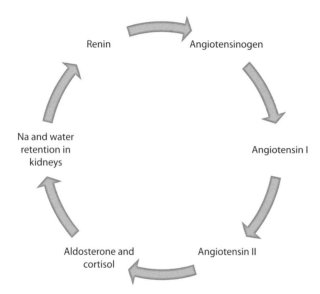

FIGURE 13.8 Renin-angiotensin cycle.

Diagnosis

Electrolyte disturbances such as hypernatremia, hypokalemia, metabolic alkalosis.

Check renin levels. May be high or low, primary corresponding to low renin, high corresponding to secondary hyperaldosteronism.

Check aldosterone levels.

CT the abdomen looking for adenomas.

Treatment

For Conn's syndrome, surgery is often first line.

The classic medical therapy for hyperaldosteronism is **spironolactone** (an aldosterone receptor antagonist) for 5–8 weeks and it can both treat and help diagnose. Amiloride (Midamor), triamterene (Dyrenium), or eplerenone (Inspra) may also be helpful if hyperaldosteronism is secondary or the patient is not a candidate for surgery.

Surgery is definitive and most useful in Conn's (primary) syndrome.

Take Home Points

- Presentation is subtle. If suspected, renin levels will show abnormality (either high or low).
- Spironolactone is the classic medical treatment.
- Surgery is used commonly in Conn's syndrome as first line.

Pheochromocytoma

A primary adrenal catecholamine-producing tumor that produces norepinephrine and epinephrine.

Associated with other disorders, including multiple endocrine neoplasia (MEN) type II, and von Hippel-Lindau disease.

Symptoms

Classically, **fluctuant hypertension**, tachycardia, palpitations. Follow the rule of 5 Hs:

- Headache
- Hypertension
- Hyperhidrosis
- Hyperglycemia
- Hypermetabolism

Stimulation of the sympathetic nervous system by catecholamine release triggers characteristic symptoms.

Diagnosis

Labs: 24-hour urine collection for catecholamines (metanephrines), which are increased.
Imaging: CT is useful but only in finding tumors $> \frac{1}{2}$ inch diameter.
MRI: useful since these tumors have distinctive suprarenal appearance.

Scintigraphy: Uses ^{131}I-MIBG and can better localize extra-adrenal tumors. Newer than and not as practical as above.

Treatment

Volume expansion as needed then a combination of α and β blockers can be used. Use prazosin and phenoxybenzamine for α and propranolol for β blockade.

Then **surgery**, usually laproscopic, is the treatment of choice.

Take Home Points

- Presentation of pheochromocytoma may only be fluctuant hypertension.
- Urine collection for catecholamines is the test of choice.
- Surgery is the ultimate treatment.

Malnutrition

Protein-Energy Malnutrition

Two forms: Marasmus—lack of both **calories** and **protein**. Caused by starvation state.

Kwashiorkor—lack of **protein** with adequate calories (usually in carbohydrate form). Often seen in developing countries when young children stop breastfeeding.

Symptoms

Marasmus children tend to appear thin, short in stature, lethargic, and undernourished.

Kwashiorkor children appear edematous, ascetic, with thin arms and legs. Often with "flaky paint" dermatosis, short in stature, and enlarged fatty liver.

Diagnosis

Various vitamin deficiencies accompany both forms. Kwashiorkor patients tend to have low albumin, low essential amino acids, and low glucose. Electrolyte abnormalities often exist including hypokalemia, hypocalcemia, hypophosphatemia, and hypomagnesemia.

Treatment

First replace fluid and electrolytes. Commonly done over 24–48 hour period. Then replace macronutrients, including lipid, protein, and carbohydrate using PO forms. This process can take up to 12 weeks but is associated with better prognosis with earlier intervention.

Take Home Points

- Malnutrition commonly comes in two forms: Marasmus and Kwashiorkor.
- Replace fluids and electrolytes in the beginning then slowly give macronutrients. Overfeeding early can be fatal!

Obesity and Weight Excess

Obesity in the developed world has progressed to epidemic proportions and now rivals smoking as a key health concern. According to the National Health and Nutrition Examination Survey (NHANES) of 2003–04, 32% of Americans are obese. Risk factors include pre-adolescent/adolescent excess weight, parental excess weight, sedentary lifestyle, excess television watching, low socioeconomic status, pregnancy, and high-fat diet.

Symptoms

Symptoms are centered on morbidity and occur in direct correlation to the degree of excess weight. Exercise intolerance, low daily energy, and irritability may be associated with the mildly overweight status while the obese or morbidly obese may experience significant muscular atrophy, depression, constricted breathing, frictional or yeast dermatosis, severe exercise intolerance, and pulmonary and cardiovascular events. Psychological impact of especially morbid obesity should not be underestimated.

Diagnosis

Physical exam: Android or central obesity is commonly seen in men and includes a predilection toward central abdominal adiposity. Gynecoid obesity occurs more commonly in women and is seen as non-central abdominal adiposity mainly around the gluteal region.

Body Mass Index:

BMI = weight (kg) / (height (m))^2

TABLE 13.9 Classification of Weight Status Based on BMI

Weight Class	BMI (kg/m²)
Underweight	< 18.5
Normal	≥ 18.5–24.9
Overweight	≥ 25.0–29.9
Obesity Class I	≥ 30.0–34.9
Obesity Class II	≥ 35.0–39.9
Obesity Class III	≥ 40

Recommended classes by the National Institutes of Health (NIH) and World Health Organization (WHO).

It should be noted that BMI measurement and classification has limitations for individuals who are excessively muscular and are thus heavy without excess body weight. Also, BMI is more accurate for those of Caucasian, African, and Hispanic descent and adjustment of values may be needed for Asians or other ethnic groups.

Waist circumference measurement may indicate increased risk for most obesity-related medical conditions although accuracy for prediction of health risks is limited mainly to those classified as overweight or obesity class I. In these two classes, waist circumference > 40 in (102 cm) in men or > 35 in (88 cm) in women is considered excessive and is associated with further weight-related health risks.

Other types of evaluation include bioelectric impedance measurement, and caliper-based or water displacement-based determination of total body fat. These techniques have not been shown to have advantages above measurement of BMI when consideration of BMI limitations has been taken into account.

Labs: Very rarely is obesity/weight excess due to systemic or endocrinologic disease such as hypothyroidism, Cushing's disease, insulinoma, or hypothalamic disorders.

Treatment

The first law of thermodynamics is one of conservation of energy and states that, in a closed system, energy may neither be created nor destroyed. In application to excess weight, upon burning more calories than that which are taken in, the energy for that metabolic fuel must come from energy stores including fat and muscle. Therefore, if a patient is attempting to lose weight and is frustrated due to reduction of intake and seemingly excess exercise, caloric balance must still be maintained to remain the same weight.

Diets of various types dominate the popular media. They are basically all variations on the theme of reducing caloric intake. Some recommend macronutrient restriction such as carbohydrates. These diets work slightly differently in that they use the principle of macronutrient restriction (protein/carbohydrate/fat) to interrupt metabolism of storing energy. Thus, the used calories are actually reduced since storage of energy is interrupted. Overall, these have been thought to be a less healthy way of weight loss and have shown poor long term weight reduction, although initially effective.

Lifestyle change for sustained weight loss should be advised, including overall caloric reduction and increased caloric expenditure. The patient should be counseled that their body will adjust to the energy balance it is given; if that changes to restrictive, weight will be lost. However, if it again changes back to a previously higher energy balance, the body will adjust back, causing a "yo-yo" pattern. The generally accepted caloric deficit guideline is 500 kcal/day, which should result in a weight reduction of approximately 1 lb per week with eventual goal of 10–15% total reduction of body weight in 6 months, although this guideline should be individualized. A permanent change in energy balance should be stressed to sustain weight loss.

Medications: Silbutramine (Meridia, Reductil) works through norepinephrine/serotonin/dopamine reuptake inhibition to suppress appetite and stimulate calories burned. Orlistat (Xenecal, Alli) works through gastric and pancreatic lipase inhibition to block fat digestion and absorption and should be taken before fatty meals. Supplement patients who are on this medication with fat soluble vitamins. Short term options include sympathomemetic drugs: diethylpropion, phentermine (Adipex-P), phendimetrazine (Bontril), or benzphetamine (Didrex). Other experimental medications are under investigation but none have universally shown both a safe profile and effectiveness for weight reduction.

Surgery: Various surgical procedures, referred to as bariatric surgery (gastric bypass, gastric stapling), exist and are effective for those of BMI ≥ 40 kg/m² or ≥ 35 kg/m² with significant comorbidities. Weight loss is usually abrupt; then mild weight gain is seen followed by a plateau phase. Significant side effects include fat vitamin deficiencies, operative complications, and, rarely, gastric dumping syndrome.

Liposuction or surgical body sculpting removes and repositions fat cells and has been shown good efficacy in decreasing BMI although effects on insulin sensitivity and obesity-related health effects appears to be negligible.

Take Home Points

- Obesity and excess weight is currently of epidemic proportions in the U.S. and is increasing worldwide.
- BMI is the best and most widely used measurement calculation for assessing weight status.
- Central weight excess is associated with significantly higher health risks.
- Lifestyle changes should be stressed for weight reduction. Caloric balance and not temporary restriction should be stressed.
- Surgery should be considered in those who fail weight reduction attempts and have a BMI ≥ 40 kg/m^2 or ≥ 35 kg/m^2 with significant comorbidities.

Vitamin and Mineral Deficiencies

Vitamins

TABLE 13.10 Common Vitamin Deficiencies

Vitamin	Associations/Signs of Deficiency	Treatment
A*	Night blindness, dry eyes, scaly rash, increased infections	PO or IM replacement
D*	Rickets, osteomalacia, hypocalcemia. Low 25(OH)D$_3$, 1,25(OH)$_2$D$_3$, and PO$_4$ levels.	PO replacement
E*	Hemolytic anemia, peripheral neuropathy, ataxia	PO replacement
K*	Hemorrhage, increased PT time (INR)	PO replacement for non-emergency, IM/SC for emergency (phytonadione is generic name)
B$_1$(thiamine)	Wet beriberi (high output cardiac failure) Dry beriberi (peripheral neuropathy) Wernicke and Korsakoff syndromes Deficiency often seen in alcoholics	PO for mild cases IM, IV for moderate/severe or unknown (always give thiamine before glucose!)
B$_2$ (Riboflavin)	Angular stomatitis, dermatitis, cheilosis. Difficult to diagnose based on hx/PE alone	PO replacement can be both diagnostic and curative. IM also available
B$_3$ (Niacin)	Pellagra (3 D's-dementia, dermatitis, diarrhea), stomatitis, glossitis	Give niacinamide instead of niacin to avoid side effects. Start PO and use IM/SC if needed. May also use niacin but watch for common side effects.
B$_6$ (Pyridoxine)	Meds: Hydralazine, isoniazid, penicillamine, OCPs. Seborrheic dermatitis, anemia (normo/microcytic) peripheral neuropathy, glossitis, cheilosis, lymphopenea, and convulsions in infants.	Correct the underlying cause of medication. PO replacement in adults and IM/IV in infants.

(continued)

TABLE 13.10 Continued

Vitamin	Associations/Signs of Deficiency	Treatment
B$_{12}$ (Cobalamin)	Macrocytic anemia plus neurologic symptoms. Look for pernicious anemia, infection with *D Latum* (fish tape worm)	PO or IM/SC replacement
Folate	Macrocytic anemia without neurologic symptoms. Occurs much quicker than vit B12 in alcoholics. Look for pregnancy and neuro tube defects in infants.	PO replacement
C	Scurvy (bleeding gums, opening of old wounds, petechiae), poor wound healing, bone pain. Associated with "tea and toast" diet seen in elderly.	PO replacement

* indicates lipid soluble vitamins

Minerals

TABLE 13.11 Common Mineral Deficiencies

Mineral	Associations/Signs of Deficiency	Treatment
Iron	Microcytic anemia. Most common mineral def in the world. May see pica. Order iron panel for better look at status. **Ferritin** is best test to eval.	PO FeSO$_4$ supplements if mild/mod. IV iron for severe cases. Give stool softener for common SE of constipation.
Iodine	Diffuse goiter, cretinism, hypothyroidism.	Iodine supplement (usually supplied in iodized salt in the developed world.) at about 10 times normal maintenance dose × 2–3 weeks.
Zinc	Slow wound healing, anorexia, slowed growth, delayed sexual maturation, dermatitis, impaired taste, alopecia.	PO replacement.
Copper	Rare; associated with malnourished states, infantile diarrhea, diet limited in milk, sprue, prolonged total parenteral nutrition use.	PO replacement.
Selenium	Rare; cardiomyopathy, myalgias.	Selenomethionine supplement PO.
Chromium	Rare; glucose intolerance, peripheral neuropathy. Associated with TPN use.	PO replacement.

Phenylketonuria (PKU)

A congenital lack of the metabolic enzyme responsible for breaking down the dietary amino acid phenyl-alanine, phenylalanine hydroxylase, resulting in toxic levels of phenylalanine.

Symptoms

Mental retardation evident often after the infant stage and most often severe. Seizures and abnormal EEGs develop later. May also tend to have lighter skin, hair, and eyes. **"Mousy odor"** of the breath may also be present.

Diagnosis

PKU screen routinely done on every child born in U.S. within 72 hours. Child is fed normal diet of milk and if PKU is present, phenylalanine levels will rise in the blood and become detectable. In infants with family history of PKU and normal screen, check urine after 4–6 weeks and periodically until one year of age. Screening tests must be confirmed by further testing if positive.

Treatment

Restriction of phenylalanine in the diet as early in life as possible is paramount. This prevents retardation. Lofenalac is the phenylalanine-free formula of choice and is widely available in the U.S. Other foods with limited phenylalanine are becoming more widely available and food makers have started placing warnings on food that contains phenylalanine (such as artificial sweeteners, dairy).

Take Home Points

- PKU often results in mental retardation.
- Dietary intervention must occur early to save the child from neural damage.

Disorders of Mineral Metabolism

Calcium

TABLE 13.12 Calcium Derangement

	Hypo	Hyper
Associations	Tetany, muscle cramps, QT prolongation, psychosis. Physical exam shows Chvostgek's and Trousseau's signs.	"Bones, Stones, Groans, Psychotic overtones" for fractures/osteopenia, nephrolithiasis, abdominal pain/pancreatitis, depression/mental status changes.
Etiology	Parathyroid removal (often mistake with thyroidectomy), DiGeorge's syndrome, pancreatitis, short bowel syndrome, Vitamin D deficiency, low magneisium	C- Calcium excess H- **Hyperparathyroid**/hyperthyroid I- Thiazide diuretics M- Metastases/Milk Alkali syndrome P- Paget's disease of the bone A- Addison's disease N- Neoplasm Z- Zollinger-Ellison syndrome E- Excess Vit D E- Excess Vit A S- Sarcoidosis
Treatment	Correct serum calcium for Albumen! Measure ionized Calcium. IV or PO replacement	IV fluids and Lasix to increase excretion. Treat underlying cause. Calcitonin, bisphosphonates including zoledronic acid (Zometa) or pamidronate (Aredia), may be useful depending on level of abnormality. Dialysis if severe.

Magnesium

TABLE 13.13 Magnesium Derangement

	Hypo	Hyper
Associations	Tetany/increased deep tendon reflexes (DTRs), arrhythmias, constipation, other electrolytes (especially K, classically hard to correct)	Too much $MgSO_4$ given to preeclamptic woman in labor! Decreased deep tendon reflexes (DTRs), CNS depression, respiratory failure.
Etiology	Diarrhea/vomiting, celiac disease, renal failure, alcoholism, malnutrition, diabetic ketoacidosis, pregnancy, pancreatitis	Exogenous MgSO4 given in labor! Renal failure.
Treatment	IV/PO replacement (monitor for over correction!)	IV calcium, insulin and glucose, Lasix, dialysis if severe

Phosphorus

TABLE 13.14 Phosphorus Derangement

	Hypo	Hyper
Associations	General muscle weakness, diaphragmatic weakness	Metastasis, hypocalcemia
Etiology	Diabetic ketoacidosis, calcium derangement	Renal failure, parenteral overadministration
Treatment	PO or IV replacement	Calcium carbonate

Electrolyte and Fluid Disorders

Hyponatremia

Low plasma sodium level. Sodium < 135 mEq/L.

Symptoms

Commonly asymptomatic, especially if it has existed for long term. Mental status change may be short or long term. Muscle cramps, lethargy, and seizures can occur acutely.

Diagnosis

Measurement of plasma sodium. Remember to correct for glucose level!

Plasma osmolarity then will help further diagnostic division.

Hypertonic hyponatremia:

- Due to increased osmols from glucose or hypertonic infusion of glucose, mannitol, or glycine.

Isotonic hyponatremia:

- Due to pseudohyponatremia from osmols present because of hyperlipidemia, hyperproteinemia, or isotonic infusions of glucose, mannitol, or glycine.

Hypotonic hyponatremia:

- Further consideration of volume status needed (biggest and most tested group).

- FENa (fractional excretion of sodium) will help tell if the kidney is appropriately conserving sodium.

- Obtain FENa labs (UNa/UCr)/(PNa/PCr) x 100 = FENa.

TABLE 13.15 FENA Results

FENa	Source of Derangement	Etiology
< 1%	Pre-renal	Renal salt conservation
> 2%	Intrinsic renal	Renal salt wasting

*Hypo*volemic hypotonic hyponatremia:
Etiologies: Dehydration, diarrhea/vomiting, diuretics, nephropathies, partial urinary tract obstruction, diabetic ketoacidosis, or adrenal insufficiency.
*Eu*volemic hypotonic hyponatremia:
Etiologies: **SIADH**, psychogenic polydipsia, hypothyroidism, or beer potomania.
*Hyper*volemic hypotonic hyponatremia (edematous states):
Etiologies: CHF, liver disease, nephrotic syndrome, or advanced renal failure.

Treatment

If mental status changes are extreme, consider "hot salts" (3% NaCl solution) over 6 hours.

In hypertonic or isotonic hyponatremia, correct the underlying cause (stop infusions, lower lipids, etc.). In hypotonic hyponatremia, consider volume status. Treatment often involves administration of IV Na-containing fluid but be careful to not correct over 12 mEq/L per day to avoid the dreaded **central pontine myelinolysis.**

Hypovolemic hypotonic hyponatremia: Administer isotonic (normal) saline with close monitoring of sodium level.

Euvolemic hypotonic hyponatremia: Fluid restrict only.

Hypervolemic hypotonic hyponatremia: Fluid restrict and diuretics as needed.

Take Home Points

- First, measure serum osmolality, then classify hyponatremia based on volume status.
- Hypotonic hyponatremia is the most common form of hyponatremia.
- Correct the hyponatremia slowly especially if the patient has been in this state for a long time.

Hypernatremia

Increased blood sodium levels. Sodium > 145 mEq/L.

Common etiologies include dehydration, diuretic use/abuse, diabetes insipidus, diarrhea, renal disease, or dementia causing lack of water intake.

Symptoms

Similar symptoms to hyponatremia: mental status change, confusion, seizures, hyperreflexia. Oligouria or polyuria may be present depending on etiology.

Diagnosis

Often caused by dehydration, so check urine output and plasma osmolarity, BUN/creatinine.

Consider evaluation for diabetes insipidus (water deprivation test).

Treatment

Treat the underlying cause.

Dehydration: IV NS until rehydrated then hypotonic solution may be administered until sodium is normal.

Treat diabetes insipidus if present.

Don't correct plasma sodium too rapidly in order to avoid **cerebral edema.**

Take Home Points

- Dehydration is the most common cause.

Hypokalemia

Plasma potassium < 3.5 mEq/L. Etiologies are broad, but common ones include diabetic ketoacidosis, hypomagnesemia, laxative abuse, vomiting, adrenal derangement, and acid/base disturbances.

Symptoms

Fatigue, muscle weakness, **muscle cramps**, ileus, hyporeflexia, flaccid paralysis if severe. Cardiac arrhythmias may present as chest pain, palpitations, presyncope, or syncope.

Diagnosis

ECG: ECG shows **T-Wave flattening** and possibly U-waves. May progress to ST depression, AV block and cardiac arrest.

Labs: Plasma potassium, urine potassium, plasma pH

- Urine potassium high (> 20 mEq/L) → renal potassium losses

  - Lactic or ketoacidosis, hyperaldostronism, Cushing's syndrome, hypomagnesemia, or meds (amphotericin, diuretics, gentamicin).

- Urine potassium low (< 20 mEq/L) → nonrenal potassium causes

  - Transcellular shift from insulin, β-Blockers, alkalosis or GI losses from diarrhea, laxative abuse, vomiting, or NG suctioning.

Treatment

Treat the underlying disorder.

Remember to replace magnesium!

As an inpatient, give IV KCl (often as a "K rider" to another isotonic crystalloid fluid) and monitor closely, then switch to PO. Typical inpatient infusion is often 10 mEq/L. Do not exceed 20 mEq/L intravenously.

If mild hypokalemia, give supplement in pill form or replete with dietary sources, which include oranges, bananas, cantaloupe, prunes, raisins, beans, apricots, and squash.

Take Home Points

- Presentation may involve muscle cramps or cardiac abnormalities.

- Replace magnesium if needed or potassium will be resistant to repletion.

- Monitor ECG during treatment.

Hyperkalemia

Serum potassium > 5.0 mEq/L. The most common cause is spurious hyperkalemia from hemolysis caused by sitting in the vial too long. Non-spurious causes include renal failure, mineralcorticoid deficiency, cellular shifts from insulin deficiency, and tumorlysis. Meds are also a major category and include effects from: spironolactone, triamterene, ACE-Is, heparin, pentamidine, amiloride, arginine, trimethoprim, NSAIDs, succinylcholine, digitalis effect, and β-blockers.

Symptoms

Ventricular fibrillation, intestinal colic, areflexia, weakness, paralysis, parasthesias.

Diagnosis

Recheck the blood draw! Order repeat K and electrolytes to include Mg.

ECG: Peaked T waves, PR prolongation. Later, hyperkalemia may lead to widening of the QRS complex and **loss of p waves** which may potentially progress to sine waves (**torsades de pointes**) then to cardiac arrest!

Place on continuous cardiac monitoring.

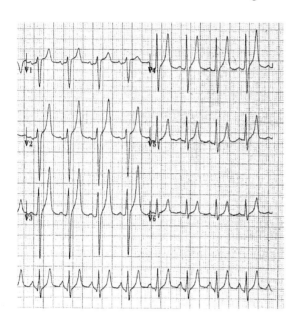

FIGURE 13.9 Hyperkalemaia. Note tall, peaked T waves. Reprinted with permission from Cox NLT, Roper TA. *Clinical Skills*. 2005, Oxford University Press.

Treatment

For mild derangement not evident clinically on ECG, may give PO treatment and correct underlying cause. Sodium polystyrene sulfonate (Kayexalate) PO/NG or retention enema.

For clinically apparent derangement or ECG changes:

- Acutely: Calcium gluconate to stabilize cardiac muscle
- Consider albuterol breathing treatment
- IV glucose + insulin to shift K into cells
- Furosemide IV to increase excretion
- Dialysis as last resort

Remember to replace Mg if needed.

Take Home Points

- Make sure the lab value is not due to hemolysis before initiating treatment.
- Start ECG monitoring as soon as hyperkalemia is discovered.

Hypovolemia

Lack of adequate intravascular volume.

Symptoms

Poor skin turgor, dry mucous membranes, low urine output, concentrated urine, tachycardia. Children may show fluid inadequacy by lack of tears, lethargy, and increased fussiness.

Diagnosis

Hypovolemia remains a clinical decision.
Labs: Urine specific gravity, BUN/creatinine; FENa < 1%.

Treatment

Fluids vary by type.

Crystalloid fluids will directly replace volume themselves, such as normal saline or lactated ringer.

Colloid fluids will exert osmotic action from the intravascular space to pull fluid from the extravascular space, thus expanding the intravascular fluid volume. Examples include hetastarch (Hextend) or albumin solution.

Common crystalloid therapy includes normal saline or lactated ringer by bolus then switching to maintenance rate for adults. See table below for guidance for children.

Adults can commonly be returned to a normovolemic state by simply providing fluid boluses of crystalloid solution followed by maintenance fluids. The rule of thumb is to provide crystalloid fluids by bolus or rapid infusion until the patient urinates. This does not apply to certain disease states like renal failure or CHF.

Children have a somewhat more complex requirement:

Bolus

LR or NS

TABLE 13.16 Bolus in Children

Small children	20 mL/kg (2% body wt)
Adolescents	10 mL/kg (1% body wt)

Deficit

$D_5 0.45NS + 20mEq/L$ K
Based on estimate 5% mild, 10% moderate, 15% severe
Two different methods (see table below)

TABLE 13.17 Deficit Replacement by Two Different Methods*

	Combined Deficit and Maintenance	Sequential Deficit and Maintenance
First 8 hours after bolus	½ remaining deficit + ⅓ daily maintenance	Remaining deficit (after bolus)
Next 16 hours	½ remaining deficit + ⅔ daily maintenance	Daily maintenance

*These methods are considered equal in efficacy.

Maintenance Calculation

$D_5 0.2NS + 20$ mEq/L K

Holliday-Segar formula

TABLE 13.18 Maintenance Fluid Calculation

Weight (kg)	Kcal/d or mL/d	Kcal/h or mL/h
0–10 kg	100/kg per day	**4 mL/kg/hour**
11–20 kg	1000 + (50 mL/kg/day above 10)	**40 + (2 mL/kg/hour above 10)**
> 20 kg	1500 + (20 mL/kg/day above 20)	**60 + (1 mL/kg/hour above 20)**

Take Home Points

- Fluid replacement should be done with a combination of boluses, deficit replacement, and maintenance fluid administration.

- Crystalloid solutions are, by far, more common but colloid solutions may be more useful in situations of needing rapid volume expansion.

Hypervolemia

The state of having too much fluid in the body. This fluid is often shunted to a "third space," meaning a place within the body that acts to isolate the fluid volume from the intravascular space (this may be a pleural effusion or ascetic fluid).

Symptoms

Depending on the reason: weight gain, edema, increasing belt or waistband size, JVD, rales/crackles in lungs, or hypertension.

Diagnosis

Clinical assessment
Labs: Urine specific gravity, BUN/creatinine.
Imaging: Chest x-ray showing pulmonary edema/effusion.

Treatment

Diuresis with furosemide (Lasix) or dialysis if severe.

Surgical drainage of a "third space" fluid reservoir may be indicated, e.g. pleurocentesis, peritoneal tap, etc.

Take Home Points

- Hypervolemia is most commonly caused by CHF or renal abnormalities.
- Diuretics are the mainstay of therapy and are adequate in the vast majority of cases.

14 Neonatal Medicine

Conditions Originating in the Perinatal Period

TABLE 14.1 Congenital Anomalies

Anomaly	Associations/Diagnosis	Treatment
Cleft lip/palate	Abnormal development of labial groove. Poor feeding and recurrent otitis media.	Surgical repair.
Gastroschisis	Intestines extrude outside of abdominal wall—**WITHOUT** a surrounding membrane. Often associated with **polyhydramnios** during pregnancy.	NG tube to suction. Sterile gauze dressing with immediate primary surgical closure. May require staged procedures.
Omphalocele	Intestines extrude outside of abdominal wall—**WITH** a surrounding membrane.	Staged surgical repair.
Tracheosophageal fistula	Different types but most common ends in blind esophageal pouch. Presents with severe feeding problems and copious oral secretions.	Suction of pouch and surgical repair.
Diaphragmatic hernia	Abdominal cavity contents herniated through diaphragm into pleural cavity. Respiratory distress and **scaphoid abdomen**. > 95% on left side.	Intubation to improve ventilation. Surgical repair.
Hirschprung disease	Intestinal wall absence of ganglion cells in one specific area. Leading to relative constriction of bowel during development. After birth, abdominal distention and vomiting are seen.	Diversion with colostomy until > 6 months old, then resection of segment and reanastimosis.
Choanal atresia	Cyanosis when feeding that is relieved by crying. Inability to pass nasogastric tube is pathognomonic.	Surgery.

Fetal Growth Restriction (FGR)

A term used to describe fetal growth restriction occurring before birth; generally defined as ≤ 10% of expected size for gestational age. There are three classes of etiologies, each with their own causes, including fetal, placental, and maternal.

TABLE 14.2. Etiologies of FGR

Fetal	Placental	Maternal
Genetic (trisomies, autosomal deletions, ring chromosomes, etc.)	Single umbilical artery	Poor nutrition
Multiple gestation	Velamentous umbilical cord insertion	Prothrombotic states
	Bilobate placenta	Hypoxemia
	Placental hemangioma	Hypertension and vascular disease
	Placenta previa	EtOH, cigarette smoking, and substance abuse
	Abruptio placenta	Infection (TORCHES)
	Confined placental mosaicism (CPM)	Toxins or medications (warfarin, anticonvulsants, etc)

Diagnosis

Physical exam: Often large discrepancy in fundal height for gestational age (after 20 weeks). There are other techniques for determining inappropriate size including abdominal circumference, etc. These are used less often in practice than fundal height measurement.

Imaging: Ultrasound is the gold standard. May need level II (advanced) ultrasound to confirm. Oligohydramnios may be present.

Key points to look for are symmetric vs. asymmetric growth restriction.

Asymmetric often occurs with placental problems or malnutrition states. Head is relatively spared from abnormal growth and is apparent later in pregnancy. Associated with better prognosis and "catch up" growth post partum.

Symmetric often occurs with congenital infection or genetic problems. Head is symmetrically included in abnormal growth. Poorer prognosis for normal growth after birth.

Treatment

Largely depends on the cause. For asymmetric growth restriction, proper nutrition and close, frequent follow up is warranted. For symmetric, investigation of possible causes is needed and treatment should be aimed at etiology. Often, prevention and good prenatal care is the best approach.

Take Home Points

- Etiologies include three categories of problems, fetal, placental, and maternal.
- Diagnosis is best done by ultrasound.
- Asymmetric vs. symmetric FGR is key in determining prognosis. Asymmetric is better.

Post-Term Infant

Any infant born after 42 + $^0/_7$ weeks after the first day of the last menstrual period. A main risk is of being hypoglycemic or macrosomic with accompanying risks including birth trauma, e.g., shoulder dystocia, Erb palsy, etc. Overall neonatal mortality also increases beyond the point of post-term gestation.

Diagnosis

Establish dates of pregnancy!
Check for birth trauma and hypoglycemia.
Meconium aspiration is more common with later pregnancy.

Treatment

Prevention with induction and augmentation of labor should be offered and discussed at 41 weeks gestation. If macrosomia is considered a significant risk, consider Cesarean section.

Take Home Points

- Post-term pregnancy is that gestation extending beyond 42 + $^0/_7$ weeks.
- Risks include hypoglycemia, birth trauma, and increased overall mortality.
- Offer induction of labor at 41 weeks gestation.

Birth Trauma

See Chapter 9: Pregnancy and Childbirth for shoulder dystocia discussion.

TABLE 14.3 Conditions Associated with Birth Trauma

Trauma	Diagnosis/Associations	Treatment
Cephalhematoma	Subperiosteal hemorrhage **limited by skull sutures**. Often associated with vacuum delivery. Exam will differentiate from other trauma such as subgaleal hemorrhage.	None necessary. May cause hyperbilirubinemia from blood breakdown as it resolves. Rarely can show calcifications.
Subgaleal hemorrhage	Trauma to subgaleal vessels and is an emergency. **Crosses the skull sutures**. Felt as a generalized boggy scalp.	Surgical evacuation of blood.
Erb's palsy	Upper brachial plexus (C5-C6) injury. Adduction/internal rotation of shoulder with pronation of wrist. "Waiter's tip" position.	Bracing close to body and monitoring for likely improvement.
Klumpke's palsy	Lower brachial plexus (C7-T1) injury. Paralysis of the hand and wrist. May be in "claw hand" position.	Bracing and passive physical therapy. Likely improvement.

Neonatal Respiratory Distress Syndrome (Hyaline Membrane Disease)

Respiratory distress syndrome (RDS) is primarily due to lack of mature surfactant in the lungs at birth. Because of this lack of surfactant, surface tension in the alveoli is much greater leading to micro and macro airspace collapse. As the disease progresses, pulmonary inflammation develops leading to epithelial injury and pulmonary edema, causing a further difficulty of blood oxygenation.

Symptoms

Newborn with nasal flaring, cyanosis, tachypnea, and cyanosis, grunting, or intercostal and subxiphoid retractions (accessory muscle use for respiration). Usually the newborn is difficult to calm and fussy. History of premature birth is very commonly present.

Diagnosis

Physical exam: Crackles throughout lung fields, low O_2 saturation, and high breathing rate.

Labs: ABG shows low PO_2 and high PCO_2 although this does respond to supplemental oxygen. Hyponatremia may develop later in the course.

Imaging: CXR often shows diffuse **"ground glass"** appearance indicating atelectasis as well as air bronchograms.

Treatment

Start with supplemental oxygen therapy and quickly move to "oxyhood" (sometimes called oxygen tent) over baby's head to better deliver oxygen. Consider positive pressure ventilation or intubation and mechanical ventilation. Transfer to the neonatal ICU in this case.

Artificial surfactant, beractant (Survanta) given through endotracheal tube is the gold standard.

If risk factors such as prematurity and GDM are present during pregnancy and labor starts prematurely, prevention of RDS with maternal parenteral administration of steroids may be life saving.

Take Home Points

- RDS is the result of lack of mature surfactant in the lungs.
- Commonly seen in premature infants.
- Give artificial surfactant via endotrachial tube for treatment.
- Prevent RDS in high risk pregnancies by the use of parenteral steroids.

Meconium Aspiration

Pneumonitis caused by neonatal inhalation of meconium-containing amniotic fluid. This occurs with a higher frequency the later the pregnancy gets, presumably due to the higher proportion of meconium at the later gestational age. Meconium aspiration should be clinically distinguished from pneumonia, TTN, or other types of early respiratory problems.

Symptoms

Newborn with nasal flaring, cyanosis, grunting, or intercostal and subxiphoid retractions (accessory muscle use for respiration). Usually difficult to calm and fussy. The baby is often born with meconium-stained amniotic fluid.

Diagnosis

Physical exam often reveals prominent crackles throughout lungs. If air trapping occurs from proximal bronchial obstruction, "barrel chest" appearance may result. Obtain O_2 saturation and breathing rate. Look for signs of tension pneumothorax.

Labs: ABG shows low PO_2 and high PCO_2.

Imaging: CXR often shows diffuse opacities in lungs or atelectasis. Should not show consolidation.

Treatment

In delivery room, DeLee suctioning may be used to clear nose, mouth, pharynx. If baby has not cried yet when transferred to the resuscitation team, consider suctioning below the vocal cords with an endotrachial tube (not DeLee suction). If baby has cried, simply clear the fluid from mouth, nose, and pharynx with simple suction. Passing an NG tube and suctioning the contents of the stomach may also act to decompress the pleural cavity. If baby still exhibits signs of respiratory distress, start supplemental oxygen and consider positive pressure ventilation or intubation and mechanical ventilation.

Take Home Points

- Meconium aspiration causes pneumonitis, not pneumonia (in early stages).
- Distinguish between meconium aspiration pneumonitis and other types of respiratory problems.
- "Suctioning below the vocal cords" is only useful before the baby takes its first breath.

Pneumomediastinum/Pneumothorax

The pathologic state of extrapulmonary air in the pleural cavity in the case of pneumothorax and air in the mediastinal area in pneumomediastinum. These commonly occur together in the neonate and may be treated in similar fashion, thus, will be discussed together here. Causes vary but use of positive pressure ventilation or mechanical ventilation after birth is the leading risk factor.

Symptoms

Signs of respiratory distress and tachypnea. May have loss of lung sounds in one field on exam. Exam may reveal anterior superior subdermal emphysema.

Diagnosis

Physical exam: Low O_2 saturation, high breathing rate, and clinically in respiratory distress. **Transillumination** may reveal "flash" of light at end of expiratory cycle indicating abnormality.
Labs: ABG may show low pO_2 and high pCO_2.
Imaging: CXR shows increased, sharp heart border and lack of vascular markings extending to the sides of lung fields. Consider that CXRs are taken in babies while in the supine position, thus, differ from the upright PA/lat appearance in adults.

Treatment

If infant is in otherwise unresponsive respiratory distress, a chest tube may be placed. If oxygenating well (with or without O_2 supplement) defect may be observed and followed without treatment. The vast majority resolve on their own.

Take Home Points

- Use of positive pressure ventilation or intubation after birth is an important risk factor for pneumothorax.
- Transillumination with the finding of a "flash" at the end of expiration shows pneumothorax.
- Treatment with chest tube may not always be necessary.

Transient Tachypnea of the Newborn (TTN)

A lung disorder characterized by pulmonary edema resulting from delayed resorption and clearance of fetal alveolar fluid. Risk factors include prematurity, Cesarean section delivery, gestational diabetes, and maternal asthma.

Symptoms

Fast breathing and fussiness that most commoqnly presents within 2 hours of delivery.

Diagnosis

Physical exam: Respiratory rate ≥ 60 breaths/min. Low O_2 sats, mild respiratory distress symptoms of nasal flaring, intercostals and subxiphoid retractions, grunting, tachypnea, and possibly cyanosis.
Labs: ABG may show low pO_2, high pCO_2.
Imaging: Chest x-ray will show hyperinflated lungs with streaky perihilar markings, giving the appearance of a **shaggy heart border** with clear lung peripheries.

Treatment

Oxygen support therapy. Intubation and mechanical ventilation are rarely needed.
Duration is usually 12–24 hours but may last as long as 72 hours.

Take Home Points

- Eliminate other causes of newborn respiratory distress before diagnosing with TTN.
- Support with oxygen is the standard treatment, course is typically short.

Neonatal Sepsis

Sepsis and systemic inflammatory response occurring in the newborn. Bacteremia with a variety of organisms is commonly present, including group B streptococcus.

Symptoms

Respiratory distress (tachypnea, grunting, intercostals and subxiphoid retractions, nasal flaring, etc.), temperature instability (**more often lower than normal temp rather than fever**), and low blood glucose. Risk factor assessment may reveal prolonged rupture of membranes (PROM) or known maternal group B strep infection.

Diagnosis

Labs: Obtain C-reactive protein (more sensitive/specific if not obtained until 12 hours after delivery), blood cultures, and CBC with manual differential. Expect absolute white count to be elevated, which is normal. With manual diff, calculate the I/T ratio.

$$\frac{I}{T} = \frac{Immature}{Total} = \frac{Bands}{Bands + seg's + other\ immature\ cells}$$

Normal is < 2–2.5. If above 2.5, this indicates sepsis.
Imaging: Chest x-ray. Look for opacity indicative of pneumonia for a possible sign of infection.

Treatment

Move baby to warmer to support body temperature.
Start antibiotics. Classically, ampicillin and gentamicin.

Obtain peripheral IV access and consider starting fluids.
Monitor with periodic heel stick glucoses and repeat labs in 6–12 hours.
Monitor closely.

Take Home Points

- Use the $^I/_T$ ratio for aid in diagnosis.
- Have a low threshold for starting antibiotics due to the rapid deterioration of newborns with sepsis.
- Monitor closely for development of respiratory distress.

Hemolytic Disease due to Rh Isoimmunization

Erythroblastosis fetalis: The increased production of erythroblasts of the fetus in response to destruction and hemolysis by maternal antibodies.

Hydrops fetalis: A condition of severe hemolytic disease from maternal antibodies. Not compatible with life.

The Rh negative mother has had previous exposure to Rh positive blood, either in previous pregnancy or other exposure. Pregnancy may be associated with polyhydramnios or history of previous miscarriage or stillborn.

Symptoms

The newborn may range from fairly asymptomatic to pale, with scalp edema, cardiomegaly, hepatomegaly, pleural effusions, and ascites. Often babies continue to develop jaundice secondary to hemolytic antibodies.

Diagnosis

Labs: If the mother is Rh negative, check the father—this disease may only occur if he is Rh positive.

Before birth, amniotic fluid sampling for bilirubin levels may help determine if and what degree hemolytic disease has affected the newborn. At birth, cord blood sample must be taken to determine fetal blood type. Do direct Coomb's test and bilirubin level on this blood. If the blood is Coomb's positive, obtain fetal hemoglobin/hematocrit and reticulocyte count.

Treatment

For mild cases, may range from no treatment with close follow up to regular transfusions. For moderate to severe disease, **exchange transfusion** is indicated. This may be done early with partial exchange or later with double exchange depending on severity of hemolysis. Phototherapy may decrease fetal bilirubin levels transiently but isn't treatment for the hemolytic disease. Also correct acidosis and accompanying disorders, e.g. heart failure etc.

Transfer to the neonatal ICU.

Remember to give mother RhoGAM at 72 hours postpartum.

Take Home Points

- Rh maternal-fetal incompatibility will cause fetal blood hemolysis.
- This disease only occurs in Rh negative mothers previously exposed to positive RBC Rh antigen (with resultant formation of antibodies).
- Spectrum of disease in the newborn is wide.

Perinatal Jaundice

Jaundice may occur for a variety of reasons in the newborn but treatment is critical to avoid long term neurologic damage; termed kernicterus.

Symptoms

Yellow appearance to the skin and eyes. Jaundice tends to occur from the head down.

Diagnosis

Physical exam: May approximate degree of jaundice by correlation anatomic level of jaundice with level of bilirubin. This is only an approximation.

Labs: Obtain total, indirect (unconjugated), and direct (conjugated) bilirubin levels from serum. Bilirubin levels physiologically should peak in range of 12–15 mg/dL at day 2–5 and may be associated with mild jaundice. Higher levels or jaundice appearing < 24 hours of life are always pathologic. Otherwise, bilirubin levels are compared to established nomograms to determine levels appropriate for time after birth. If abnormal, obtain a second level and calculate the hourly rate of rise. A linear relationship then may be assumed and used to extrapolate possible rise in bilirubin in the future (although a linear relationship admittedly does not exist). Follow increased levels of bilirubin until they trend downward.

TABLE 14.4 Causes of Perinatal Jaundice

Disorder	Associations	Treatment
Physiologic	Mild jaundice appearing in term or preterm infants with levels peaking at 2–5 days and not exceeding 15 mg/dL.	Phototherapy if at all.
Breast milk jaundice	Occurring in breastfed infants and usually peaking at approximately 20 mg/dL at 2–3 weeks of age.	Treatment is to switch to bottle feeding and monitor for resolution.
Illness	Infection and sepsis, hypothyroidism, liver toxicity, cystic fibrosis, and others may induce a hyperbilirubin state.	Correct the disorder.
Hemolysis due to maternal Rh antibodies	May present as erythroblastosis fetalis or milder form of hemolysis.	See above for treatment.
Metabolic derangement	Immaturity or genetic disorder of hepatic conjugating enzymes. May include Criggler-Najjar, Gilbert syndrome, or Dubin-Johnson syndrome.	Phototherapy or none.
Biliary atresia	May be accompanied by grayish, clay-colored stools.	Treat with surgery.
Medications	Sulfa drugs.	Stop offending agent.
Kernicterus	Often bilirubin levels > 25 mg/dL (although may occur lower if comorbidity present). Clinically may have spasticity, seizures, lethargy, and other neurologic signs.	Neurologic damage often permanent. Prevention is key. Prompt phototherapy and exchange transfusion is treatment.

Treatment

May depend on degree of hyperbilirubinemia. Mild to moderate disease may be treated with phototherapy "bili-lights." This conjugates bilirubin through the skin.

Severe cases may be taken to neonatal ICU for exchange transfusion.

Take Home Points

- Kernicterus is the pathologic and permanent state that may result from hyperbilirubinemia.
- The vast majority of cases may be treated with phototherapy.

Feeding Problems in Newborns

Feeding problems may be due to several difficulties including breastfeeding incompatibility, structural problems such as choanal atresia and neonatal heart failure, infant intolerance to formula or breast milk, and maternal complications such as breast abscess. New breastfeeding mothers often develop significantly uncomfortable nipples due to the mechanical suction of the infant but should be encouraged to continue breastfeeding as this will often resolve in a short period of time.

Symptoms

In the infant, excessive fussiness, spitting up, lethargy, or lack of suck reflex.

Diagnosis

If breast fed, observe mother and child breastfeeding, make sure latch is correct and beneficial as this is the most common breastfeeding problem.

Milk allergy is suspected and diagnosis is supported after feeding problems resolve after switch to soy-based formula. Other allergies can be discovered after switch to hypoallergenic formula.

Initial milk from mother is colostrum and should be replaced with normal breast milk after about 3 days of breastfeeding postpartum. Time to secretion of normal milk is lessened with each delivery.

Remember, ≤ 10% weight loss in newborns is normal. Return to birth weight is expected by the second week of life.

Treatment

If breastfeeding is a problem, consider a lactation consult for breastfeeding training by licensed, experienced breastfeeding nurse.

For milk or formula allergy, switch to soy or hypoallergenic formula. Remember to choose iron fortified formula.

Take Home Points

- Mothers should be encouraged to breastfeed despite minor complications, due to the proven health benefits to babies.
- If milk allergy is suspected, soy or hypoallergenic formula may be tried.

Eye Injuries

Foreign Body in the Eye

Any foreign body may cause a clinical syndrome of irritation and possible abrasion. Conjunctivitis is common and distinction should be made between traumatic symptoms and those caused by retention of foreign body. Commonly, these elements are sand, dust, metal filings, wood splinters, etc.

Symptoms

Degree of pain may range from the extreme caused by corneal abrasion to the mild sensation of general irritation. Tearing, hyperemia, and photophobia are common. Obvious bleeding and, rarely, ruptured globe are obvious. History often reveals metal work, welding, wood shop work, or other activity with high risk for particulate projectiles.

Diagnosis

Physical exam: Look for rust ring which usually forms in about 48 hours.

Fluorescein eye drops with Wood's lamp is very useful in detecting foreign body or abrasion. Slit lamp is also mandatory if abrasion or foreign body is found. Evert the eyelid to evaluate for hidden lid foreign bodies.

Imaging: Consider a CT of the orbits. DO NOT ORDER AN MRI unless absolutely sure no metal is in the eye!

Treatment

Copious ocular irrigation for 15 minutes is the standard of care and should be done as soon as possible after the injury.

With slit lamp or magnification, use a cotton swab or small tissue forceps to extract any bodies that are immediately visible. If very small, attempt to use a large bore needle to remove them but this technique should be reserved only for the very experienced!

Topical anesthetic (e.g. proparacaine 0.5% Ophth (Alcaine)) is certainly warranted. Give erythromycin, tobramycin, or bacitracin-polymixin B eye drops for antibacterial coverage. Give systemic opioids for pain relief. Avoid contact lens use and consider a 24–72 hour eye patch. Follow up with ophthalmologist in 1–2 days.

Take Home Points

- Look for an occupational risk factor in the patient with unexplained eye irritation.
- Use fluorescein eye drops for screening.
- Copious irrigation should be done ASAP after the injury.

Chemical Burns of the Eye

Chemical injuries are common in occupational scenarios and may occur secondary to direct contact or fume exposure. Alkali burns are especially destructive due to the depth of penetration.

Symptoms

Exquisite pain is present usually following obvious splash, spray, or other exposure to noxious chemicals. Profuse tearing, hyperemia, photophobia, swelling, and pain are almost always present. Obtain history for alkali or acidic burn. Don't forget, chemical fumes can cause burns as well.

Diagnosis

Immediately flush the eye for 15–30 minutes without delay or pause for diagnosis.

Carefully examine the eye with slit lamp or magnification after applying topical anesthesia such as proparacaine 0.5% Ophth (Alcaine).

Treatment

Initially, flush with copious amounts of water or normal saline for 15–30 minutes. Do not delay flushing for diagnosis.

Give topical anesthetic for complete eye exam with magnification or slit lamp.

Consider cycloplegic (e.g. Atropine 1% ophth) to reduce iritis and iris spasm which may be very painful.

Give topical antibiotics.

Treat with generous oral pain meds.

Follow up with an ophthalmologist in 24 hours.

Take Home Points

- Alkali burns tend to be deeper and cause more severe injuries than acid burns.

- Irrigate copiously with water upon presentation.

- Mace personal protective spray, "tear" gas, or pepper spray may cause significant irritation but rarely permanent damage.

Blunt Trauma to the Eye

Direct trauma to the eye may result in various types of injury from globus rupture to corneal abrasion to optic nerve avulsion.

Symptoms

Pain, swelling, hyperemia, photophobia, tearing, and contusion will be obvious. History of event should reveal exact mechanism.

Diagnosis

Physical exam: Do a superficial exam of the bony orbits to evaluate for fracture. Examine for extraocular movement dysfunction. Positive exam or lack of eye movement suggests possible orbital fracture or globe injury.

The eye itself may show corneal abrasion, scleral defect, lens displacement, mydriasis, anterior rupture, anterior or posterior humor leak, commotio retinae (white, patchy areas on the retina indicating eyelid edema), or retinal hemorrhage.

Never forcibly open the eyelids since this may aggravate a globe injury.

Generously anesthetize with systemic agents such as hydromorphone (dilaudid) or morphine and do a complete eye exam. Stop the exam if significant anterior chamber hemorrhage (hyphema), or globe rupture is found.

Imaging: Consider CT of the head to evaluate for fracture.

Evaluate and treat for foreign bodies as above.

Treatment

Initially, control pain with hydromorphone (dilaudid) or morphine. IM/IV is more effective than PO route because of short time to onset.

Dilate the pupil with short acting mydriatic such as cyclopentolate 1% ophth (Cyclogyl) and phenylephrine 2.5% ophth (Neo-Synephrine ophthalmic).

Topical antibiotic drops should be started according to regimen for foreign bodies.

Referral to ophthalmologist in < 24 hours is often needed. Consider stat consult and transport if significant injury or globus rupture.

Treatment of anterior chamber hemorrhage (hyphema) includes measurement of intraocular pressure and administration of a carbonic anhydrase inhibitor (acetazolamide) if needed.

Use of aminocaproic acid (Amicar) may reduce recurrent bleeding.

Avoid NSAIDs in anesthetic regimens as this may cause further bleeding.

Eye patch/shield until evaluation by ophthalmology or 72 hours in mild injury.

Take Home Points

- Evaluate for global rupture and internal eye damage.
- Consider CT scan to assess the bony orbit.
- Pain control is very important.

Wounds and Bites from Animals

Wounds and bites from various creatures often cause significant local trauma and commonly are the source of inflammation and infection.

Symptoms

Obvious bleeding or laceration. Signs of superficial infection such as erythema, swelling, red streaking up extremity (lymphangitis), pain, and decreased range of motion.

Diagnosis

Physical exam: Evaluate for drainage tract or fluctuance which may indicate abscess.

If bite is in the hand, consider tensynovitis (see Chapter 12: Orthopedics and Rheumatology).

Wound culture/sensitivities of any expressible fluid from infected-looking wound.

Consider blood cultures.

Imaging: Plain x-rays on any wound that is suspected of having foreign body or crush fracture.

Consider bone scan and plain x-rays to evaluate for underlying osteomyelitis if wound is significantly infected.

Treatment

Generously irrigate. This alone may help most against future infection.

Take into account the time course the patient presents from injury. Determine the level of cleanliness of the wound. Follow recommendations for tetanus and rabies prophylaxis in Chapter 3: Diseases of the Nervous System.

If wound appears infected, consider debridement of the surrounding tissue.

Tetanus and rabies prophylaxis as indicated.

Antibiotics: See table for common bites. Give amoxicillin/clavulanate (Augmentin), trimetheprim-sulfamethoxazole (TMP-SMX) DS, or clindamycin (Cleocin). Erythromycin or clarithromycin (Biaxin) are second line.

Referral is indicated for deep hand infections or tensynovitis for immediate operative debridement.

Closure may be completed with skin adhesive, suture, or staples. However, consider primary closure vs. secondary vs. delayed primary closure based on likelihood of infection and cosmesis desired. In high tension areas, consider mattress suturing for strength; in deep wounds consider multiple layer closure. Consider referral to plastic surgery if large laceration on face. Never close a dirty or infected wound!

Take Home Points

- Look for signs of infection.
- If the wound is dirty, difficult to irrigate, or with irregular mechanism consider "delayed primary closure" in which the wound is sutured only after several days.
- Amoxicillin/clavulanate (Augmentin) is the antibiotic of choice for most wounds and bites.

TABLE 15.1 Bites by Animals

Creature	Likely Organism	First Line Treatment
Human	*Viridans Strep, S. epidermidis, S. aureus*, elkenella, bacteroides	Early: amoxicillin/clavulonate (Augmentin) Late: ampicillin/sulbactam (Unasyn)
Cat	*Pasteurella multocida, S. aureus*	Amoxicillin/clavulanate (Augmentin)
Dog	*Pasteurella multocida, S. aureus, Bacteroides* sp	Amoxicillin/clavulanate (Augmentin)
Rat	*Spirillum minus, Streptobacillus moniliformis*	Amoxicillin/clavulanate (Augmentin)

Foreign Bodies

TABLE 15.2 Treatments and Associations by Common Locations of Foreign Bodies

Location	Associations/Treatment
Ear	Straighten the external ear canal by pulling the tragus or pinna. Irrigation is first step. Extract with alligator forceps, ear probes, or glue on end of Q-tip if possible.
Nose	Have patient try to hold one nostril and blow object out. Consider sedation for young, combative patients. Topical vasoconstrictor/anesthetic such as tetracaine/cocaine may help to dislodge object. Extract with forceps when possible.
Bronchus	Decreased/absent breath sounds on one side of chest or wheezing on exam. Cough may or may not be present. Order a CXR to visualize. Attempt to dislodge with abdominal thrusts. Bronchoscopy with extraction is gold standard.
Pharynx/larynx	Protect the airway! If occluded, attempt abdominal thrusts on children and adults or back blows/abdominal thrusts on infants. Look for cyanosis, inability to make noise, decreased consciousness. Consider cricothyroidotomy if significant time passes without breathing.
Esophagus or GI tract	Determine if blunt or able to pass through the gut. Order CXR, acute abdominal series. Endoscopy if object may be extracted from above. Consider surgery if past the stomach, causing active bleeding, embedded in wall of gut, not passing over time, or obstructing. Consider watchful waiting if object is small, blunt, and rapidly passing down the gut by serial x-rays.

Food Poisoning

A spectrum of illnesses causing gastroenteritis related to consuming tainted food. History usually reveals eating questionable food or sharing meal with other sick contacts. Look for recent meals of leftover rice (*B cereus*), undercooked poultry (*Salmonella*), undercooked hamburger (*E Coli* 0157:H7), or raw oysters (*Shigella*).

Symptoms

Nausea, vomiting, diarrhea (bloody or not), fever, malaise, anorexia, and abdominal cramps are common.

Diagnosis

Labs: Stool hemoccult testing may show positive if diarrhea is bloody, although may have false positive due to frequent wiping. CBC for leukocytosis or lymphocytosis. Chem 7 for electrolyte levels.

Stool studies such as C *difficile* toxin, ova/parasites, leukocytes, reducing substances, and culture are indicated.

Blood cultures if admitted to the hospital.

Treatment

Often, empiric therapy is based on history. Bismuth subsalicylate (Pepto) may be tried first and provide some anti-inflammatory action.

Antibiotics are controversial and not proven effective. Consider only if prolonged illness state, known or highly suspected susceptible organism, or other treatments have failed.

Ciprofloxacin (Cipro) has broad spectrum coverage. TMP-SMX (Bactrim, Septra) also active against many likely organisms.

Do not give loperamide (Imodium) or antiemetics too soon as it may worsen the course if the etiology is a toxin-producing organism such as *Shigella*, *C Perfingens*, or *B Cereus*. Give antibiotics in later course of illness if dehydration is suspected.

Hydration is the standard treatment. Orally if tolerated or IV if needed.

Take Home Points

- True food poisoning may be due to bacteria or bacterial toxin.
- Most etiologies aren't fully determined.
- Treat conservatively at first, reserve antibiotics for later stages or after definite diagnosis.

Poisonings

The syndrome that develops after toxic levels of a known harmful agent are reached.

Symptoms

Almost any presentation is possible, but often symptoms include loss or decreased consciousness, lethargy, coma, altered breathing, altered vision, or other patterns of symptoms referred to as "toxidromes." See table below.

TABLE 15.3 Common Toxidromes

Poison	Toxidrome
Cholinergic (insecticides)	Salvation, lacrimation, diaphoresis, n/v, urination, muscle fasciculations, bronchorrhea, bradycardia, seizures, respiratory failure, paralysis.
Anticholinergics	Altered mental status, mydriasis (dilation), dry/flushed skin, urinary retention, decreased bowel transit, hyperthermia, dry mucous membranes, seizures, arrhythmias, rhabdomyolysis. Classic pneumonic: "Hot as a stove, fast as a hare, red as a beet, dry as a bone, mad as a hatter."
Salycylates	Altered mental status, metabolic acidosis, tinnitus, hyperpnea, tachycardia, diaphoresis, n/v.
Hypoglycemia	Altered mental status, diaphoresis, tachycardia, hypertension, paralysis, slurring of speech, seizures.

(continued)

TABLE 15.3 Continued

Poison	Toxidrome
Serotonin syndrome	Altered mental status, increased muscle tone, hyperreflexia, **hyperthermia**, intermittent whole body twitch.
Tricyclic antidepressants	Altered mental status, slurred speech, dry mucous membranes, myoclonus, hyperreflexia, decreased bowel sounds, respiratory depression, respiratory failure, seizure, pulmonary edema. **Cardiac effects** include tachycardia, **prolonged QRS**, PR, and QT intervals, conduction delay, SVT, PVCs, ventricular tachycardia.

SVT = superventricular tachycardia, PVCs = periventricular contractions

Diagnosis

Obtain information such as duration of exposure, time since exposure, amount of exposure, other medications or poisons that may affect presentation, any metabolic derangements, and treatment since exposure.

Labs: Drug screen is one of the first steps. Chem 7 and CBC.

EKG for arrhythmias and placement of cardiac monitoring.

Treatment

Above all: Remember your ABCs! Intubate if necessary.

If agent is identified and an antidote exists, give it. See table above.

- Activated charcoal is first line and absorbs many substances excluding heavy metals. Most effective if given < 1 hour from ingestion. May show greater benefit in substances that are in sustained release form, undergo entero-hepatic circulation (digoxin), or are slow to transit the gut, e.g. tricyclic antidepressants and opiates.

- Bowel irrigation with polyethylene glycol may be considered but is rarely used because of long time course and unsure absorption of toxin. May be useful in heavy metals or drug "mules."

- Emesis is rarely if ever the right answer. Contraindicated in caustic or inflammatory agents or if patient is seizing or with impaired gag reflex. Short time course required from ingestion to be effective.

- Gastric lavage if short time course from ingestion (< 30–60 min) and patient is awake with intact gag reflex or intubated. May be used in suicide attempts with pill ingestion but make sure pills will fit in the lavage tube.

- Alkalization of blood/urine is used generally for aspirin, phenobarbital, and tricyclic antidepressants. Improves elimination.

- Hemodialysis is definitive treatment. Used after significant amount of time passed from ingestion or significant toxic effect occurring. Use with theophylline, methanol, lithium, barbiturates, or ethylene glycol.

Take Home Points

- Poisoning may occur with almost any substance, dose is often the issue.

- History may be the most revealing part of the toxic workup.

- Treatment should be started as soon as possible for the maximum effect.

Toxic Effects of Substances of Common Use/Abuse

TABLE 15.4 Effects of Common Illicit Drugs

Class	Examples	Effects
Hallucinogens	LSD, "magic mushrooms," PCP (phencyclidine), peyote	Psychosis, audio/visual hallucinations, delusions, paranoia, arrhythmias
Depressants	EtOH, marijuana, "moonshine," benzodiazepines, barbiturates	Depressed mood, altered consciousness, relaxed feeling, paranoia, amotivational syndrome
Stimulants	Amphetamines, "ice", cocaine, crank, PCP (phencyclidine)	Stimulation and elevation of mood, erratic/dangerous behavior, psychosis, aggression, delusions (of grandeur), paranoia, tachycardia, mydriasis (dilation), hypertension
Opioids	Heroin, narcotics, RX pain medications	Pain control, high feeling, euphoria, respiratory depression, miosis (constriction), constipation, chronic sensitization
Inhalants (huffing)	Glues, fuel vapors, paint vapors (especially metallic colors)	Euphoria, dizziness, slurred speech, ataxia, respiratory depression, arrhythmias

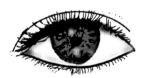 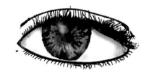

FIGURE 15.1 Bilateral miosis. Reprinted with permission from Cox NLT, Roper TA. *Clinical Skills.* 2005, Oxford University Press.

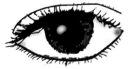 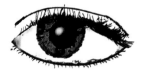

FIGURE 15.2 Bilateral mydriasis. Reprinted with permission from Cox NLT, Roper TA. *Clinical Skills.* 2005, Oxford University Press.

Treatment of Nonmedicinal Substance Ingestion

TABLE 15.5 Treatment of Nonmedicinal Substance Ingestion

Substance	Treatment
Heavy metals including lead, mercury	EDTA or dimercaprol
Iron	Deferoxime
Acetone	Removal from source, GL, O_2 and fluids
Carbon monoxide	100% O_2
Cyanide	Emesis or lavage; amyl nitrite→sodium nitrite→sodium thiosulfate
Ethylene glycol (automobile antifreeze), methanol	Ethanol drip (or PO), fomizole

TABLE 15.5 Continued

Substance	Treatment
Ethanol	Emesis or GL; IV glucose, fluids, consider dialysis
Benzene	Respiratory support, benzodiazepine for seizures, transfusion if anemia severe (may cause long term effects)
Organophosphates (herbicides/insecticides)	2-PAM (pralidoxime) or atropine
Rat poison	Vitamin K

GL = gastric lavage

Adverse Effects of Specific Medicinal and Biologic Substances

TABLE 15.6 Effects of Common Medicinal and Biologic Substances

Substance	Effect	Substance	Effect
Acetaminophen	Liver damage	HMG CoA reductase inhibitors (statins)	Muscle aches, rhabdomyolysis, liver toxicity
Alpha-1 blockers	Orthostatic hypotension (first dose)	Isotretinoin (Acutane)	Suicidal tendencies, pregnancy-teratogen
Aminoglycoside	Oto/renal toxicity	INH (isoniazid)	Peripheral neuropathy, lupus, vit B6 deficiency
Amiodarone	Pulmonary fibrosis, thyroid problems	Lithium	Hypothyroidism, diabetes insipidus
Aspirin	GI bleed	Loop diuretics	Hypokalemia, hypocalcemia,
Beta blockers	Asthma exacerbation, depression, alopecia	MAO-inhibitors	Reaction with wine, aged cheese, many drug/drug interactions
Bupropion	Seizures	Metronidazole	Photosensitivity, abd cramping, flushing/nausea with EtOH
ACE-inhibitors	Cough, pregnancy-renal agenesis	Metformin (Glucophage)	Lactic acidosis
Calcium channel blockers	Heart block	Methotrexate	Myelosupression, pulmonary fibrosis
Chloramphenicol	Aplastic anemia, gray baby	Niacin	Flushing
Clindamycin	Psudomembranous colitis (*C difficile*)	Oxytocin	SIADH
Carbamazapine (Tegretol)	SIADH, aplastic anemia, agranulocytosis	Phenytoin (Dilantin)	Pregnancy-Teratogen

(continued)

TABLE 15.6 Continued

Substance	Effect	Substance	Effect
Colchicine	GI upset, nausea/vomiting, Diabetes Insipidus	Progesterone	Spotting, weight gain, depression
Cimetidine	Inhibits hepatic enzymes, gynocomastia, Inc warfarin effect	Sildenafil (Viagra)	Blue vision, contraindication with nitrates
Cyclosporine	Nephrotoxicity	SSRIs	GI upset, delayed ejaculation, insomnia
Allopurinal	Gout flare, GI upset, rash, Stevens-Johnson syndrome (rare)	Tetracycline	Pregnancy-teeth staining, photosensitivity
Digoxin	GI upset, bradycardia, arrhythmia	Thiazide diuretics	Hypercalcemia, gout exacerbation
Finastride	Pregnancy-male genital malformation	Trazodone	Priapism
Fluoroquinolones	Pregnancy-cartilage damage in fetus, tendon rupture	Rifampin	Orange tears/urine/sweat
Heparin	Heparin-induced thrombocytopenia	Phenergan	Dystonic reaction
Ketoconazole	Gynecomastia	Warfarin (Coumadin)	Warfarin skin necrosis, birth defects, occult bleeding, GI bleeding, bruising
Meperidine (Demerol)	Seizures, coma, toxic metabolite build-up	Vancomycin	"Red man" syndrome
Disulfiram (Antabuse)	Severe nausea/vomiting, flushing on EtOH use	Valproic acid (Depokene)	Hepatotoxicity, pancreatitis, teratogen
Estrogen/progesterone contraceptives	Hypercoagulability	Opioids	Respiratory depression, CNS depression, addiction, constipation

Rape and Sexual Assault

Alleged sexual assault is often a sensitive legal issue as much as a medical one. Strict witnessed exams and collection of evidence with a controlled evidence "chain of custody" is required. As this is best dealt with in an ER or other appropriate facility, it is often referred to specifically trained personnel (SANE personnel). A team approach is needed with the inherent significant emotional and legal implications.

Diagnosis

History must include last menstrual period, time of last consensual coitus, contraceptive status.

Rape kits should be sought and include necessary bags, probes, culture media, etc. to successfully handle samples from victim and victim's clothing.

Document patient's mental state and the recount of the event in their own words as accurately as possible. Do not assume anything and do not ad lib.

Collect patient's clothing.

Speculum exam with non-lubricated, water-moistened speculum.

Collect samples from vagina, rectum, mouth, under the fingernails, and locations of obvious trauma. Analyze samples by wet mount for presence of sperm.

Pregnancy test immediately and in two weeks.

Obtain gonorrhea and chlamydia testing and RPR or VDRL for syphilis immediately and at 6 weeks after the event.

HIV blood testing immediately, at 90 days, and 120 days after the event.

Hepatitis panel immediately, at 6 weeks, and at 6 months after the event.

Wood's lamp can be used to evaluate for seminal fluid.

EtOH and drug screen.

Depending on the state and circumstances, a "**chain of custody**" of evidence may be needed. As a general rule, give the evidence to the local authorities after placing each sample in a separate, sealed, and labeled container.

Treatment

Obtain history in a very non-threatening, non-confrontational manner.

Consult trauma/sexual assault counselor.

Offer emergency contraception.

Prophylaxis for gonorrhea/chlamydia and syphilis with ceftriaxone (Rocephin) IM x1, azithromycin PO x1, and penicillin G IM x1.

Treat bacterial vaginosis, if found, with metronidazole (Flagyl).

Consider Hep B immunoglobulin (HBIG) if exposure known to be high Hep B risk.

HIV prophylaxis is controversial and generally not recommended unless exposure known to be high risk.

Treat physical pain/nausea/sleep disturbance as needed.

Ensure extensive support network of patient.

Ensure patient's physical safety if discharged from hospital.

Close follow up is absolutely necessary.

Take Home Points

- Remain objective, do not make alliances.

- Test for and address pregnancy, STDs, and physical trauma.

- Collect all evidence and clothing and establish a chain of custody.

- Follow up the patient with further testing and counseling.

Traumatic Brain Injury (TBI)

The clinical syndrome caused by acute focal or generalized forces upon the head that lead to scalp, skull, or neurologic injury. This injury may not be obvious upon presentation and may only present symptoms well after the injury.

Symptoms

Clinical presentation may be obvious but injury may have also occurred hours/days ago. Loss of consciousness (LOC) and decreased consciousness are common as well as seizures, focal disturbances, ataxia, apraxia, decreased concentration, vomiting, headache, and amnesia of the event. Trauma to the spinal cord may cause paraplegia or quadriplegia that correlates with a certain spinal level.

Diagnosis

Classify injury as mild, moderate, or severe per Table 15.7. Further classify mild TBI by risk category for intracranial bleeding.

Physical exam: Note any bruising or skull bone crepitus indicative of fracture. Do not manipulate the temporal bones too much to avoid laceration of the middle meningeal artery if fracture is present. Raccoon eyes and Battle's sign (mastoid ecchymosis) may indicate basilar skull fracture. Do a good ear exam for hemotympanum. Note CSF rhinorrhea or otorrhea. Examine the optic discs for "blurring" indicating increased ICP. Exam should include checking entire spinal column for step offs or deformities. In-line stabilization should be used during exam.

Neurologic exam should include general mental state, motor, and sensory exams.

Record Glasgow Coma score (GCS), which should be used for classification.

Imaging: Plain skull x-ray may show fracture. To evaluate cervical injury: Obtain a cross table cervical spine x-ray. Make sure you see T1, which constitutes an adequate study. If inadequate, CT the neck to "clear" it.

Obtain a head CT (if warranted) for bleeds, although slow ones may not immediately be seen. Look for signs increased ICP or midline shift of ventricles. Consider repeating hours later.

TABLE 15.7 Classification of TBI by GCS Score

Degree of TBI	Maximum GCS
Mild	14–15
Moderate	9–13
Severe	< 9

Ideally, GCS is taken < 30 min after injury.

TABLE 15.8 Mild TBT Risk of Intracranial Bleeding According to Clinical Features

Risk Category	Features
Low risk	GCS 15. No history of LOC, amnesia, vomiting, or headache.
Moderate risk	GCS 15. One or more of the following: LOC, amnesia, vomiting, headache.
High risk	GCS of 14–15. Skull fracture and/or neurologic deficits. Predisposition such as coagulopathy, drug or EtOH consumption, previous neurosurgical abnormalities, seizure disorder, age ≥ 60 years.

Mild TBI of the low risk group may or may not require neuroimaging.

Mild TBI of the moderate or high risk group should have neuroimaging evaluation.

Moderate and severe TBI should have neuroimaging evaluation. Admission for at least 24 hours is required.

Treatment

Remember your ABCs at first.

Admission/neurosurgical consult is optional depending on study result and clinical presentation.

Scalp lacerations often bleed profusely but are not your first priority.

Consider mannitol, hypertonic saline, or Lasix to decrease ICP, but these medications may be tricky in shock. Rely on neurosurgery to help.

IV steroids and hyperventilation have fallen out of favor and are no longer recommended. Rely on neurosurgery to help.

Mild or more severe traumatic brain injuries may have lasting symptoms despite negative imaging and testing, counseling or psychiatric/neurologic consultation may be needed later in the course. Rates of continued effects are higher if coupled with post traumatic stress disorder (PTSD).

See Chapter 3: Diseases of the Nervous System on related topics.

Take Home Points

- GCS score is pivotal in the evaluation of TBI.
- Make sure to evaluate for increased ICP.
- Effects of traumatic brain injury may be long lasting.

Internal Injuries, Abdomen and Pelvis

Traumatic injury of any abdominal or pelvic tissue or organ with or without surface defect. Commonly, this includes bleeding, making urgent surgery a priority.

Symptoms

Pain in the abdomen or pelvis is usually present but the patient may have impaired sensation or consciousness. Look for hypotension, decreasing blood pressure, decreased/decreasing consciousness, expanding abdomen, peritoneal signs, and dependant bruising.

Diagnosis

Physical exam: "There should be a finger or tube placed in every orifice" to check for bleeding or fluid drainage. Evaluate for pelvis fracture by manual manipulation but limit this maneuver to only once.

Imaging: Pelvic fractures should have a plain AP x-ray. Remember, it is hard to break a pretzel in one place—the same is true of the pelvis—always look for the second fracture site if one is found.

Patients with penetrating abdominal injuries, including gunshots and penetrating knife wounds, should go directly to laparotomy.

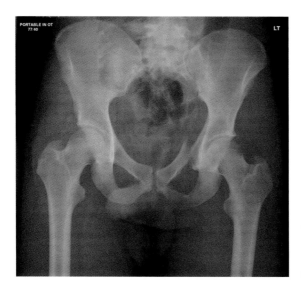

FIGURE 15.3 X-ray showing fractured pubic rami on the left. Note fracture of both the superior and inferi or pubic rami. Reprinted with permission from Thomas J, Monaghan T. *Oxford Handbook of Clinical Examination and Practical Skills.* 2007, Oxford University Press.

Otherwise, see table below.

TABLE 15.9 Diagnostic Methods for Assessing Internal Bleeding

	DPL	Ultrasound (FAST exam)	CT Scan
Advantages	• Early diagnosis • Performed rapidly • 98% sensitive • Detects bowel injury	• Early diagnosis • Noninvasive • Performed rapidly • Repeatable	• Most specific for injury • Sensitive: 92–98% accurate
Disadvantages	• Invasive • Low specificity • Misses injuries to diaphragm and retroperitoneum	• Operator-dependent • Bowel gas and subcutaneous air distortion • Misses diaphragm, bowel, pancreatic, and solid organ injuries	• Cost and time • Misses diaphragm, bowel, and some pancreatic injuries • Transport required

DPL = Diagnostic peritoneal lavage
FAST ultrasound- Focused assessment with sonography in trauma
Reprinted with permission from the American College of Surgeons.

Treatment

If internal disruption of the organs is confirmed by the above testing, celiotomy is indicated. If tests above are negative but hypotension continues and bleeding into the peritoneum or retroperitoneum is suspected, celiotomy is indicated. In short, have a low threshold for taking to the OR.

Before pelvis fracture is fixed, stabilize it by pelvic braces or a simple, tightly drawn sheet around the pelvis. Consider angiography to evaluate for circulation/DVTs around pelvis.

Take Home Points

- Occult internal hemorrhage may be the reason for acute decompensation.
- It's hard to break a pretzel in one place; the same is true for the pelvis.
- Urgent surgical consult is often needed.

Frostbite

A localized injury to an exposed body part (commonly fingers, hands, toes, feet, nose, etc.) resulting from extreme cold exposure causing freezing of tissue and resultant tissue dehydration, protein breakdown, metabolic insufficiency, and necrosis. Research has shown that most damage occurs during a freeze/thaw, freeze/thaw cycle, thus refreezing after frostbite has occurred causes more injury than waiting until one complete thaw can be accomplished.

Symptoms

When frostbite occurs, appendage becomes hard, white, without signs of circulation, and anesthetic. Pain is not a symptom until later, but may indicate "frostnip."

Diagnosis

Generally a clinical diagnosis, but as rewarming starts, various methods to evaluate microcirculation damage exist: thermography, angiography, digital plethysmography, and radioisotope vascular and bone scanning. These are generally helpful for the surgeon to make decisions about what and where to cut.

Blistering often starts 4–6 hours after rewarming. Proximal bloody blisters are a negative prognostic indicator and indicate deep tissue damage. Distal serum filled blisters are better and may indicate only superficial damage.

Treatment

Make sure patient is in no danger of refreezing the appendage as this may cause much more damage. If still in the high-risk environment, do not thaw the appendage!

Slow (over 20–30 minutes) rewarming with use of warm (40°C, 104°F) water should be done. Expect tissue to turn pink and blotchy. It is advisable to monitor heart function for arrhythmias during this procedure if possible. Do not rub or massage the tissue.

Give opioid analgesics during rewarming since it can be very painful.

The appendage should be kept warm and dry after rewarming. Blisters should remain intact for 7–10 days.

Give tetanus prophylaxis as indicated.

No antibiotics are warranted unless infection is noted.

No nicotine or other vasoconstrictors.

Referral to surgery is usually indicated at some stage.

Take Home Points

- Do not thaw the affected part unless risk of refreezing is minimal.
- Give anesthesia during rewarming.
- Slowly rewarm the affected part.

Hypothermia

The bodily state of core temperature ≤ 95°F (35°C). All body systems are affected by this decrease in temperature, eventually leading to failure.

Symptoms

Wide variations of clinical presentations exist. Commonly, mental status change (ataxia, amnesia, apathy, and dysarthria), loss of consciousness, psychiatric disturbance (delusions), and shivering. History is often suggestive of cold exposure, lack of clothing, drugs/EtOH exposure, infection, hypothyroidism, recent anesthesia, or immobility.

Diagnosis

Physical exam: Best temperature taken is rectal. Low BP may also be present and the patient may be in shock.

Labs: CBC, metabolic panel, hepatic function tests, TSH, glucose, illicit drug screen, EtOH level, ABG, and blood cultures.

ECG: Characteristic J (Osborn) waves indicating delayed repolarization are classic. Arrhythmias such as A fib and bradycardias are also common. The lethal arrhythmia is usually ventricular fibrillation.

Imaging: None specific for hypothermia, but consider CXR for pulmonary infection, etc.

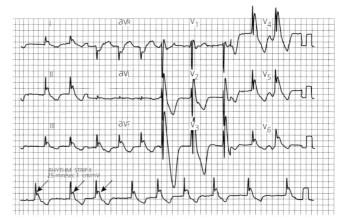

FIGURE 15.4 Hypothermia ECG showing rhythm disturbance of atrial fibrillation and slow ventricular response, prolongation of QRS, and delayed repolarization (J waves) (arrows). Reprinted with permission from Brown J. *Oxford American Handbook of Emergency Medicine.* 2008, Oxford University Press.

Treatment

Start with ABCs and CPR as needed. Remember to check pulse for one full minute before declaring death. "No one is dead until they're warm and dead."

Mild cases may be treated with passive rewarming techniques including removal of wet clothing and application of blankets, etc.

Moderate to severe cases require active rewarming, which includes warm humidified O_2, heated IV fluids, and possibly, peritoneal lavage. Extreme cases with cardiac arrest may benefit from cardiopulmonary bypass rewarming although this is very impractical.

Take Home Points

- Defined as body temp ≤ 95°F (35°C).
- Monitor ECG for J (Osborn) waves.
- Recognize those patients needing passive vs. active rewarming.
- "No one is dead until they're warm and dead."

Heat Injury

TABLE 15.10 Spectrum of Heat Injury

Term	Features
Heat syncope	Syncope associated with exposure to environmental heat stress, dehydration, and orthostatic changes. Core body temperature is normal or near normal.
Heat exhaustion	Associated with exposure to environmental heat stress. Acute symptoms including flushing, lightheadedness, nausea/vomiting, diaphoresis, and *mild* altered mental status. Core body temperature is between 100.4°F (38°C) and 104.0°F (40°C).
Exertional heat stroke	May occur in the setting of exertion with or without extreme environmental heat stress. Alteration of mental status is severe and may include loss of consciousness. Core body temperature is > 104°F (40°C).
Classic heat stroke	Associated with exposure to environmental heat stress without extreme exertion. Alteration of mental status is severe and may include loss of consciousness. Body's thermoregulation does not function properly and skin is often sweatless. More commonly occurs in the elderly.

Symptoms

Heat stress may be reported by the patient, with reports of feeling tired, dizzy, lightheaded, nauseous, or hot. Patient often has evidence of lack of thermoregulatory control in severe cases. Mental functioning is often acutely impaired. Note history of recent anesthetic gas exposure such as halothane or succinylcholine.

Diagnosis

Physical exam: Evidence of end organ damage may include RUQ pain, arrhythmia, hematuria, etc. Always obtain temperature per rectum!

Labs: Transaminases (AST/ALT) in heat stroke may show > 3 x normal but may be normal at acute presentation, **creatinine kinase** elevation indicating muscle damage, increased BUN/creatinine indicating kidney damage, urine **myoglobin** indicating saturation of kidneys with myoglobin. Electrolytes often show dehydration and hypernatremia, hyperchloremia. In severe heat stroke, phosphorus and calcium are altered. CBC may show hemoconcentration indicating dehydration. Coagulation profile may show increased PT/aPTT and INR indicative of liver damage. Obtain arterial blood gas for Ph and metabolic acidosis. LDH levels may be taken early and show some correlation to short term prognosis.

Monitor cardiac function for arrhythmias.

In heat stroke, watch for other problems that may develop, such as fulminate hepatic failure, respiratory failure, kidney failure, DIC, and eventual brain death.

Imaging: None specifically indicated although individual organ systems may need imaging as the course progresses, e.g. chest x-ray for decreased respiratory functioning.

Treatment

Immediate cooling with wet blankets, fans, cold water, ice packs to axilla and groin if possible.

IV fluids (multiple boluses plus at least 2x maintenance) to increase and maintain vigorous urine output.

Intubate if necessary.

Treat seizures with benzodiazepines as needed.

Manage concurrent organ damage and its effects.

DIC may be an indication of eminent crash, be vigilant.

In moderate to severe cases, hold out of sports or vigorous activity for the entire heat season. Decreased activity is warranted for the next heat season as well. A re-injury may be fatal!

Take Home Points

- Heat injury is a spectrum of illness, with heat stroke a potentially fatal condition at the extreme of that spectrum.

- Admission to the ICU may be warranted in the extreme case.

Complications of Surgery

TABLE 15.11 Complications of Surgery by System

Complication	Symptoms	Associations	Management
CNS	Acute decrease in mental status, obtundation, or lack of arousal from surgery	Anesthesia effects/side effects, hypoxic brain injury, hypothermia, hypoglycemia, electrolyte disturbances	Check glucose level and correct, naloxone as needed, give O_2, check temperature and provide warmth, replete electrolytes (don't forget the Mg)

(continued)

TABLE 15.11 Continued

Complication	Symptoms	Associations	Management
Respiratory	Respiratory distress or failure, desaturation and hypoxemia	Pulmonary embolism (thrombo, air, fat), atelectasis, pneumonia, aspiration pneumonitis, pulmonary edema, pneumonia	Oxygen, mechanical ventilation as needed, diagnosis of PE and anticoagulation, incentive spirometer post op, antibiotics and pneumonia treatment as needed.
Gastrointestinal	Constipation, nausea, vomiting, bleeding, abdominal pain.	Paralytic ileus, ischemia, perforation, anesthetic effects/side effects, adhesion formation and resultant obstruction.	NPO status, NG tube as needed, stool softeners, antiemetics, tincture of time, or reevaluation for surgery and possible laparotomy.

Hemorrhage Complicating Surgery

Diagnosis

Frank bleeding around surgical site or other wound area. Generally this often fairly obvious but may be seen as decreased blood pressure, increased heart rate, and hypovolemic shock symptoms. The wound may also be hiding blood in body cavities ("third spacing").

Labs: Hemoglobin/hematocrit usually won't change in the acute setting. If after surgery, a relative decrease may be seen compared to pre op status.

Treatment

Prophylactic prevention is the best weapon and includes stopping warfarin (Coumadin) dosing and switching to real heparin before surgery, then turning it off the day before the procedure. Stop all aspirin/herbals/NSAIDs, clopidogrel (Plavix), or other blood thinners before surgery.

Direct pressure on the bleeding location if obvious. Other techniques include use of Bovie electrocautery, suturing the bleeder, and tourniquet.

Reverse warfarin (Coumadin) effect with vitamin K if in the acute setting if patient has good hepatic function. Consider fresh frozen plasma (FFP) if bleeding is profuse.

Fluids and blood products as needed. Generally, one unit of packed red blood cells will raise the hematocrit 3 points.

Treat with presser agents as needed.

Take Home Points

- Hemorrhage may occur during the procedure or afterward, causing symptoms but not necessarily obvious blood loss.
- A rule of thumb for blood replacement is one unit packed RBCs = 3 hematocrit points.

Postoperative Fever

Infection occurring acutely or subacutely in conjunction with surgery.

Symptoms

Generalized **fever**, local pain, swelling, oozing/drainage from wound, and erythema. Patients may also exhibit symptoms of infection in places other than the surgery site. The mnemonic to remember: "Wind, water, walking, wound, and wonder drugs" are the 5 Ws of surgery. They stand for the sources of post op fever and include respiratory (pneumonia, atelectasis), urine or UTI, DVT or PE, surgery site infection, or anesthetic or drug effect, respectively.

Diagnosis

Always examine the wound for signs of infection.

Labs: U/A and urine culture for UTI especially after long indwelling catheter.

Imaging: Consider CXR for pneumonia. Doppler U/S of the legs if suspicious for DVT vs. infection or cellulitis.

Draw blood cultures if still uncertain of site.

Treatment

Usually, first generation cephalosporin or penicillin is given intraoperatively for infection prophlylaxis. Consider continuing treatment after procedure if infection is highly likely (dirty wound) or confirmed infection. Otherwise, tailor antibiotics to specific sensitivities and recommendations for location.

Take Home Points

- "Wind, water, walking, wound, and wonder drugs" are the 5 Ws of surgery.

Other Complications of Surgical Procedures

TABLE 15.12 Complication of Surgical Site

Complication	Association/Diagnosis	Treatment
Hematoma	Noninflammatory mass under the wound. U/S may be used to confirm presence of blood clot.	Either watchful waiting for reabsorption if mild without adverse mass effect, or open evacuation.
Dehiscence	Separation of closed wound site. May be caused by necrosis of wound edges, underlying hematoma, infection, excess tension on suture line, or lack of undermining and suturing of wound.	Remove sutures and reclose if uncomplicated or allow healing by secondary intention.
Suture abscess	Usually small local abscess at suture site. Caused by retained stitch.	Incision and drainage of abscess. Treat local cellulitis as indicated. Remove the suture.
Hypertrophic scar formation and keloid	More common in dark-skinned individuals. Complication of late healing.	Steroid injection, radiation therapy, dermabrasion, pressure dressings, or surgical removal and debulking.

Burns

Diagnosis

TABLE 15.13 Burn Classification

Classification	Association	Level of Injury
Superficial	Sunburn or mild hot water. Skin is red without blisters.	Epidermis only.

(continued)

TABLE 15.13 Continued

Classification	Association	Level of Injury
Superficial partial thickness	Often surrounded by redness with blister formation. Capillary refill is present.	Epidermis and papillary dermis. Deep dermis, hair follicles, and sweat glands are spared.
Deep partial thickness	Blistering and white appearance of injury area with blister formation. Capillary refill is usually absent.	Epidermis, reticular (deep) layer of dermis. Sweat glands, hair follicles, capillaries, and nerve fibers are burned.
Full thickness	Charred, pale, painless, and leathery skin. No capillary refill. No blistering.	Through the epidermis and dermis and possibly into the subcutaneous tissues.

Determine body surface area (BSA) according to the rule of 9's:

- Face and scalp 9%
- Back 18%
- Front 18%
- Perineum 1%
- Arm each 9%
- Leg each 18%

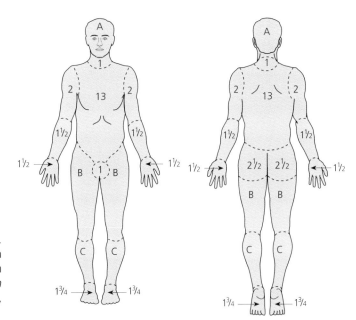

FIGURE 15.5 Lund and Browder chart. Assessing the extent of burns by estimation of body surface area. Reprinted with permission from Brown J. *Oxford American Handbook of Emergency Medicine.* 2008, Oxford University Press.

TABLE 15.14 Relative Percentage of Body Surface Area by Age

Area	Age 1 Year	Adult
A = ½ of head	8 ½	3 ½
B = ½ of thigh	3 ¼	4 ¾
C = ½ of one lower leg	2 ½	3 ½

Determine if the patient is at risk for inhalational injury. Have a low threshold for treating.

Labs: Obtain screening Chem 7, CBC, albumin, calcium, ABG for pH, and U/A.

Imaging: Consider CXR if pneumonitis or ARDS from inhalation is suspected.

Treatment

Admission criteria (or transfer to a local burn center) are as follows:

    Lightning or electrical burns

    Full thickness burn > 1% estimated BSA

    Deep partial thickness burn over > 10% estimated BSA

    Full thickness burn on hand, feet, face, perineum

    Circumferential burns

    Coexisting inhalational injury

Superficial partial thickness burns should be cooled by rinsing with cool water/saline irrigation.

    If minor, dress with Epilock or Elasto-Gel and monitor as outpatient. May recommend aloe-containing OTC preparations for pain relief.

    If more serious:

- Remove all clothing and jewelry, including rings and watches that are remotely near burned area
- Give O_2
- Tetanus prophylaxis
- Do not apply ice to burned area
- Do not rupture blisters unless infected or overtly large
- Systemic or topical antibiotics are indicated in some 2nd and all 3rd degree burns
- Systemic pain relief to include opioids

In severe burns:

- Place NG tube, Foley catheter, 2 large bore IVs
- IV fluids with rate > maintenance for first 24 hours
- ECG monitoring for first 24 hours
- Monitor electrolytes
- NPO status initially, then, high protein diet
- Consider TPN if NPO status expected > 5 days
- Possible escharotomy if circumferential and causing breathing restriction or pseudocompartment syndrome of extremity
- Skin (usually split-thickness) grafting
- Daily debridement and redressing of wounds
- Consultation or transfer to burn center

During initial resuscitation, the **Parkland formula** for fluid repletion can be used.

    LR (lactated ringer) mL = 4 mL/kg × (% body surface area burned), the first half should be given over the first 8 hours, and the second half over the next 16 hours.

    Topical preparations include silver sulfadiazine (Silvadene), silver nitrate, mafenide (Sulfamylon).

    Important side effects of topicals include:

    Silver nitrate: May leach Na, Cl, and K out of wound and cause deficiency.

    Mafenide: Metabolic acidosis and possible renal tubular acidosis.

Take Home Points

- Determine the thickness of the burn to help guide treatment.
- Determine if the patient should be admitted or not.
- Fluid resuscitation is very important in burns, use the Parkland formula.

16 Hematology and Immunology

Lymphoma

Hodgkin Lymphoma

A hematologic cancer involving neoplastic B-cells (Reed-Sternberg cells) set in an inflammatory background. According to the World Health Organization (WHO), two categories exist: Classic HL and nodular lymphocyte predominant HL (NLPHL). Classic HL is further subdivided into: nodular sclerosis, mixed cellularity, lymphocyte depleted, and lymphocyte predominant. Etiology is unknown but theories predominate about relation to viral infection (EBV) and predisposing immunologic links. There is a characteristic bimodal age incidence although, curiously, ages differ between developed and developing countries.

Symptoms

Presentation varies widely and may include new onset fever, night sweats, weight loss, fatigue, anorexia or pruritus. Alcohol-induced pain in areas of lymphoma. Patients may also notice prominent lymphadenopathy. Obtain a complete family history.

Diagnosis

Diagnosis is made by biopsy of an enlarged lymph node. **Reed-Sternberg cells** are pathognomonic and have "owl eye" or "mirror" appearance under microscope.

Physical exam: Cervical or supraclavicular lymphadenopathy, weight loss, increased temperature. Hepatosplenomegaly may be prominent.

Labs: CBC with manual differential for lymphocytic abnormalities, normocytic anemia, CRP/ESR often increased, LFTs and transaminases may indicate liver involvement.

Imaging: Chest x-ray, CT of chest, abdomen, and pelvic areas for staging. Ultrasound may be useful, as well as MRI for staging. Gallium scan or PET scan may also be used.

Staging involves using the **Ann Arbor staging system**, which consists of classification based on lymph node involvement and anatomic spread.

Obtain bone biopsy, especially for higher stage disease.

Treatment

Radiation therapy, chemotherapy, or a combination of both is commonly effective. Radiation is the treatment for localized disease of early stage. Chemotherapy, consisting of quadruple cyclic cocktail of adriamycin, bleomycin, vinblastine, and dacarbazine (ABVD) is used for higher stages.

Cell transplant may also be added for recurrent disease or to improve initial survival.

Take Home Points

- Hodgkin lymphoma (HL) is a disease of neoplastic B-cells with background inflammation.
- Staging uses the Ann Arbor staging system for lymphatic spread.
- Treatment consists of local radiation or chemotherapy.

Non-Hodgkin Lymphoma

A heterogeneous group of lymphomas characterized by the absence of Reed-Sternberg cells on biopsy. NHL may present with similar symptoms including night sweats, weight loss, fever, fatigue, anorexia, and lymphadenopathy. It tends to spread in more unpredictable ways than HL, however, and is harder to stage. Diagnosis is similar to HL in that biopsy is the gold standard with histologic grade most important. Treatment decisions should be made by an experienced oncologist but often involve various cyclic regimens of chemotherapy and/or radiation.

Multiple Myeloma

A carcinoma of the plasma cells, multiple myeloma, consists of monoclonal tumor cell proliferation and monoclonal protein in the serum and urine.

Symptoms

Bone pain (backache common), lethargy, weakness, dyspnea, pallor, palpitations, recurrent infections, and common bleeding episodes. This disease is associated with conditions including carpal tunnel syndrome, macroglossia, diarrhea, symptoms of hyperviscosity (eye sight difficulties, headaches, etc.) or symptoms of hypercalcemia ("stones, bones, groans, and psychotic overtones").

Diagnosis

Physical exam: Bone tenderness, pathologic fractures, pallor, and increased temperature.

Labs: Serum and urine protein electrophoresis (**SPEP and UPEP**) are essential and show IgM M-spike and increased **Bence-Jones proteins,** respectively. CBC may show normocytic anemia with rouleaux formations prominent, neutropenia and thrombocytopenia. High ESR is common. Serum calcium and ionized calcium are often high (despite normal alkaline phosphatase). Renal function often shows increased BUN and creatinine indicating renal failure.

Imaging: Obtain full body radiographic scan (*not* scintiography) and look for **"punched out"** lesions. MRI may be helpful to visualize bone involvement.

Bone marrow biopsy characteristically shows **plasma cell predominance**.

Diagnosis is made by the presence of the following criteria:

1. Monoclonal protein in serum or urine electrophoresis.

2. Plasma cell infiltration of the bone marrow.

3. Presence of end organ damage felt related to the plasma cell proliferation (hypercalcemia, lytic bone lesions on x-ray, renal failure, etc.).

Treatment

Chemotherapy is effective and regimens vary. These often include either melphalan (Alkeran) or cyclophosphamide. Thalidomide may be useful although use in combination with dexamethasone (Decadron).

Stem cell transplant, especially in younger patients, has shown good effect but falls short of cure.

Local radiation therapy is effective and is often used in areas of pathologic fracture.

Renal failure is treated with aggressive oral hydration. Hypercalcemia is treated with aggressive hydration and bisphosphonates such as pamidronate (Aredia).

Anemia is treated with either transfusion or erythropoietin (Epogen).

Monitor for infections and treat them early. Remember to vaccinate.

Take Home Points

- Multiple myeloma is a plasma cell malignancy with monoclonal protein overproduction.

- Hypercalcemia is often an accompanying syndrome.

- The mainstay of treatment is chemotherapy although radiation and bone marrow transplant may be used in some cases.

Leukemia

TABLE 16.1 The Leukemias

	Acute Lymphocytic Leukemia (ALL)	Acute Myelogenous Leukemia (AML)	Chronic Lymphocytic Leukemia (CLL)	Chronic Myelogenous Leukemia (CML)
Associations	Children; viral-like prodrome and refusal to walk. Bone pain, bruising, and fever.	Adults; exposure to smoking, benzene, radiation, or may occur *de novo*. Bruising, fatigue, dyspnea, fever, petechiae.	Older adults; Slow progression of disease. Lymphadenopathy, fatigue, hepatosplenomegaly, easy bruising.	Middle-aged adults; stable chronic phase that progresses to acute **"blast crisis."** Symptoms include fatigue, fever, malaise, weight loss, and night sweats. Blast crisis has fever, bone pain, weight loss, and splenomegaly.
Diagnosis	Lymphadenopathy and splenomegaly. CBC shows anemia, decreased platelets and variable WBCs. Increased LDH, uric acid. Obtain bone marrow biopsy and LP for leukemic cells. CXR for mediastinal involvement.	Gingival hypertrophy. Peripheral smear shows **Auer rods**. Decreased leukocyte alkaline phosphatase (LAP). **DIC** may be seen in coagulation studies. CBC shows anemia, decreased platelets, and marked leukocytosis.	Lymphocytosis prominent with **"smudge cells"** on smear. CBC shows anemia, thrombocytopenia. Bone marrow biopsy shows infiltration with lymphocytes. LDH increased. Genetic analysis often helpful. Expression of CD5 and CD23 on cell surface is characteristic.	CBC shows prominent leukocytosis and anemia. Decreased LAP, increased vitamin B12 levels. Genetic analysis for **Philadelphia chromosome, t(9,22)** is diagnostic.
Treatment	Good prognosis; Phases of chemo include remission induction, consolidation, and remission maintenance. Regimens vary and may be used with radiation.	Treat DIC if present, cyclic chemotherapy is the treatment of choice. Supportive care as needed for side effects.	Supportive care often used since disease has typical indolent course. Chlorambucil or fludarabine are the classic chemotherapy agents. Supportive care for complications or side effects. May eventually need splenectomy.	Hydroxyurea and interferon-α are classic to suppress blast crisis in the chronic phase. Bone marrow transplant may also be successful. When in blast crisis, **imatinib (Gleevec)**, a receptor tyrosine kinase (RTK) inhibitor is very effective.

Anemias

Anemias (Hgb < 13.8 g/dl or Hct < 41% for males Mgb, < 12.1 g/dl or Hct < 36% for females) may show classes based on cell size, color, or other physical characteristics of the red blood cell. These characteristics often suggest etiology based on known patterns. Common anemias are presented here.

Symptoms

Pallor, tachypnea, tachycardia, palpitations, fatigue, dyspnea on exertion, chest pain, pica, and poor exercise tolerance. History may be pertinent for chronic or acute blood loss, chronic blood loss, dietary deficiency/malnutrition, sensitivity to certain foods, exposure to chemicals, or family history.

Microcytic Anemias

Iron deficiency anemia. May be caused by malabsorption, malnutrition, or, commonly, chronic blood loss. Look for sources of bleeding including the urine or GI tract. Exam may show spooning of nails, glossitis, or angular stomatitis around the mouth. Although hemoccult stool testing is not intended for this purpose, it may be useful if positive. Serum ferritin (low in IDA) is the single most useful test in diagnosis; it is also an acute phase reactant so may be falsely elevated in the setting of illness. Obtain an iron panel including serum iron (low), total iron binding capacity (high), and transferrin (high). Replace with oral iron.

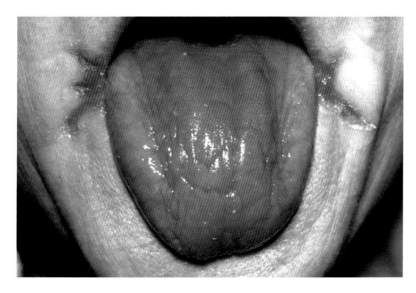

FIGURE 16.1 Patient with chronic iron deficiency anemia causing angular stomatitis and glossitis. Reprinted with permission from Cox NLT, Roper TA. *Clinical Skills.* 2005, Oxford University Press.

Thalassemia. Autosomal recessively inherited group of abnormalities involving formation of α and β hemoglobin chains. More common in those of Mediterranean descent, severity of illness related to the state of one or both genes being defective (although a wide spectrum of severity exists). The test of choice is hemoglobin electrophoresis which will reveal if disease is α or β thalessemia and heterozygous or homozygous. Peripheral smear shows target cells, nucleated RBCs and diffuse basophilia. Skull x-ray shows "hair on end" appearance. Treat with transfusions as necessary and iron chelation therapy to prevent resultant iron overload.

Lead poisoning. Often seen in children, due to chronic exposure. History may reveal residence in house with lead paint or parental occupational exposure to lead. Blood lead levels taken for screening usually are capillary and need to be confirmed by venous sample if positive. Peripheral smear shows characteristic "basophilic stippling." Serum erythrocyte protoporphyrin level is increased and should be cross-confirmed with blood lead level. Plain radiographs reveal metaphyseal "lead lines" in children chronically exposed. Treatment is chelation therapy with oral succimer (Chemet) or parental dimercaprol (BAL) + Ca EDTA (calcium edentate disodium). Monitor for seizures during chelation.

Normocytic Anemias

Acute blood loss. Produced by acute injury or recent blood loss will produce a normocytic anemia only after volume replacement or some time for recovery. Do not rely on blood studies to determine amount of blood loss or threshold for transfusion in the acute setting.

Anemia of chronic disease. May be normo or microcytic. Patient is often in chronically ill state which may contribute to symptoms. Reticulocyte index (normal 0.5–2.0%) is often inappropriately low, indicating decreased response to anemia. Erythropoietin (Epogen) may improve the patient's condition. Treat the underlying disease if possible. Iron is not helpful.

Hemolytic anemias. Etiologies of hemolytic disease are many and diverse and include autoimmune (lupus, lymphoma, ABO incompatibility in newborns), extrinsic (drugs such as penicillin, cepha-losporins, and α-methyldopa), intrinsic (hereditary spherocytosis, pyruvate kinase deficiency, hereditary elliptocytosis), or infection (mycoplasma or Epstein-Barr virus). Common laboratory findings are commonly increased unconjugated bilirubin, low haptoglobin, increased LDH, and increased reticulocyte count. Specific tests including osmotic fragility test and direct/indirect Coomb's test (for warm or cold agglutinins). All hemolytic anemias should have microscopic exam of the RBCs. Treatment depends on cause. Surgical splenectomy may be the only option for some.

Glucose-6-phosphate dehydrogenase (G6PD) deficiency. An X-linked recessive trait affecting males. Patients may experience hemolysis and hemoglobinuria after exposure to certain oxidant-containing foods or medications. Triggers commonly include fava beans, antimalarials, sulpha compounds, anti-helminths, and others. Several enzyme-linked screening tests exist including direct RBC enzyme assay. Newborns and infants may have excessive jaundice. Treat by stopping or avoiding the offending inges-tion. Hydrate to increase urine output. For infants, consider phototherapy. Transfuse if necessary.

Macrocytic Anemias

Folate/Vitamin B$_{12}$ deficiency. Commonly seen in chronic alcoholics, pregnant women, chronic gas-tritis, elderly eating "tea and toast" diet, pernicious anemia, methotrexate, or phenytoin use, fish tape worm infection (*Diphyllobothrium latum*), or patients with prior GI surgery. Often asymptomatic but may show neurologic involvement such as parasthesias, ataxia, spasticity, or delirium. Peripheral smear shows large RBCs and hypersegmented neutrophils. Check serum levels of both. A Schilling test may delineate etiology of B$_{12}$ deficiency. Replace vitamins orally if no absorption problems. Give vitamin B$_{12}$ shots every month if needed.

Take Home Points

- The next step after finding low Hgb or Hct should be evaluation of the MCV.
- Obtain an iron panel and ferritin for almost all anemias. The next step should be reticulocyte count.
- There is no specific "transfusion threshold" so base the need for transfusion on the clinical picture.
- Rule of thumb: Infusion of 1 unit packed RBCs = increase of 3 Hct points.

Sickle Cell Anemia

A chronic hemoglobinopathy that results in misshapen red blood cells (sickled RBCs) due to the pres-ence of abnormal "Hb S," resulting in polymerized long-rod hemoglobin chains when deoxygenated. These sickled RBCs are inflexible and fragile leading to various "crises" of vaso-oclusion and hemolytic anemia. Genetics show an autosomal recessive inheritance much more common in African Americans and Hispanics.

Symptoms

Sickle cell patients are asymptomatic until crisis. Vaso-occlusive crisis is often very painful and occurs commonly in the hands and feet but may occur anywhere in the body. Triggers such as **cold weather, hypoxia, or infection** tend to be triggers.

Visceral sequestration caused by sickling within organs may be life threatening. Splenic sequestration/infarction often occurs in younger patients and repeated events lead to autosplenectomy.

Acute chest syndrome (ACS) is life threatening and has symptoms of severe chest pain, dyspnea, hypoxia, and air hunger.

Aplastic crisis occurs particularly associated with **parvovirus B19** infection and is characterized by a drop in HCT and reticulocyte count.

Other complications are stasis ulcers, shortened fingers/toes (due to repeated infarction), pigment gallstones, and osteomyelitis (commonly *Salmonella* spp.).

Diagnosis

Labs: CBC for H/H, which are typically low. Search in history for baseline values and compare to determine if patient is in acute crisis. Leukocytosis and thrombocytosis often present. Peripheral smear shows sickled cells and commonly "Howell-Jolly" bodies indicating splenic damage. Reticulocyte index often very elevated. "Sickledex" test positive. Bilirubin is high and haptoglobin is low. LDH is elevated. Hemoglobin electrophoresis will show increased Hb S and is the definitive test.

Imaging: Chest x-ray to evaluate for acute chest syndrome, CT/MRI if indicated to evaluate for CVA. Bone scan is mandatory if suspected osteomyelitis.

Treatment

Vaccinate known sicklers (Haemophilus, Pneumococcus, Meningococcus).

Avoid triggers such as exposure to cold weather, dehydration, hypoxia, smoking, certain medications, etc.

Oral penicillin or amoxicillin recommended for children 2mos–5yrs. Continue until puberty if frequent crises or indication.

Prevent crisis with folic acid supplement and hydroxyurea (Droxia).

In acute crisis, give oxygen, aggressive IV hydration, and warmth.

Treat acute crisis with NSAIDs, Tylenol, keterolac (Toradol), or tramadol (Ultram) when possible. Elevation to narcotic analgesics such as morphine or meperidine (Demerol) may be needed.

Transfuse if necessary.

Exchange transfusion may be needed in severe crisis or acute chest syndrome.

Treat any infection aggressively and early. Educate family to monitor for fever and respond quickly to avoid crisis.

Monitor for narcotic pain dependence/seeking on presentation. This is often a fine line but be aware many sicklers also commonly have comorbid narcotic dependence.

Take Home Points

- Sickle cell crisis triggers include cold exposure, hypoxia, or infection.
- Major complications include acute chest syndrome (ACS), visceral sequestration and autosplenectomy, and aplastic crisis.

- Give penicillin or amoxicillin to children 2 months–5 years old.
- Commonly, adults become opiate dependent and tolerant.

Septicemia

A spectrum of systemic inflammation caused by response to infection or global inflammatory state. Although infection does not need to be present in SIRS, the entities of sepsis and septic shock are associated with an infectious agent of some type. Multiple organ dysfunction syndrome (MODS) is the consequential disease state that develops as a result of the global insult and is responsible for most mortality in this disease.

Diagnosis

TABLE 16.2 Sepsis Spectrum

Term	Criteria
Systemic inflammatory response syndrome (SIRS)	1. Elevated or decreased temperature 2. Elevated heart rate > 90 beats per minute 3. Elevated respiratory rate > 20 breaths per minute 4. WBC count > 12,000/mm³ or < 4000/mm³ or > 10% band form Two or more of the above need to be present for SIRS
Sepsis	SIRS + documented infection (typically bacterial)
Septic shock	Sepsis-induced hypotension and end organ hypoperfusion

Treatment

Initiate ABCs as needed.

For SIRS, treat underlying cause which may or may not be bacterial.

Blood cultures should always be taken before beginning antibiotics.

Start empiric broad spectrum antibiotics. These may include gentamicin + 3rd generation cephalosporin (such as ceftriaxone (Rocephin)). Add vancomycin if Gram-positive organisms are suspected or metronidazole (Flagyl) if anaerobic organisms are suspected.

Fluid resuscitate if shock is present. Add a pressor agent such as dopamine or norepinephrine (Levophed) if needed.

Consult surgery if septic focus thought to be abscess. Will need immediate incision/drainage.

Take Home Points

- SIRS is often a precursor to sepsis and should be recognized by its four characteristic features, two of which need to be present for diagnosis.
- Look for the source of inflammation and treat as soon as possible.
- Systemic antibiotics are needed in almost all cases.

Polycythemia Vera

A myeloproliferative state that leads to the clonal proliferation of red blood cells (RBCs) with variable cell maturities and hematopoietic efficiency. This production of RBCs may be associated with clonal overproduction of other cells including WBCs or platelets. Genetic linkage is able to be demonstrated in the vast majority of cases and involves a mutation in the JAK2 gene.

Symptoms

Symptoms often stem from hyperviscosity and include headache, dyspnea, blurred vision, pruritus particularly to hot water, gout, dizziness, tinnitus, and facial plethora.

Diagnosis

Physical exam: Facial plethora, epistaxis, retinal venous engorgement, hepatomegaly, weight loss, and **splenomegaly**.

Labs: CBC showing **increased red cell mass** and hemoglobin and hematocrit. WBCs and platelets are often increased above normal. Neutrophil alkaline phosphatase (NAP) is increased, as is vitamin B12 levels. Erythropoietin level is low. Uric acid often increased contributing to gout comorbidity.

Treatment

Serial phlebotomy is the mainstay of treatment. Goal is hematocrit < 45%.
  Hydroxyurea (Hydrea) may reduce frequency of phlebotomies.
  Low dose aspirin to reduce platelet function.
  Interferon α is under investigation for this purpose and shows promise.

Take Home Points

- Genetic mutation in the JAK2 gene is highly associated with polycythemia vera.
- Characteristic labs are increased RBC mass, increased Hgb/Hct, and low erythropoietin.
- Phlebotomy is the cornerstone of treatment.

Hereditary Hemochromatosis

An autosomal recessive disease whereby the intestinal absorption of dietary iron is in excess and as a result accumulates in internal tissues and organs which further causes dysfunction. Classic areas of accumulation include heart muscle, pancreas (causing "bronze diabetes"), liver, and skin. Hereditary hemochromatosis is the most common genetic disease in Caucasians.

Symptoms

Symptoms commonly may be seen as skin hyperpigmentation, arthralgias, fatigue, impotence in men, premature amenorrhea in women, or symptoms of heart failure or diabetes mellitus. History may reveal a family member with the same symptoms/disease.

Diagnosis

Physical exam: May reveal skin hyperpigmentation in a global pattern, findings of heart failure including edema, ascites, etc., hepatomegaly, splenomegaly, jaundice, testicular atrophy, or weight loss.

Labs: Fasting transferrin saturation (serum iron/TIBC) is increased and ferritin is high. Genetic testing for mutation in the HFE gene, specifically C282Y and H63D mutations, can be done by PCR and used to further screen in family members. Confirmation of disease may be found by liver biopsy. Liver AST/ALT, PT, aPTT, albumin levels may show liver cirrhosis or hypofunctioning. Testing of glycemic levels for diabetes are also warranted if advanced stage is suspected. Creatinine and BUN may show kidney damage.

Treatment

Early screening in high risk populations is warranted.

Early treatment is essential in preventing end organ damage from iron overload.

Phlebotomy is the mainstay of treatment and is most useful if started early in the disease. Reversal of end organ damage is not possible but prevention of further damage may be lifesaving.

If phlebotomy is not possible or in the presence of severe heart disease, deferoxamine (Desferal) is an iron chelating agent that may be used.

Avoid excess Vitamin C.

Take Home Points

- Hereditary hemochromatosis is the most common genetic disease of Caucasians.
- Key labs include fasting transferring saturation and ferritin, both of which will be abnormally high.
- The cornerstone of treatment is phlebotomy.

Transfusion Reaction

TABLE 16.3 Transfusion Reactions

Reaction	Associations	Diagnosis	Treatment
Immediate	Chills, anxiety, fever, flushing, tachycardia, hypotension, or pain. Wrong blood type or Rh antigen in previously sensitized patient.	Coombs test (positive), low haptoglobin, elevated serum bilirubin, UA shows hemoglobinuria. Repeat type and cross of donated blood and recipient blood.	Stop transfusion. Maintain BP and urine output (goal ≥ 100 cc/hour). Use IVFs, furosimide (Lasix) and/or dopamine as needed.
Delayed	2–14 days after transfusion. Symptom of jaundice, anemia, and fever.	Unexpected drop in H/H well after transfusion. Decreased haptoglobin. Hyperbilirubinemia.	Supportive care. Usually is self limited.
Allergic reaction	Due to unknown allergen in donor blood. Often occurs on short term basis. Pruritis or urticaria may develop.	No signs of hemolysis upon laboratory investigation.	Antihistamine (diphenhydramine (Benadryl)) or, if severe, epinephrine. Transfusion may be resumed.
Transfusion related acute lung injury (TRALI)	Caused by antibodies to donor WBCs. Respiratory symptoms such as dyspnea, tachypnea, chest pain, and cough develop. Occurs 1–6 hours after transfusion.	Chest x-ray shows non-cardiogenic pulmonary edema. Wheezing or rhonchi may be heard.	Supportive care with oxygen or intubation if needed.

Hypercoagulable States

The abnormal inherited or acquired tendency of blood to clot inappropriately.

Reasons for Hypercoagulability

Inherited disorders—Factor V Leiden deficiency, protein C or S deficiency, antithrombin III deficiency, homocystinemia.

Acquired disorders—Prolonged immobilization, tissue damage from surgery or fracture, DIC, hyperlipidemia, multiple myeloma, lupus anticoagulant (antiphospholipid syndrome), nephrotic syndrome (leading to loss of protein C/S), smoking, malignancy, oral contraceptive use, or pregnancy.

Symptoms

Patients are generally asymptomatic until an event heralds diagnosis or thrombosis. Events may include deep venous thrombosis (DVT), pulmonary embolus (PE), superficial thrombophlebitis, cardiac ischemia, or stroke.

Diagnosis

Labs: CBC for platelet level, coagulation panel (PT/aPTT, and calculated INR), protein C and S levels, thrombin level, antithrombin III level, bleeding time. Obtain genetic testing as needed and ANA for lupus. Consider a 50:50 mixing study to determine if anticoagulant present. If present, test for lupus, which would indicate thrombotic tendency, not antithrombotic. Test for β-HCG.

Imaging: Obtain imaging of head (CT, MRI) if suspected CVA. Doppler flow ultrasound if DVT suspected. See Chapter 5: Cardiovascular Disease for other tests available.

Treatment

Anticoagulation with heparin or low molecular weight heparin, enoxaparin (Lovenox) is indicated initially. This prevents further clot formation but does not treat the current clot. After 2–3 days, warfarin (Coumadin) may be started for oral anticoagulation. Keep the INR between 2 and 3. The duration of treatment varies depending on defect. Lifelong anticoagulation may be indicated but courses may be as little as 3 months if condition is found to be acquired and corrected.

Thrombolytics are controversial and of limited proven benefit.

Treat any condition that is possible such as lupus or renal failure.

Take Home Points

- Hypercoagulable states may be inherited or acquired.
- Major causes of mortality include PE, cardiac ischemia, and ischemic stroke.
- Heparin or LMWH should be started 2–3 days before warfarin due to a theoretic hypercoagulable state caused by initiation of warfarin.

Disseminated Intravascular Coagulation (DIC)

A serious condition that occurs by systemic deposition of fibrin and consumption of coagulation factors. Causes vary but are classically due to Gram-negative sepsis, amniotic fluid embolus, abruptio placenta, liver failure, and malignancy.

Diagnosis

Usually seen in the very ill, DIC may first be seen as bleeding at IV sites, ecchymosis, purpura, and distal limb discoloration. Bleeding may become brisk and occur from GI tract or surgery site.

Labs: When suspected, immediately obtain coagulation studies for PT/aPTT which are both prolonged. Thrombin time is markedly prolonged. CBC shows decreased platelets. Fibrin split products are very high while fibrinogen is low. Above are the most important labs acutely but the following may also be abnormal: D-dimer positive, increased bleeding time, schizocytosis, leukocytosis, increased LDH, decreased antithrombin III, decreased factors V, VIII, X, XIII, hematuria, and occult blood in stools.

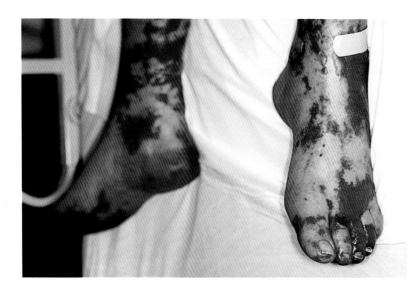

FIGURE 16.2 Gangrenous ecchymoses in an individual with DIC. Reprinted with permission from Warrell DA, Cox TM, et al. *Oxford Textbook of Medicine*, 4th edition. 2003, Oxford University Press.

Treatment

Admit the patient to the ICU.

Treat the underlying cause. Consider high dose broad spectrum antibiotics until infection is ruled out.

Replace acutely lost blood with transfusion.

Give fresh frozen plasma (FFP) for clotting factors. Cryoprecipitate is an alternative.

Give antithrombin III if FFP fails.

Administration of platelets is not useful as they are destroyed due to systemic coagulation.

Heparin may be considered if complications from clotting are suspected, *but never give after head injury.*

Take Home Points

- Look for subtle signs of onset such as bleeding from IV sites and distal limb discoloration.
- PT/aPTT are both prolonged in DIC.
- Give FFP, cryoprecipitate, or antithrombin III for treatment.

Hemophilia

Hemophilia is an X-linked recessive hypocoagulable state leading to lifelong excess bleeding with minor trauma and commonly joint deformity due to repeated hemarthrosis. Hemophilia A and B are reflections of genetically deficient factors VIII, and IX, respectively. Hemophilia A is 5 times more common than B.

Symptoms

Since this is an X-linked disorder, almost all affected are males. Degrees of severity exist and depend on levels of the missing factor: < 1% severe, < 5% moderate, and > 5% mild. First episodes of bleeding often from either minor trauma or circumcision. Further bleeding occurs with minor cuts or scrapes and may be profuse, even life threatening. Hemarthroses are a common complication and can be disfiguring due to calcium deposition and deformity.

Diagnosis

Labs: Coagulation studies show increased aPTT but normal PT. CBC may show anemia and normal platelet count. Bleeding time is only sometimes prolonged. Factor VIII is low in hemophilia A, factor IX is low in hemophilia B. Female hemophilia A carrier state may be diagnosed by comparison of factor VIII level and Von Willibrand factor (VWF). PCR and genetic testing is also effective in detecting carriers.

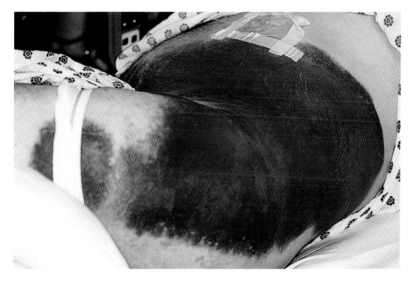

FIGURE 16.3 Mild to moderate blunt trauma induced left flank and hip ecchymosis and hematoma in a patient with severe hemophilia A. Reprinted with permission from Warrell DA, Cox TM, et al. *Oxford Textbook of Medicine*, 4th edition. 2003, Oxford University Press.

Treatment

Recombinant and immunoaffinity-purified forms of both factor VIII and IX are now available. These may be given at hemophilia centers, ERs, or refrigerated at home. Patients may now use home infusion if involved in minor trauma or hemarthrosis.

Target factor activity following minor bleeding episode is > 20%. Before surgery, target should be 100% with > 50% maintained until healing completed.

Desmopressin (DDAVP) is also effective in acutely raising factor VIII levels and may be used in mild hemophiliacs.

Vaccinate for hepatitis B at the time of diagnosis. Regular visits to hemophilia specialist are recommended.

Genetic counseling as indicated.

Take Home Points

- Hemophilia A is due to lack of factor VIII, hemophilia B is due to lack of factor IX.
- Hemarthrosis and resulting joint deformity may be profound and debilitating.
- Replacement of the missing factors is the cornerstone of treatment.

Idiopathic Thrombocytopenic Purpura (ITP)

An acute or chronic disease of thrombocytopenia without a specific etiology to account for a change in platelet level. Pathogenesis is unknown but theories involve immunologic destruction of existing platelets and suppression of platelet production involving platelet-specific antibodies.

Symptoms

Petechial hemorrhages, purpura, easy bruising, gingival bleeding, GI bleeding, recurrent and brisk nose bleeds, or spontaneous bleeding if platelet count < 20,000. History may be positive for recent minor viral disease.

Diagnosis

Strictly a diagnosis of exclusion.

Physical exam: petechiae, purpura, multiple ecchymoses, conjunctival hemorrhage, bleeding from minor trauma sites.

Labs: CBC shows normal WBCs and low platelets. Platelets may be significantly decreased to < 20,000 although these drastically low platelet counts are more highly associated with acute ITP. Bleeding time often prolonged. PT/aPTT normal. Positive bound platelet associated antibody (PA-IgG).

Imaging: CT head for possible intracranial bleeding if indicated.

Treatment

Commonly self limited to < 2 months in younger patients. More common to progress to chronic form in older patients.

Platelet transfusion only indicated for acute, profuse bleeding.

Treat with corticosteroids (IV or oral) if platelet count < 20,000 or < 50,000 with symptoms. IVIG is used if steroids are not effective. Anti Rho(D) immune globulin (RhoGam) may also be tried instead of or including IVIG.

Splenectomy is a last resort and generally reserved for chronic form which has failed other treatment.

Take Home Points

- ITP is a result of isolated thrombocytopenia without other reason for this state.
- Give steroids if mild, step up to IVIG if needed.
- Most disease is self limited and nonprogressive.

Thrombotic Thrombocytopenic Purpura and Hemolytic Uremic Syndrome (TTP/HUS)

These two closely related syndromes are likely disorders on the same clinical spectrum. Pathophysiology in both disorders involves thrombocytopenia and microangiopathic hemolytic anemia without apparent cause, leading to microthrombi deposition causing end organ damage.

Classic associations:

HUS: Triad of hemolytic anemia, thrombocytopenia, and acute renal failure (ARF).

TTP: Pentad of HUS triad + fever and neurologic signs.

Symptoms

Symptoms are much the same as other thrombocytopenic disorders with petechial hemorrhages, purpura, easy bruising, gingival bleeding, GI bleeding, recurrent and brisk nose bleeds, or other spontaneous bleeding if platelet count is decreased. Neurologic symptoms can include subtle changes such as confusion or severe headache. Focal, objective abnormalities are less frequent, but grand mal seizures and coma can occur. Age is often a clue to the disorder as HUS mainly occurs in children. Other past medical history may be disease specific as follows:

HUS: Recent viral illness or infection with *E coli* 0157:H7 or *Shigella*.

TTP: Pregnancy, HIV disease, or OCP use.

Diagnosis

Labs: CBC shows anemia and thrombocytopenia (often 35,000–100,000 range). LDH is elevated. Haptoglobin is decreased. Bilirubin is elevated. Peripheral smear may show schistocytes, burr cells, or helmet cells. BMP often reveals renal failure (especially in HUS). Urinalysis may show blood, increased RBCs, or RBC casts.

Treatment

Admission to the hospital or ICU is often needed.

Supportive care with fluids and control of blood pressure is mandatory.

Consider dialysis for significant renal failure.

Mainstays of therapy include plasma exchange, fresh frozen plasma (FFP), or cryosupernatant.

In refractory cases (or TTP) consider corticosteroids, vincristine, IVIG, rituximab (Rituxan), aspirin, and immunosuppresion with azathiprine or cyclophosphamide.

DO NOT give platelet transfusion in TTP/HUS, as it is contraindicated.

Take Home Points

- TTP/HUS are linked by the triad of features including hemolytic anemia, thrombocytopenia, and ARF.

- Plasma exchange, FFP, or cryosupernatant are cornerstones of therapy.

Immunity Deficiency

B-Cell

TABLE 16.4 B-cell Disorders

Disorder	Associations/Diagnosis	Treatment
X-linked (Bruton) agammaglobulinemia	B-cell deficiency in boys. Pseudomonas infections in infancy. Quantitative Ig levels (specific subclasses) are low	IVIG and prophylactic antibiotics
IgA deficiency	Most common immunodeficiency. Recurrent infections, URIs	None/unnecessary

T-Cell

TABLE 16.5 T-cell Disorders

Disorder	Associations/Diagnosis	Treatment
DiGeorge syndrome (thymic aplasia)	Tetany (from hypocalcemia) in first days of life. Dx with absolute lymphocyte count, mitogen stim response, and skin testing.	Bone marrow transplant (BMT) and thymus transplant has showed success.
Ataxia-telangiectasia	Oculocutaneous telangiectasias, progressive cerebellar ataxia. Likely shortened life span to < 30 years.	IVIG and antibiotics may help acutely. Ultimately no treatment.

Combined

TABLE 16.6 Combined Immunodeficiencies

Disorder	Associations/Diagnosis	Treatment
Severe combined immunodeficiency (SCID)	Lack of both B and T cells. Chronic, severe, infections including fungal and others.	BMT and stem cell transplant. IVIG. Prophylaxis for PCP. Gene therapy in future?
Wiskott-Aldrich syndrome	Eczema, thrombocytopenia, ↑ IgE, IgA, ↓ IgM. X-linked.	BMT, splenectomy, continuous antibiotics, IVIG. Prognosis poor with death before 15-year-old if no BMT.

Complement

TABLE 16.7 Compliment Deficiencies

Disorder	Associations/Diagnosis	Treatment
Hereditary angioneuroctic edema (C1 esterase deficiency)	Autosomal dominant. Repeated episodes of possibly life threatening angioedema commonly brought on by stress or minor trauma. Diagnose with compliment levels.	Daily danazol for prophylaxis.
Terminal compliment deficiency (low C5-C9)	*Neisseria* infections. Gonococcal infections.	Vaccinate against *Neisseria* and antibiotics as needed.

Intestinal Infections

TABLE 17.1 Common Intestinal Infections

Etiology	Associations	Treatment
Viral (adenovirus, rotavirus, Norwalk-like virus, etc.)	Low grade fever, nausea/vomiting, non-bloody diarrhea, abdominal cramps. Look for history of sick contacts.	Hydration is key. Either orally or IV. Bismuth-subsalicylate.
Campylobacter infections	Subtypes denote common location, i.e. pylori, jejuni, coli, etc. Cause nausea/vomiting, diarrhea, abdominal cramps. May rarely see **Guillain-Barré** after illness.	Rehydration Azithromycin, Ciprofloxacin, or erythromycin.
Clostridium difficile	Severe diarrhea, fever, abdominal cramps. History often positive for hospital stay, recent antibiotic use. Send a stool sample for *C difficile* toxin if suspected.	Isolate the patient! Rehydration Metronidazole is first line, Vancomycin is second. Wash hands after leaving the room to prevent spread!
Food poisoning/ gastroenteritis (*Shigella, Salmonella, E coli* species (0157-H7, enterotoxigenic, etc.), *V parahaemolyticus, C perfringens, Y Enterocolitica, S aureus, B cerius*)	Obtain history relating to suspected meal time, < 24 hours-likely toxin, > 24 hours-likely invasive bacteria. Symptoms commonly fever, abdominal cramps, diarrhea (bloody or not), nausea/vomiting. History may reveal illness in individuals who shared the suspected meal.	Rehydration Treatment is controversial. Do not treat *E. Coli* 0157-H7 with antibiotics! Loperamide (immodium) is controversial as it may make disease worse if toxigenic. If antibiotics indicated, use Ciprofloxacin, TMP/SMX, or other broad spectrum.
Giardia lamblia	Bloating, flatulence, nausea/vomiting, loose/greasy/foul smelling stools, weight loss. History of time spent outdoors. Check stool for ova/parasites.	Rehydration Tinidazole (Tindamax) Metronidazole (Flagyl) Nitazoxanide (Alinia)

Streptococcal Pharyngitis

Strep-caused pharyngitis is a focus of therapy due to its tendency to cause rheumatic sequelae if left untreated (not to shorten course of symptoms of pharyngitis). The basis of rheumatic problems is thought to be due to antigenic mimicry of the heart valve and renal glomerular cells, leading to rheumatic heart disease (and fever) and post-streptococcal glomerulonephritis. Other complications follow more acute courses and include peritonsillar abscess, otitis media, septicemia, sinusitis, pneumonia, meningitis, as well as others.

Symptoms

Sore throat, decreased oral intake, malaise, fever, tender anterior cervical lymph nodes, halitosis. History often reveals sick contacts or daycare exposure.

Diagnosis

Physical exam: Fever, anterior cervical lymphadenopathy, exudative tonsillitis, and posterior pharyngeal erythema.

TABLE 17.2 Clinical Tool for Determining Chances of *Strep* Throat Infection

Risk Factor	Points
Anterior cervical lymphadenopathy	1
Fever	1
Tonsilar exudate	1
Absence of cough	1
Age younger than 15 years	1
Age 15–45 years	0
Age > 45 years	-1

Scoring:
–1 or 0 points: streptococcal infection ruled out (2%)
1 to 3 points: order rapid test and treat accordingly
4 to 5 points: probable streptococcal infection (52%); consider empiric antibiotics.
Warren J. McIsaac, MD, MSc; David White, MD David Tannenbaum, MD; Donald E. Low, MD, A clinical score to reduce unnecessary antibiotic use in patients with sore throat, Can Med Assoc J, JAN. 13, 1998; 158 (1)

Rapid strep tests (antigen agglutination) from tonsillar swab have good sensitivity and specificity. Some practitioners prefer to back up negative results with throat cultures.

Throat culture is the gold standard but takes 2–3 days for result.

Mono spot for mononucleosis is often warranted.

Treatment

Penicillin is the standard. Oral Pen V if compliant, IM Pen benzathine G if not.

Macrolides such as erythromycin or azithromycin are second line or considered in pen-allergic patients.

If given amoxicillin and a rash develops, the patient likely has mononucleosis and not strep throat.

NSAIDs have been shown most effective for the pain of sore throat and myalgias; otherwise, lozenges, throat sprays, and rest may help symptoms.

Take Home Points

- Strep throat is treated to prevent rheumatic heart disease, rheumatic fever, and poststrep glomerulonephritis.

- Diagnosis can be reasonably made by use of a clinical tool and point system.

- If a rash appears after giving amoxicillin, mononucleosis is the diagnosis!

Streptococcal Infections

TABLE 17.3 *Streptococcal* Infections

Disease	Prototypic Antibiotic
Cellulitis	Pen G
Necrotizing fasciitis	Incision/drainage procedure + Pen G + clindamycin
Impetigo	Antibacterial ointment (Mupiricin)

(continued)

TABLE 17.3 Continued

Disease	Prototypic Antibiotic
Wound infection after trauma	TMP/SMS DS or clindamycin
Strep toxic shock syndrome	Pen G + clindamycin
Pneumonia	Azithromycin
Scarlet fever	Penicillin
Intrapartum GBS prophylaxis	Penicillin or ampicillin
Meningitis	Ceftriaxone or cefotaxime + vancomycin + dexamethasone
Otitis media	Amoxicillin
Sinusitis	Amoxicillin or amoxicillin/clavulonate (Augmentin)

Staphylococcal Infections

TABLE 17.4 *Staphylococcal* Infections

Disease	Prototypic Antibiotic
Endocarditis	(Nafcillin + gentamycin) or vancomycin
Osteomyelitis	Vancomycin
Mastitis	Continued nursing + dicloxicillin or TMP/SMX DS
Toxic shock syndrome	Remove tampons (common source), nafcillin, IVIG, +/– vancomycin
Cellulitis (nonMRSA)	Penicillin or dicloxacillin
Scalded skin syndrome	Nafcillin
Hordeolum (stye)	Hot packs +/– nafcillin/oxacillin (if internal)
Conjunctivitis	Ophthalmic drops of gatifloxacin, levofloxacin, or moxifloxacin

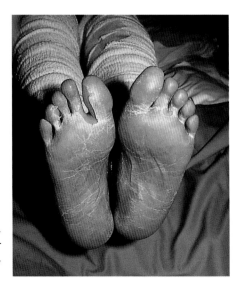

FIGURE 17.1 Desquamation of the feet in toxic shock syndrome. Reprinted with permission from Humphreys H, Irving WL. *Problem-Oriented Clinical Microbiology and Infection*, 2nd edition. 2004, Oxford University Press.

Escherichia coli Infections

TABLE 17.5 *E. coli* Infections

Disease	Prototypic Antibiotic
Urinary tract infection	TMP/SMX DS (Bactrim, Septra) or ciprofloxacin
Gastroenteritis 0157:H7	No antibiotics
Gastroenteritis—traveler's diarrhea	Azithromycin or ciprofloxacin, loperamide (Imodium), bismuth subsalicylate

Haemophilus Influenzae Infection

TABLE 17.6 *H influenzae* Infections

Disease	Prototypic Antibiotic
Epiglottitis	Ceftriaxone (Rocephin)
Otitis media	Amoxicillin
Pneumonia	Azithromycin

Pseudomonas Infection

TABLE 17.7 *Pseudomonas* Infections

Disease	Prototypic Antibiotic
Otitis externa (swimmer's ear)	Ofloxacin ear drops
Contact lens wearer's conjunctivitis	Gentamycin eye drops + piperacillin eye drops to infected eye around the clock
Cystic fibrosis—pneumonia	Tobramycin + piperacillin
Cystic fibrosis—pneumonia suppression	Inhaled tobramycin (1 month on, 1 month off)
Sepsis related to burns	Vancomycin + amikacin + pipercillin, debridement

HIV Infection and AIDS

Human immunodeficiency virus (HIV) is a double-stranded RNA retrovirus which uses its gp120 antigen to attach to cell surface CD4 receptors and gain access to the cell. Cells affected are mainly helper T-lymphocytes, but others include monocytes, macrophages, and neural cells. Millions of cases exist in the world with over half of victims residing in Africa. Since 1999, more heterosexual transmission has occurred than homosexual.

Symptoms

After early transmission, patients are most commonly asymptomatic for a period of weeks. When antibodies form, an acute viral-like illness with generalized malaise, low grade fever, and myalgias may be reported. After seroconversion, an asymptomatic period with generalized lymphadenopathy may last a variable amount of time. After which, "class B" conditions may appear, such as oral/vaginal candidiasis, herpes zoster, oral hairy leukoplakia, peripheral neuropathy, cervical dysplasia, fever/diarrhea > 1 month, idiopathic thrombocytopenic purpura, etc. After progression of disease to include the diagnosis of AIDS (see below), almost any symptom/sign may be seen and usually is indicative of one of the AIDS-defining illnesses.

Diagnosis

Perform a complete physical exam and document any abnormal findings.

According to the Centers for Disease Control and Prevention (CDC) recommendations, AIDS is present in those patients with CD4 counts < 200 mm^3 or one or more AIDS-defining illnesses (commonly pneumocystis pneumonia, Kaposi sarcoma, candidiasis of the esophagus, trachea, bronchi, or lung, toxoplasmosis of the brain, etc.).

Labs: ELISA antibody testing for screening. If reactive, confirm with second ELISA. If still reactive, obtain Western blot analysis. ELISA seroconversion typically takes 4–10 weeks after infection for a positive result.

CD4 count is key to therapy and prognosis. Obtain accompanying viral load.

Obtain screening labs such as CBC, Complete chemistry, hepatitis panel, CMV antibodies, toxoplasmosis antibodies, RPR/VDRL, PPD, etc.

Imaging: CXR for pneumonia, CT head for toxoplasmosis (ring-enhancing lesion). Other imaging as clinically necessary.

Treatment

Treat HIV directly with **highly active antiretroviral therapy (HAART)**. Regimens consist of multiple (commonly 3–4) drug combinations. Drugs include zidovudine, lamivudine, efavirenz, fosamprenavir, ritonavir, nelfinavir, abacavir, nevirapine, and others.

TABLE 17.8 When to Start HAART in HIV+ Patients

CD4 Count	HIV Symptoms Present?	Start HAART?
Any	Yes	Yes
< 200mm^3	Yes/no	Yes
> 200, < 350 mm^3	No	Offer
> 350 mm^3 (viral load > 100,000 cop/mL)	No	Consider
> 350 mm^3 (viral load < 100,000 cop/mL)	No	No

TABLE 17.9 Prophylaxis in HIV+ Patients

Indication	Disease	Prophylaxis
HIV +	Influenza	Annual vaccination
HIV +	Pneumococcal pneumonia	Vaccination
HIV +	Hep B virus	Vaccination
HIV +	Hep A virus	Vaccination

(continued)

TABLE 17.9 Continued

Indication	Disease	Prophylaxis
HIV + with no history of exposure/vaccination	Chickenpox or varicella zoster	Vaccination
CD4 < 200 mm³	*Pneumocystis Carini* pneumonia	TMP/SMX daily or dapsone or aerosolized pentamidine
CD4 < 100 mm³ and Toxoplasmosis IgG positive	*Toxoplasmosis Gondii*	TMP/SMX DS daily
CD4 < 50 mm³	Mycobacterium avium complex (MAC)	Azithromycin weekly
HIV + and PPD ≥ 5 mm diameter or contact with person with active TB	Tuberculosis	INH + pyridoxine for 9 months

Follow disease with serial visits and CD4/viral load counts every 3–6 months.

All pregnant women should be screened for HIV status and placed on zidovudine (AZT) if positive. Refer to infectious disease specialist.

Take Home Points

- HIV/AIDS is now at pandemic levels although antiretroviral medications have significantly improved quality and quantity of life.

- Back up positive ELISA with repeat testing and Western blot analysis.

- CD4 count and viral load are the most important labs to follow.

- Prophylax with appropriate medications at certain CD4 counts.

Pneumocystis Pneumonia (PCP)

A pneumonia caused by *Pneumocystis carinii* most commonly infects immunocompromised patients. Source of immunocompromise is often HIV, but others include chemotherapy, immunodeficiencies, and transplant patients. This is a common AIDS-defining illness and often occurs with CD4 count < 200 mm³.

Symptoms

Insidious onset of dyspnea on exertion, weakness, fatigue, malaise, fever/chills, and scantly productive cough. Comorbidity in the immunocompromised patient includes oropharyngeal candidiasis and other opportunistic infections.

Diagnosis

Physical exam: Diffuse rhonchi and possible rales if effusion is present. Tachypnea may be present.

Labs: Obtain ABG if hypoxemia is suspected, LDH levels are often increased. Diagnosis is often by saline-induced sputum sample and Gram staining, although bronchoalveolar lavage may be necessary; *P carinii* cysts will be seen. Check HIV if not previously diagnosed (see above); obtain CD4 count.

Imaging: CXR reveals diffuse perihilar infiltrates and interstitial shadowing. Rarely, a consolidation is seen. Effusion, abscesses, cavitations, or pneumothorax may also be seen depending on degree of disease.

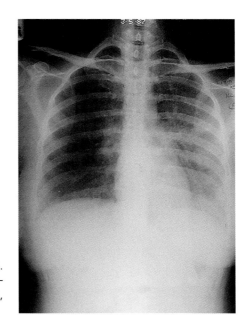

FIGURE 17.2 Chest X-ray showing Pneumocystis carinii pneumonia. Reprinted with permission from Humphreys H, Irving WL. *Problem-Oriented Clinical Microbiology and Infection*, 2nd edition. 2004, Oxford University Press.

Treatment

Prevention is the standard and should include TMP/SMX (Bactrim, Septra), dapsone, or aerosolized pentamidine (Pentam) if CD4 < 200 mm³.

Give oxygen.

Give steroids if patient is acutely ill and hypoxemic. Prednisone is a good choice and is proven to decrease mortality.

TMP/SMX or dapsone/TMP are first line antibiotics. Treatment course is 21 days.

D/C prophylaxis if CD4 rises > 200 mm³ for greater than 3 months.

Take Home Points

- If PCP is diagnosed, look for the source of immunodeficiency.
- Prophylaxis with TMP/SMX, dapsone, or pentamidine at CD4 < 200 mm³.

Kaposi Sarcoma

A disease caused by human herpes virus 8 and is most often found in the immunocompromised (HIV positive), endemic (African) form, or elderly men. This neoplasm is characterized by vascular tumors of the skin and viscera (any organ may be affected) and derives from capillary endothelial cells or fibrous tissue associated with the causative virus, HHV8.

Symptoms

Often presents with reddened or purple vascular skin or mucosal lesions. KS tends to affect the head, neck, and trunk in HIV patients or feet and lower extremities on older men. Tumors may be tender or pruritic and can also occur on mucous membranes, in lymph nodes, or viscera.

Diagnosis

Physical exam: Multicentric red-blue violaceous tumors on the skin. Lesions may occur in skin, mucous membranes, viscera, or lymph nodes.

Labs: HIV testing as above, biopsy is the gold standard. HHV8 antibody testing is usually positive and **Southern blot** analysis or PCR should be done on the biopsy to confirm diagnosis.

Imaging: Obtain CXR and CT for disseminated disease.

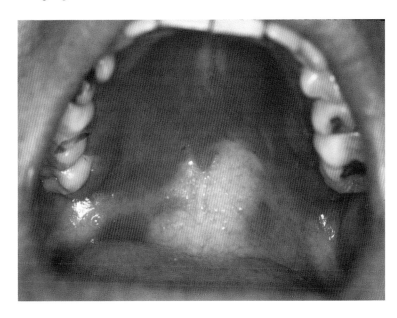

FIGURE 17.3 Kaposi sarcoma. Reprinted with permission from Humphreys H, Irving WL. *Problem-Oriented Clinical Microbiology and Infection*, 2nd edition. 2004, Oxford University Press.

Treatment

Treat HIV infection as indicated.

Local disease may be amenable to surgery, radiotherapy, CO_2 laser, cryotherapy, or intralesional chemotherapy. Generalized disease may be treated with chemotherapy such as doxorubicin and daunorubicin (liposomal forms), bleomycin, vinblastine, interferon, etc. Anti-viral medications (foscarnet, ganciclovir, cidofavir) are still unproven but show promise.

Take Home Points

- Kaposi sarcoma is a neoplasm affecting the immunocompromised, older men, and select Africans caused by HHV 8.

- Local disease may be treated by surgery, radiotherapy, or other local treatments. Generalized disease may respond to chemotherapy.

Varicella (Chickenpox)

Varicella is a syndrome caused by the double-stranded DNA virus varicella-zoster (human herpes virus 3). Commonly, this disease is a childhood exanthem but may reactivate later after a dormant period spent in nerve ganglia. Spread is thought to be both direct contact and respiratory droplets, occurring about 48 hours before appearance of the rash until the final lesions have crusted over.

Symptoms

Commonly in children, symptoms include vesicular, erythematous, pruritic lesions starting on the trunk and moving toward extremities (centripetally). Low grade fever and malaise is common. Vesicles finally rupture and crust over (indicating end of contagious stage).

Reactivation varicella (called zoster or shingles) usually presents with similar lesions but are confined to a single dermatome. This reactivation is commonly preceded by localized pain of the dermatome affected. After acute illness, shingles may leave residual pain termed "post-herpetic neuralgia."

Diagnosis

Physical exam: Lesions are vesicular papules with erythematous base. Rupture of vesicle with development of a crusted top is usual. Appearance is of a "dew drop on a rose petal."

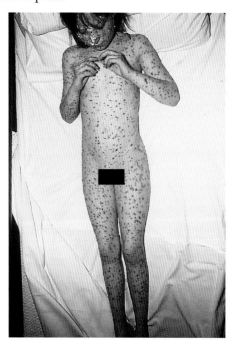

FIGURE 17.4 Primary varicella rash in 8-year-old female. Reprinted with permission from Humphreys H, Irving WL. *Problem-Oriented Clinical Microbiology and Infection*, 2nd edition. 2004, Oxford University Press.

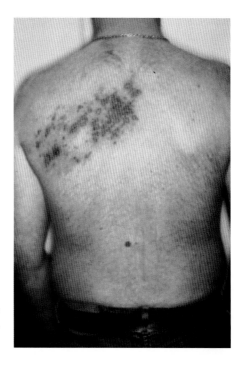

FIGURE 17.5 Characteristic varicella zoster distribution demonstrating thoracic nerve root involvement. Reprinted with permission from Humphreys H, Irving WL. *Problem-Oriented Clinical Microbiology and Infection*, 2nd edition. 2004, Oxford University Press.

Most often clinical diagnosis is adequate, although multinucleated giant cells may be present on Tzanck smear of scrapings (rarely done).

Treatment

For children < 12 years, supportive care and treatment of symptoms is adequate. (To avoid the risk of Reye syndrome, do not give aspirin.)

Post-exposure prophylaxis should be initiated in high risk patients (such as pregnant, immunocompromised, or > 15 years w/o history of disease) with varicella-zoster immunoglobulin (VZIG) within 96 hours of exposure.

Treat adolescents (≥ 12 years), immunocompromised, or pregnant patients with **acyclovir (Zovirax)** or **valacyclovir (Valtrex)** to shorten the course.

Live attenuated vaccine is routinely recommended for children and adults who have a nonreliable history of primary disease or are sero-negative, to avoid the development of primary disease. However, do not vaccinate pregnant women with this live vaccine!

Zoster (shingles) should be treated with anti-viral medications such as acyclovir (Zovirax), famciclovir (Famvir), or valacyclovir (Valtrex) within 72 hours of eruption. Give oral steroids to control symptoms in those > 50 years old. Topical capsaicin or topical lidocaine (Lidoderm) may be effective for acute pain relief.

Post-herpetic neuralgia may be treated with NSAIDs, capsaicin (Zostrix), TCA antidepressants such as amitriptyline (Elavil), lidocaine patch, pregabalin (Lyrica), and gabapentin (Neurontin).

Take Home Points

- Varicella-zoster virus causes chickenpox and shingles.
- Treatment for children < 12 years is supportive; high-risk populations should get antiviral medications.
- The major complication associated with shingles is post-herpetic neuralgia (PHN).

Herpes Simplex

Herpes simplex virus (HSV) is a DNA virus which produces recurrent vesicular lesions in several areas, commonly the oral, ocular, and genital areas. When not active, the virus resides in a latent phase in the basal ganglia of the infected nerve. History may reveal triggers such as stress, excessive light exposure, trauma, menstruation, or fever.

HSV—1 usually perilabial.

HSV—2 usually genital.

These may often be switched.

Symptoms

Fever blisters are commonly preceded by 3–5 days of characteristic pain or tingling in the affected area, then an ulcerated lesion forms and often crusts over.

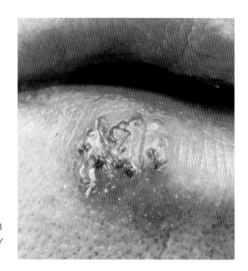

FIGURE 17.6 HSV-1 lesion on lip. Reprinted with permission from Humphreys H, Irving WL. *Problem-Oriented Clinical Microbiology and Infection*, 2nd edition. 2004, Oxford University Press.

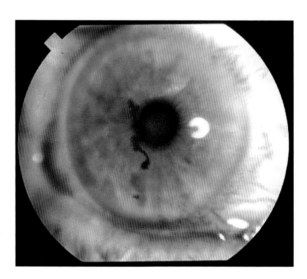

FIGURE 17.7 Dendritic herpetic keratitis. Reprinted with permission from Humphreys H, Irving WL. *Problem-Oriented Clinical Microbiology and Infection*, 2nd edition. 2004, Oxford University Press.

Diagnosis

Tzanck smear reveals multinucleated giant cells.

Pap smear may reveal suspicious giant cells.

Viral culture, EIA, or PCR (more sensitive) may be done on fluid from the lesion.

Serology:

Direct fluorescent antibody (DFA), ELISA, radioimmunoassay (RIA), and complement fixation testing may be done on scrapings of the lesion but don't distinguish HSV types. However, primary HSV confers a ≥ 4 fold increase in titer over the convalescent baseline. Recurrent infection has no increase over the convalescent baseline, thus, the titer increase may be able to distinguish primary from recurrent lesions.

Type-specific serologic antibody testing (immunoblot, Western blot, and glycoprotein-G blocking RIA) is available and can show the presence of IgM and IgG antibodies to HSV I and II. However, the clinical utility is limited since HSV I and II may occur either on the oral area or genitals. Because of this, the results should be interpreted with consideration that only 85–90% of genital herpes lesions are of type II.

Indications for obtaining type-specific serology:

- Evaluation and surveillance of asymptomatic long-term sexual partners of infected individuals, especially if pregnant
- Recurrent, undiagnosed genital lesions
- Differentiation of primary vs. recurrent disease
- Screening of high risk groups (semen donors, candidates for immunosuppresion, high risk HIV persons, frequent STD clinic patients)

Treatment

Symptomatic care and pain reduction is usually adequate for oral labial lesions. Use capsaicin topical (Zostrix) or NSAIDs as needed for pain.

If severe (or history of severe attacks), consider treatment within 72 hours of onset with antivirals. Use acyclovir (Zovirax) or valacyclovir (Valtrex) or famciclovir (Famvir).

Suppressive therapy for genital disease reduces number of outbreaks and may give psychological benefit.

Pregnant patients with history of genital disease should be placed on suppressive therapy with valacyclovir (Valtrex) at the end of pregnancy. Perform C-section if active lesions on genital tract while in labor.

Take Home Points

- HSV may occur on the oral labia, genitals, eye, body (herpes gladiatorum), or fingers/hands (herpetic whitlow).
- Diagnosis is best by analysis of vesicular fluid or lesion scrapings but serology may be useful in certain situations.
- Treat early with antiviral medications or with suppressive therapy for genital disease.

Measles (Rubeola)

An acute viral skin disease caused by a single-stranded RNA paramyxovirus which may occur in epidemic fashion. In the U.S., cases of measles are very rare, but worldwide it remains a major cause of vaccine preventable death, especially to children. Vaccination continues to be the best and most reliable strategy for preventing illness.

Symptoms

A classic triad of symptoms occurs before the appearance of rash and includes **cough, coryza, and conjunctivitis**. These are commonly accompanied by fever, malaise, photophobia, and **Koplik's spots** on oral mucosa. Rash appears generally on the head and spreads down. Onset of rash is about 2 weeks after exposure and patient remains contagious until about 4 days after the onset of rash.

Diagnosis

Physical exam: Increased temperature common and resolves 2–3 days after rash onset. Red, morbilliform, blanching rash begins as discrete lesions on head or neck that then coalesce. Pharyngitis and lymphadenopathy may be present. Koplik's spots usually appear on oral mucosa 2 days before the skin rash and are minute, whitish spots which increase in number and eventually coalesce.

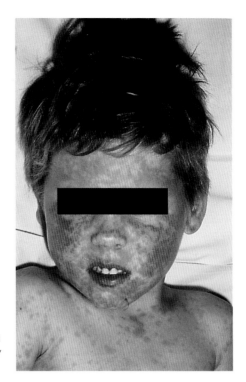

FIGURE 17.8 Primary measles infection. Reprinted with permission from Humphreys H, Irving WL. *Problem-Oriented Clinical Microbiology and Infection*, 2nd edition. 2004, Oxford University Press.

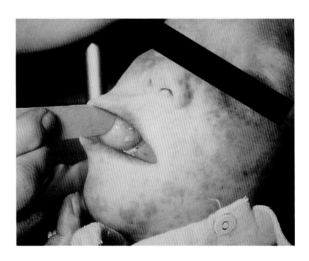

FIGURE 17.9 Koplik's spots on oral buccal mucosa. Reprinted with permission from Humphreys H, Irving WL. *Problem-Oriented Clinical Microbiology and Infection*, 2nd edition. 2004, Oxford University Press.

Labs: Serologic testing for IgG and IgM is the most widely-used technique for diagnosis and involves diagnosing specific peaks in these antibodies. Viral culture of the lesions requires special facilities, but may also be used. CBC may show leukopenia, lymphopenia, or thrombocytopenia.

Imaging: Obtain CXR for possible lung involvement.

Associated condition that develops years later is **subacute sclerosing panencephalitis (SSPE)** which is often life threatening.

Treatment

Supportive care with antipyretics, antitussives, and NSAIDs.

High risk individuals (pregnancy, HIV, immunosuppressed, etc.) may benefit from postexposure prophylaxis, including measles immunoglobulin or live-attenuated measles vaccine. However, do not give MMR or live virus vaccine to pregnant women!

Give vitamin A in endemically vitamin A-deficient areas.

Report to local health department!

Take Home Points

- Measles is very rare in the U.S. but is a major cause of vaccine preventable death worldwide.
- A life-threatening complication is subacute sclerosing panencephalitis (SSPE).
- Treatment is largely supportive.

Childhood Exanthems

TABLE 17.10 Common Childhood Exanthems

Disease	Associations	Rash	Diagnosis	Treatment
Rubella	Commonly vaccinated for in MMR. Intrapartum infection causes **"congenital rubella syndrome"** in the baby and includes cataracts, PDA, VSD, hearing loss, etc.	Descending **"blueberry muffin"** rash of infant is pathognomonic.	Serum IgM and IgG testing. Viral culture may also be used.	Postnatal infection: symptomatic treatment only. Congenital rubella: Supportive treatment and contact isolation. Vaccinate to prevent. Do not vaccinate pregnant women with MMR (live virus).
Roseola	Abrupt, moderate-high fever. After fever, rash appears.	Appearance of maculopapular, nonpruritic, blanchable rash on the trunk, arms, and neck. Short course of hours to days.	Serum antibody testing or serum PCR for HHV-6/HHV-7 may also be indicative.	Symptomatic care with antipyretics, etc. Self limited illness.
Erythema infectiosum (Fifth disease)	Associated with only mild fever, pruritus, and mild arthralgias. Rare complications include transient **aplastic crisis**, significant joint involvement, and chronic anemia. Hydrops fetalis may occur if acquired during pregnancy.	"Slapped cheek" appearance of facial rash. Rash develops into reticulated, lacy pattern on trunk and extremities. Once rash appears on face, patient is no longer infectious.	IgM antibody indicates acute infection. Less commonly but more reliable is testing viral DNA in fetal blood.	Symptomatic as needed. IVIG in refractory cases or those with significant complications.
Kawasaki disease (mucocutaneous lymph node syndrome)	Fever ≥ 5 days, bilateral conjunctivitis, cervical lymphadenopathy, characteristic "strawberry" tongue, hand/foot swelling and desquamation. **Coronary artery aneurysms** are the main concern.	Polymorphous rash which may appear as scarlatiniform, morbilliform, or erythema multiforme. Rash may desquamate in groin area.	Clinical diagnosis. Labs may show leukocytosis, thrombocytosis, anemia, elevated CRP, ESR. Obtain ECG and echocardiogram to evaluate possible aneurysms.	High dose aspirin. Consider IVIG to decrease the incidence of cardiac abnormalities. Follow up echocardiograms.

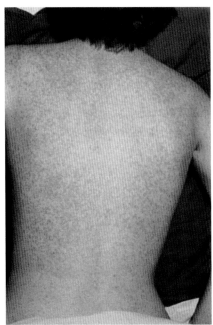

FIGURE 17.10 Characteristic rubella rash in adult female. Reprinted with permission from Humphreys H, Irving WL. *Problem-Oriented Clinical Microbiology and Infection*, 2nd edition. 2004, Oxford University Press.

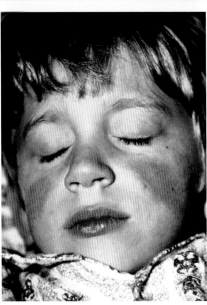

FIGURE 17.11 "Slapped cheek" appearance of erythema infectiosum. Reprinted with permission from Warrell DA, Cox TM, et al. *Oxford Textbook of Medicine*, 4th edition. 2003, Oxford University Press.

Syphilis

A sexually transmitted spirochetal disease caused by *Treponema pallidum*. This disease has historically been the most lethal STD before the emergence of HIV; however, it is now controlled well in the U.S. (although recent rise has been noted).

Symptoms

Primary—**Painless** chancre (or ulcer) on the genitals. Lasts 2–6 weeks then heals with scarring.

Secondary—Often overlaps with chancre stage; nontender rash appears usually on **hands and soles of the feet**. Rash is contagious if break in skin present. Accompanied by patchy alopecia, condyloma lata (gray-white lesions on mucous membranes), generalized lymphadenopathy, anorexia, and headache.

Tertiary—Involves other organ systems such as CNS (neurosyphilis), cardiac, bones, and skin.

Diagnosis

Primary—Darkfield microscopy of fluid from chancre may demonstrate spirochete. Screening non-treponemal tests are VDRL or RPR. Positive result should be confirmed with treponemal testing: fluorescent treponemal antibody absorption (FTA-ABS) or microhemagglutination treponemal pallidum (MHA-TP). Follow disease with VDRL or RPR titers, since FTA-ABS/MHA-TP turn positive for life after disease.

Secondary—Positive serologic testing and clinical signs of rash, condyloma lata, characteristic symptoms, generalized lymphadenopathy, or hepatomegaly.

Latent—Asymptomatic stage often between secondary and tertiary.

Tertiary—Involvement of extragenital organ systems. CNS involves neurosyphilis, which may be seen as **tabes dorsalis**, **Argyll-Robertson pupils** (constricted pupil nonreactive to light but reactive to accommodation), characteristic gait, paresis, paralysis, visual or hearing disturbance. Cardiac involves presence of murmur, aneurysms, or valvular abnormalities. Bones may show Charcot joints, osteomyelitis. Skin shows gummas (destructive granulomatous pockets) and possible secondary infections. Serologies may be negative in this stage. Consider lumbar puncture if tertiary stage suspected. VDRL may be performed on CSF along with treponemal tests.

Congenital—Can lead to meningitis, **saber shins**, **Hutchinson teeth**, and **interstitial keratitis**.

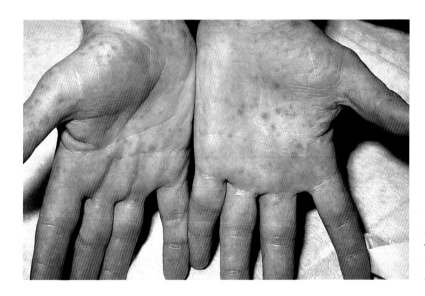

FIGURE 17.12 Typical rash of secondary syphilis on hands. Reprinted with permission from MacKie, RM. *Clinical Dermatology*, 5th edition. 2003, Oxford University Press.

Treatment

Classic and still very effective is **penicillin G** IM. Alternatives include doxycycline or azithromycin.

Primary and secondary syphilis should get 2.4 million units IM × 1.

Tertiary or latent syphilis > 1 year should receive pen G 2.4 million units q/week × 3 weeks.

Neurosyphillis is very difficult to treat and should get 3–4 million units q4 hours × 10–14 days.

Watch for **Jarisch-Herxheimer reaction** of acute febrile illness sometimes seen at beginning of treatment due to destruction of spirochetes.

Congenital syphilis should be treated with aqueous crystalline pen G for 14 days.

Follow with quantitative VDRL/RPR.

Take Home Points

- Syphilis has several stages: primary, secondary, latent, neurosyphilis, congenital, and tertiary.
- Diagnose with both a nontreponemal and treponemal testing.
- Penicillin is the most effective and appropriate medication.

Sexually Transmitted Diseases

TABLE 17.11 Common STDs*

Disease	Associations	Diagnosis	Treatment
Gonorrhea	Urethritis/epididymitis in men, urethritis, cervicitis, or PID in women. Disseminated form possible as well as pauciarticular septic arthritis.	Gram stain of purulent fluid for gm-negative diploccoci. DNA probes and PCR also widely used and sensitive. Culture possible but special medium needed.	Ceftriaxone IM or cefixime PO. Always treat for chlamydia as well. "Gut and butt" regimen.
Chlamydia	Urethritis/epididymitis in men, urethritis, cervicitis, or PID in women. Other forms of chlamydia produce pneumonia, trachoma, and psittacosis. Also associated with **lymphogranuloma venereum**.	DNA probes and PCR widely used. Culture and direct antigen testing also used.	Doxycycline or azithromycin. Always treat for gonorrhea as well. "Gut and butt" regimen.
Chancroid	Associated with **painful** chancre. Uncommon in the U.S.	Culture and Gram stain for organism. PCR testing also available.	Ceftriaxone IM or azithromycin.
Trichomoniasis	Frothy, green cervical discharge and fishy odor in women, often asymptomatic in men.	Wet prep slide with visualization of organism most common. "Whiff test" positive. PCR, culture, ELISA, DNA probes are also available.	Metronidazole (Flagyl) or tinidazole (Tindamax).
Genital warts (*Condyloma acuminate*)	Associated with HPV types 6 and 11, only rarely with higher risk types.	Clinical diagnosis usual. Aceto white color change positive. PCR may be done on biopsy but is rarely needed.	Excision, cryotherapy, CO_2 laser, or electrodescication are all common and effective. Imiquimod (Aldara), podophyllin, Podofilox (Condylox), and trichloroacetic acid are topical options.

*In all STDs, treat partner as well as patient.

Tinea (Dermatophytosis)

Variants of this superficial fungal infection are said to be the most common infection of the human race. These variants are many and include *T unguium*, *T capitis*, *T corporis*, *T versicolor*, *T cruris*, *T pedis*, and *T barbae*. Infection is most commonly chronic and not acute or subacute, although acute and devastating infection may occur in the immunocompromised.

Symptoms

Fungal infection of almost anywhere on the body. These have varied presentations but often involve color change, reddening of skin, flaking, alopecia, and pruritis. History is often positive for contacts with similar symptoms.

Diagnosis

Clinical diagnosis can often be made based on appearance. Rash is scaling or powdery although appearance varies from hypopigmented areas caused by *T versicolor* to areas of broken hair and decreased hair growth as in *T capitis* (black dot ringworm).

Skin scraping and examination with KOH. Branching hyphae should be seen if positive.

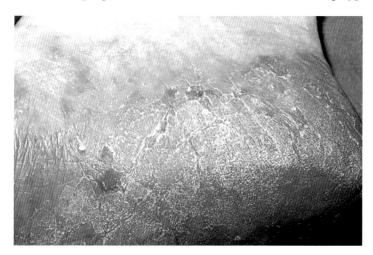

FIGURE 17.13 Tinea pedis involving the instep and heel. Reprinted with permission from MacKie, RM. *Clinical Dermatology*, 5th edition. 2003, Oxford University Press.

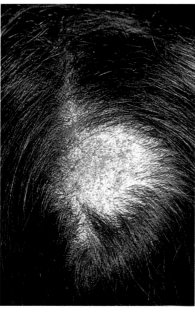

FIGURE 17.14 Tinea capitis. Brilliant green fluorescence was seen under Wood's light and *Microsporum audouinii* isolated in culture. Reprinted with permission from MacKie, RM. *Clinical Dermatology*, 5th edition. 2003, Oxford University Press.

Treatment

Topical preparations of azole medications generally effective except against *T capitis* or onychomycosis. These include miconazole (Monistat), clotrimazole (Lotrimin), and econazole (Spectazole).

Oral azoles are indicated for *T capitis*, onychomycosis, disseminated, or refractive cases. These include griseofulvin, fluconazole (Diflucan), terbinafine (Lamisil), ketoconazole (Nizoral), or itraconazole (Sporanox).

Liver function and enzyme testing should be evaluated before starting oral medications.

Expect long course of 4–6 weeks before cure.

Take Home Points

- *Tinea* infections are exceedingly common and may occur in almost any area of the body.

- Topical azoles may generally be used except in *T capitis*, onychomycosis, disseminated, and refractory cases in which systemic therapy is indicated.

Mycoses

TABLE 17.12 Common Mycoses Infections

Disease	Associations	Treatment
Histoplasmosis	**Midwestern United States**. History may show contact with birds or their droppings. Vast majority are asymptomatic. May be reactivated in immunocompromised.	Ketoconazole (Nizoral) if mild, Amphotericin-B if disseminated or severe.
Coccidiodomycosis	**Southwest United States**. Contracted by contact with dust, soil, or cave exploration. Many cases asymptomatic.	Amphotericin-B, ketoconazole (Nizoral), itraconazole (Sporanox), fluconazole (Diflucan) depending on severity.
Blastomycosis	**Mississippi and Ohio river valleys**. Soil dwelling organism. Pulmonary, skin, genital, and reactivation forms.	Itraconazole (Sporanox), ketoconazole (Nizoral), or amphotericin-B for severe disease.

Hepatitis

TABLE 17.13 Comparison of Hepatidities

Hepatitis Type	Transmission Route	Symptoms/ Associations	Diagnosis	Treatment
Hep A	Oral fecal. Occurs in outbreaks of contaminated food and during travel to Latin American or third world countries.	Acute, flu-like illness with abdominal pain and nausea. Often asymptomatic especially in the young. Never chronic!	Anti-HAV IgM positive for acute or recent infection. Anti-HAV IgG indicates past infection. Antibody is protective.	IVIG useful for prevention after exposure. Otherwise supportive care for acute infection. Vaccinate those at risk.

(continued)

TABLE 17.13 Continued

Hepatitis Type	Transmission Route	Symptoms/ Associations	Diagnosis	Treatment
Hep B	Blood or body fluid contact as through sex, drug use (needles), or perinatally.	Acute illness has fever, malaise, jaundice, anorexia, etc. Often acutely asymptomatic. May progress to chronic form and cirrhosis or liver cancer. Associated with polyarteritis nodosa.	See below.	Vaccinate! No indication to treat acute disease. Chronic form treated with lamivudine or interferon-alpha. Don't expect cure but suppression of viral load.
Hep C	Blood or body fluid contact as through sex, drug use (needles), or perinatally.	Acute illness has fever, malaise, jaundice, anorexia, etc. Fifty percent progress to chronic form. Associated with lichen planus.	Anti-HCV antibody shows prior infection. HCV quantitative RNA testing determines virus in blood. If positive, obtain genotype to match with prognosis.	Acute: Interferon-alpha to prevent progression. Chronic: Pegylated interferon-alpha 2b + ribavirin.

TABLE 17.14 Interpretation of Hep B Markers

Marker	Interpretation
HBsAg	Acute or chronic disease
Anti-HBsAg	Antibody conferring immunity
HBeAg	Indicates infectivity
Anti-HBeAg	Antibody indicating low infectivity
IgM anti-HBcAg	Antibody indicating new infection
IgG anti-HBcAg	Antibody indicating old infection

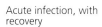
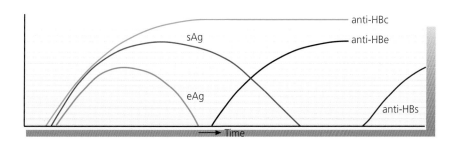

FIGURE 17.15 Acute hep B infection with recovery. Reprinted with permission from Humphreys H, Irving WL. *Problem-Oriented Clinical Microbiology and Infection*, 2nd edition. 2004, Oxford University Press.

Mumps

An acute viral condition caused by a characteristic paramyxovirus most commonly spread by respiratory droplets between children. Parotitis is the most common feature, although orchitis in adolescents may also be prominent.

Symptoms

Sore throat, fever, pain in parotids glands exacerbated by eating sour food, and malaise are usual. Orchitis is especially common in older child patients.

Diagnosis

Physical exam: Swelling of parotid gland and cervical lymph nodes. Elevated temperature common but moderate. Orchitis with tenderness may be seen. Meningismal signs including neck tenderness and nuchal rigidity are rare.

Labs: Viral isolation may be done from throat swab, urine, blood, or CSF. If mental status changes and meningismal signs, obtain spinal fluid for testing.

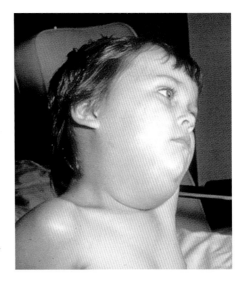

FIGURE 17.16 Parotitis of mumps. Reprinted with permission from Humphreys H, Irving WL. *Problem-Oriented Clinical Microbiology and Infection*, 2nd edition. 2004, Oxford University Press.

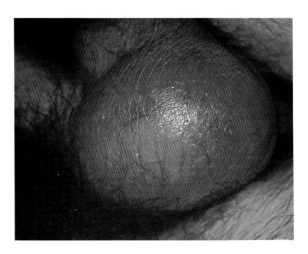

FIGURE 17.17 Orchitis of mumps. Reprinted with permission from Humphreys H, Irving WL. *Problem-Oriented Clinical Microbiology and Infection*, 2nd edition. 2004, Oxford University Press.

Treatment

Vaccinate to prevent illness with MMR at 12–15 months and 4–6 years.

Immunoglobulin is ineffective at preventing mumps.

Supportive therapy for acute illness.

Isolate and keep children home from school until 9 days after onset of symptoms (contagious period).

Even in those male patients with prominent orchitis, subfertility is uncommon and infertility is rare.

Take Home Points

- Mumps' most prominent features are parotitis and orchitis.
- Subfertility and infertility are uncommon complications.
- Vaccinate to prevent.

Hand, Foot, and Mouth Disease

Acute viral illness, usually of preschool, involving vesicular lesions of the mouth, palms of hands, and soles of feet. Cause is most often coxsackievirus.

Symptoms

Usually accompanied by low grade fever, malaise, and fussiness, this disease characteristically has vesicles on the oral buccal mucosa, tongue, and palate in conjunction with the palmar and plantar aspects of the hands and feet. History often reveals sick contacts.

Diagnosis

Physical exam: Mouth lesions or ulcers, small, vesicular lesions on palms and soles of feet.

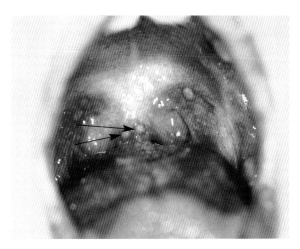

FIGURE 17.18 Typical oral lesions in hand, foot and mouth disease. Reprinted with permission from Humphreys H, Irving WL. *Problem-Oriented Clinical Microbiology and Infection*, 2nd edition. 2004, Oxford University Press.

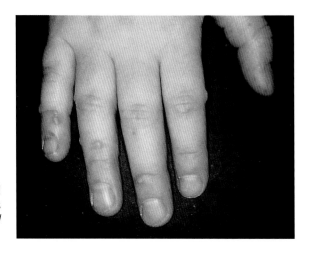

FIGURE 17.19 Typical hand vesicles in hand, foot and mouth disease. Reprinted with permission from Humphreys H, Irving WL. *Problem-Oriented Clinical Microbiology and Infection*, 2nd edition. 2004, Oxford University Press.

Labs: Virus may be isolated from lesions but is usually not done.

Treatment

Supportive with NSAIDs and acetaminophen.
 Consider isolation to prevent spread.

Take Home Point

- Hand, foot, and mouth disease is a common vesicular exanthem of childhood requiring no specific therapy other than isolation.

Infectious Mononucleosis

Mono is an acute or subacute viral disease associated with the classic triad of lymphadenopathy, pharyngitis, and fever. This disease is often caused by the Epstein-Barr virus and may be easily transmitted by oropharyngeal secretions and saliva, earning it the nickname of the "kissing disease."

Symptoms

Marked fatigue, sore throat, noticeably swollen lymph nodes, anorexia, low grade fever, and malaise. History is often positive for group living such as military recruits, college students, or campers.

Diagnosis

Physical exam: Pharyngitis with erythema and possibly tonsillar exudates. "Kissing tonsils," in which the inflamed tonsillar tissue may be so prominent as to touch in the anterior pharynx. Palpable cervical lymphadenopathy. Palpable spleen or liver may be present, indicating enlargement.

 Look for a characteristic rash that may have developed after prior misdiagnosis and treatment of strep throat with amoxicillin.

Labs: Monospot test of IgM heterophile antibodies against Epstein-Barr virus are useful in telling acute infection. Usually negative after 6 months. Positive IgG or IgM are commonly present for EBV. CBC may show lympho/leukocytosis with atypical lymphocytes and thrombocytopenia. Liver transaminases are commonly elevated.

Imaging: Splenic ultrasound may be indicated for suspected splenomegaly or to follow course. CT abdomen not needed unless recent injury makes rupture likely.

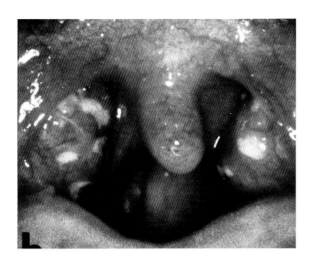

FIGURE 17.20 Tonsillar swelling in acute mononucleosis. Reprinted with permission from Humphreys H, Irving WL. *Problem-Oriented Clinical Microbiology and Infection*, 2nd edition. 2004, Oxford University Press.

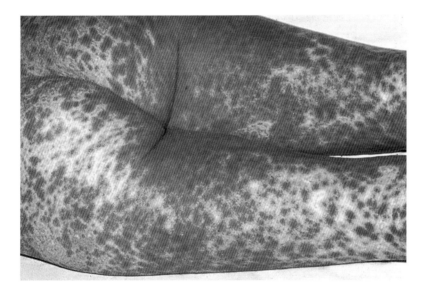

FIGURE 17.21 Morbilliform eruption caused by administration of ampicillin to a patient with infectious mononucleosis. Reprinted with permission from MacKie, RM. *Clinical Dermatology*, 5th edition. 2003, Oxford University Press.

Treatment

Supportive care.

Avoid contact sports or situations of high risk abdominal injury to avoid possible splenic injury for 3 weeks after onset of disease. If patient has had clinical documentation of enlarged spleen, follow up ultrasound before return to contact sports for resolution of splenomegaly is indicated.

Oral steroids (prednisone) are used by some clinicians and may decrease lymphadenopathy and tonsillar size, although these are commonly not indicated unless tonsils are obstructing or meningitis is suspected.

Take Home Points

- Mono is a common cause of pharyngitis and may be mistaken for strep throat.

- Monitor spleen size and restrict contact sports if patient is high risk.

- Supportive care is the treatment.

Molluscum Contagiosum

A common benign skin lesion caused by a poxvirus known for its contagiousness. Transmission is by direct contact although the virus may also survive on surfaces or in swimming pools, retaining its infectiousness for significant amounts of time.

Symptoms

Discrete, flesh-colored lesions with a characteristically umbilicated top. Often occur on children on inner thighs. Spread very easily from person to person by direct contact or sex. May be reactivated in HIV or immunocompromised patients.

Diagnosis

Physical exam: May be aided by cryotherapy revealing umbilicated top to lesion. Magnification also used. May have white core.

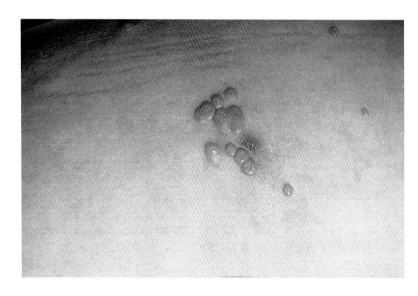

FIGURE 17.22 Molluscum contagiosum showing pearly lesions and central umbilication. Reprinted with permission from MacKie, RM. *Clinical Dermatology*, 5th edition. 2003, Oxford University Press.

Treatment

Cryotherapy, electrodessication, or excision are all effective.

Topical treatments include imiquimod (Aldara), podofilox, trichloroacetic acid, tretinoin, salicylic acid, or podophylin applied in the office. None have been researched but many are clinically used.

Take Home Points

- Molluscum is a common ailment of children.
- Umbilicated top is characteristic.
- Lesions are benign but highly contagious.

Cat Scratch Disease

An acute febrile illness with prominent lymphadenopathy caused by *B henselae*. This is a zoonotic disease transmitted by minor scratches or bites of kittens or cats.

Symptoms

The inoculation site usually presents as macule that progresses to papule or pustule. The most prominent feature then develops weeks after infection is **lymphadenopathy**, usually of head, neck, or upper extremities. Malaise and fever may be present. History often prominent for contact with cats/kittens with bite or scratch. Eye or encephalitic forms do exist.

Diagnosis

Physical exam: Significant lymphadenopathy and increased temperature.

Labs: Blood culture useful but organism *Bartonella henselae* is difficult to grow. Histopathology of inoculation site shows characteristic dermis changes, although skin testing has been replaced by serologies. Immunoflourescent antibody serologies are available and should be completed if this disease is suspected. Lymph node biopsy shows characteristic changes but is rarely needed. Look for evidence of other reasons for lymphadenopathy; lack of other disease supports cat scratch disease.

Treatment

Spontaneous resolution usually occurs in 2–4 months without treatment.

Multiple antibiotics are effective, including azithromycin, erythromycin, doxycycline, TMP/SMX, rifampin, or ciprofloxacin.

Supportive care with NSAIDs or acetaminophen as needed.

Take Home Points

- Lymphadenopathy and exposure to cats should raise suspicion of this disease.
- Treatment is with common antibiotics although resolution without treatment is usual.

Adenovirus

A common and usually febrile illness that may affect several systems including respiratory tract, eye infections, or GI infection. Although very common in the general population, this virus is often more serious in neonates or the immunocompromised.

Symptoms

Acute viral illness with cold-like symptoms is usual. Low-grade fever, malaise, chest congestion may be present. Eye infection often show hyperemia, conjunctivitis, or blepharitis. Enteritis may manifest as nausea, vomiting, diarrhea, and abdominal pain.

Diagnosis

Physical exam: Pharyngitis, anterior cervical shotty lymphadenopathy, rhinorrhea, nasal blockage, and mild fever. Eye infection may show corneal injection, hyperemia, discharge, and is usually unilateral. GI infection may show diffuse abdominal pain, normal or hyperactive bowel sounds. It is important to recognize more than one of these systems may be infected at any one time.

Labs: Viral culture from pharyngeal swab or stool possible.

Treatment

Symptomatic with NSAIDs or acetaminophen for fever.

Hydration is important.

Take Home Point

- Adenovirus is often responsible for infection involving more than one system.

Rhinovirus

A very common virus with over 90 active serotypes that are often credited with causing the common cold.

Symptoms

Common cold symptoms, including rhinitis, runny nose, sore throat, nasal congestion, facial pain, ear pain, or other minor URI symptoms.

Diagnosis

Vast majority may safely be clinically diagnosed as common cold or viral rhinitis.
    Screen for other etiologies such as bacterial sinusitis as necessary.

Treatment

Symptomatic care is the standard.
    Needless to say, antibiotics are ineffective.
    Decongestants, antihistamines, mucolytics all may be used. NSAIDs, OTC analgesics, lozenges, or throat spray all are widely used for sore throat pain. Zinc lozenges (used as treatment) failed to provide improvement in duration or symptom severity in recent trials.

Take Home Points

- Rhinovirus causes many cold-like symptoms in millions of people each year.
- No specific antiviral treatment is effective.

Toxoplasmosis

The causative organism is *T gondii*, a protozoan transmitted by ingestion of meat or food laden with cysts or oocytes which are also commonly present in cat feces. Congenital infection is passed transplacentally from newly infected mothers. Types include: congenital, ocular, acute infection in the immunocompetent, and acute infection in the immunocompromised.

Symptoms

Several different forms exist. The congenital form is worse when acquired during 1st trimester of pregnancy. This intrapartum infection may be asymptomatic, or can cause symptoms ranging from, jaundice, microcephaly, mental retardation, seizures, visual defects (**chorioretinitis**), to death in the first month of life, or symptoms can occur much later in life. Ocular form is seen as chorioretinitis and eyesight difficulties. Acute form in the immunocompromised may have CNS symptoms such as **focal neurologic deficits**, seizures, mental status changes, visual changes, encephalitis, or meningeal symptoms. Acute infection in a normal host may show symptoms of mild viral illness. Look for history of exposure to cat feces (litter boxes) or ingestion of undercooked pork.

Diagnosis

Physical exam: Presentation varies with form but often shows increased temperature, focal neurologic signs, change in mental status, signs of increased intracranial pressure (increased BP, papilledema), especially in the immunocompromised. Generalized lymphadenopathy. Retinal exam may show yellow-white, fluffy cotton patches.

Labs: Demonstration of the organism (a protozoan) in blood, body fluids, or placenta is diagnostic. ELISA and PCR testing are also useful in finding acute infection. Serologies that detect IgM and IgG are also available and may be useful to determine past infection of pregnant patients.

Imaging: CT scan of head with contrast may show intracranial **ring-enhancing lesion** and/or **intracranial calcifications**. MRI is useful, particularly if CT scan is positive. Ultrasound of fetus may show suspicion, which can be tested for by amniocentesis.

Treatment

Prevention of congenital form by instructing pregnant women to avoid litter boxes, cats, and eating raw or undercooked meat.

Otherwise, give sulfadiazine (Microsulfon), pyrimethamine (Daraprim), or leucovorin (folinic acid). Regimens include months of treatment and in immunocompromised (AIDS) may require maintenance regimen after treatment. Use TMP/SMX for prophylaxis in AIDS patients with CD4 counts < 100 and positive IgG titer. Pregnant women may start one of these drugs after 16th week.

Supportive care and admission to hospital should be considered.

Take Home Points

- Toxoplasmosis may have congenital, ocular, or acute infection in the immunocompromised or immunocompetent host.

- Transplacental transmission may occur in pregnant women that are newly infected.

- Look for a "ring-enhancing" lesion or intracranial calcifications on contrast **CT.**

West Nile Virus

The West Nile virus (WNV) was identified in Africa in the 1930s but only appeared in the U.S. in 1999 after a New York City outbreak. It is known to have a complex lifecycle involving viral amplification within a bird host then transmission to humans mainly by mosquito bites.

Symptoms

This acute flu-like illness may present with fever, flaccid paralysis, headache, neck pain, vomiting, myalgias, muscle weakness, maculopapular rash, diarrhea, or altered mental status, although this disease is often asymptomatic in most people. Presentation may resemble Guillain-Barré with localized paralysis. Timing is usually late spring. Eye pain, pharyngitis, nausea, vomiting, diarrhea, and abdominal pain can also occur.

Diagnosis

Physical exam: Encephalitis form may be severe and involve high fever, altered mental status, meningeal signs, etc. An erythematous, maculopapular rash may appear on the chest, back, and arms.

Labs: Lumbar puncture may be characteristic of viral meningitis (pleocytosis with lymphocytic predominance, increased protein). ELISA may be done on CSF. Test the serum for West Nile antibodies.

Treatment

Supportive as needed.

If severe or patient is elderly, consider admission.

Take Home Points

- West Nile virus is becoming a newly emergent threat in America.
- Encephalitis or meningitis are the worst manifestations although these only occur in a fraction of patients.
- Treatment is supportive.

Rocky Mountain Spotted Fever (RMSF)

This acute, tick-borne disease causes an acute vasculitis due to direct endothelial cell invasion by the obligate intracellular gram-negative *R rickettsii*. Despite the name, this disease occurs preferentially in the south Atlantic and southcentral U.S. although incidence is very low overall. In the U.S., two primary vectors exist: the *Dermacentor variabilis* (the American dog tick) in the eastern and southcentral states and *Dermacentor andersoni* (the Rocky Mountain wood tick) in the mountain states west of the Mississippi River.

Symptoms

Classic triad is **headache, fever, characteristic rash**. However, other symptoms include nausea/vomiting, abdominal pain, myalgias, lymphadenopathy, cough, bleeding, edema (especially in children), confusion, focal neurologic signs, and seizures. History often reveals tick bite or time in the outdoors.

Diagnosis

Physical exam: Mild fever, photophobia, rash may be macular, maculopapular, or petechial in appearance. Rash is centripetal (starts on extremities and moves toward trunk) and occurs 2–4 days after onset of fever. **Labs:** CBC may show low hematocrit and markedly low platelets. WBC count is not helpful because of common variation. Basic chemistry may show electrolyte abnormalities, especially in advanced cases.

Serology antibody testing (IFA and others) is possible but usually not helpful early (< 5 days after symptom onset) because of typical late antibody response. Skin biopsy direct immunofluorescence is possible and shows good sensitivity and specificity although results are altered by antirickettsial therapy. Cultures are not available outside large research centers.

Treatment

Antibiotics include **doxycycline** (as with most rickettsial diseases!), tetracycline, or chloramphenicol in kids. Don't wait for confirmatory testing or rash onset in candidates for therapy.

Supportive care as needed with acetaminophen and NSAIDs.

Take Home Points

- RMSF is a rickettsial infection more commonly occurring in the eastern and southcentral U.S.
- Serologies are the best way to diagnose, with skin biopsy the next most reliable.
- Diagnosis early is unreliable; thus, treat suspected patients before diagnosis.

Malaria

Malaria is a protozoan organism transmitted by the female anopheles mosquito, and historically is likely the single largest infectious killer of humanity. Types include: *Plasmodium falciparum, P. vivax, P. malariae, P. ovale*. Most severe and lethal is *P falciparum*. Types vary by endemic area although crossover is common.

Symptoms

Episodic fever, chills, malaise, fatigue, headache, and nausea. Seizures and CNS involvement may be present in severe forms, termed cerebral malaria, and are extremely serious. Look for travel to endemic areas (commonly Africa or tropical regions). If the patient is from an endemic area and has had malaria before, disease is often much milder.

Diagnosis

Physical exam: Cycles of temperature elevation occur every 36–72 hours depending on type. Hepatomegaly or splenomegaly may be appreciated on exam. If significant parasitemia, jaundice, signs of anemia, and petechiae may be present.

Labs: Malarial thin and thick blood smears examined for presence of schizonts or gametocytes. Take at least 3 samples 6–12 hours apart, best if obtained during fever spike. PCR and indirect fluorescent antibody (IFA) testing may yield type. Rapid malarial tests are in use but are limited for subspecies identification.

After diagnosis is made, follow parasitemia level every 12 hours by obtaining thick/thin smears. Otherwise, CBC likely will show anemia, leukopenia or leukocytosis, or possibly thrombocytopenia. Hepatic function panel may show elevated liver transaminases. Basic chemistry can be used to evaluate and follow renal function (renal failure present in severe cases).

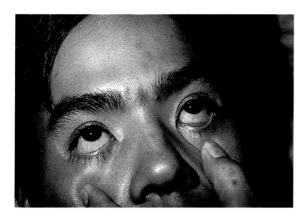

FIGURE 17.23 Deep jaundice in a Vietnamese man with severe falciparum malaria. Copyright D.A. Warrell. Reprinted with permission from Warrell DA, Cox TM, et al. *Oxford Textbook of Medicine*, 4th edition. 2003, Oxford University Press.

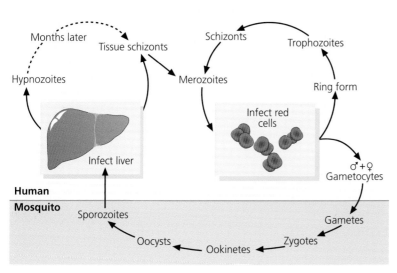

FIGURE 17.24 Life cycle of malaria parasite. Reprinted with permission from Humphreys H, Irving WL. *Problem-Oriented Clinical Microbiology and Infection*, 2nd edition. 2004, Oxford University Press.

Treatment

Avoid mosquitoes by using DEET-based repellent and barrier precautions.

Avoid the disease by taking chemoprophylaxis correctly. Mefloquine (Lariam), Malarone (atovaquone/proguanil), or doxycycline all must be started days to weeks before traveling and be continued weeks after return. Mefloquine (Lariam) is q week dosing while Malarone (atovaquone/proguanil) and doxycycline are every day.

Treatment of active disease consists of killing active protozoa and the liver stage.

Quinoline derivatives—chloroquine (in sensitive areas), hydroxychloroquine (Plaquenil), quinine, quinidine, amodiaquine, mefloquine, and primaquine—act to inhibit heme polymerase activity, resulting in the toxic build up of free heme in the malaria parasite. These are the most widely used medications and continue to be very effective in treatment or prophylaxis.

Non-quinoline derived anti-malarials—doxycycline, tetracycline, clindamycin, pyrimethamine/sulfadoxine (Fansidar), Malarone (atovaquone/proguanil), pyrimethamine, dapsone, or combinations of these—are often also very effective.

Side effects are common and include GI upset, nausea/vomiting, headache, vivid dreams, lost memory, or insomnia.

Make sure the patient doesn't have glucose-6-phosphatase deficiency before starting therapy (to avoid hemolysis), especially in quinoline derived treatment.

Consider exchange transfusion if parasitemia exceeds 10% or severe manifestations.

Admit to hospital for monitoring in non-endemic patients. Transfer to ICU if seizures occur.

Take Home Points

- Malaria is persists as a major killer even today, particularly children in Africa.
- Diagnosis is with rapid antigen detection, thick/thin smears, or serology (for type).
- *P falciparum* carries the highest mortality and requires prompt, commonly inpatient, treatment.
- Treat with a combination of medications from the quinoline and nonquinoline derived groups. Common meds include chloroquine, hydroxychloroquine, primaquine, mefloquine, doxycycline, or pyrimethamine/dapsone.

Lyme Disease

A multisystem tick borne disease caused by the spirochete *Borrelia burgdorferi*. The ixodid (deer) tick is the main vector and disease is particularly common in the northeastern, Mid-Atlantic, and north-central U.S., although all states have had reported cases.

Symptoms

Stage 1: Localized disease often with characteristic target-like rash (**erythema migrans**). Also includes acute flu-like illness with fever, headache, myalgias, and arthralgias.

Stage 2: Early disseminated disease may involve symptoms of any organ system, CNS and cardiac are most common. Look for meningitis symptoms, focal deficits, heart block, and pericarditis. Erythema migrans may occur in multiple sites, facial palsies, orchitis, hepatitis, iritis, or arthritis may also present.

Stage 3: Involves arthritis and chronic neurological syndromes. Recurrent synovitis, tendinitis, bursitis, memory loss, dementia, psychotic behavior, and depression may occur. Advanced cases may present with encephalopathy or mimic other CNS disorders such as multiple sclerosis, stroke-like syndromes, transverse myelitis, parkinsonism, etc. Peripheral neuropathies such as carpal tunnel syndrome or motor, sensory, or autonomic neuropathy may present. Ophthalmic manifestations may include iritis, keratitis, retinal vasculitis, or optic neuritis.

History often indicates tick bite, although to transmit Lyme, tick must be on for 12–24 hours.

Diagnosis

Physical exam: Increased temperature common. Target-like macular rash.

Labs: Positive ELISA serum tests for IgM or IgG to *B burgdorferi* should be followed with Western blot analysis. REMEMBER these tests may be negative in the first stage, thus, can't acutely be used for evaluation of a tick bite victim. CSF analysis with ELISA and culture may be done and is diagnostic although these may take some time.

Overall, Lyme disease remains a clinical diagnosis due to these limitations of laboratory testing, especially early in the course of disease.

(a)

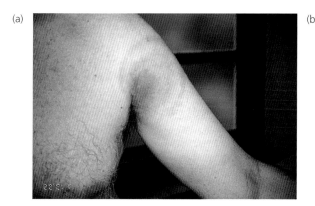

(b)

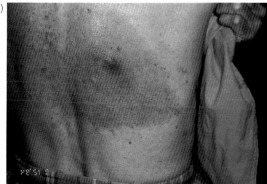

FIGURE 17.25 Erythema migrans rashes from patients with Lyme disease. (a) A rash with typical central clearing appearance. (b) A more homogenous appearing rash of EM. Reprinted with permission from Warrell DA, Cox TM, et al. *Oxford Textbook of Medicine*, 4th edition. 2003, Oxford University Press.

Treatment

All three stages can be treated with doxycycline, or amoxicillin in children, for 3–4 weeks. Consider corticosteroids in stage 2. Cefuroxime, ceftriaxone (Rocephin), or cefotaxime (Claforan) may also be used IV or IM in stages 2 or 3.

Consider ICU admission and/or cardiac monitoring in stage 2.

Consider prophylactic dose of doxycycline in all tick-bite patients.

Take Home Points

- Lyme disease is difficult to diagnose although geographic distribution, likelihood of tick exposure, and clinical presentation should be considered carefully.

- Serology confirmed by Western blot analysis will be positive in later stages.

- Main features of long term complications include arthritis and neurologic sequelae.

- Doxycycline is the pathognomonic drug.

Incubation Periods and Infectivity

Tables reprinted with permission from Wyatt, et al. *Oxford Handbook of Emergency Medicine*, 3rd edition. 2006, Oxford University Press.

TABLE 17.15 Incubation Period Usually < 1 Week

Staphylococcal enteritis	1–6 hours
Salmonella enteritis	6–48 hours (usually 12–24 hours)
Bacillary dysentery (*Shigella*)	1–7 days (usually 1–3 days)
Botulism	12–96 hours (usually 18–36 hours)
Cholera	12 hours–6 days (usually 1–3 days)
Gas gangrene	6 hours–4 days
Diphtheria	2–5 days
Gonorrhoea	1–12 days (usually 3–5 days)
Legionnaire's disease	2–10 days (usually 7 days)
Meningococcaemia	1–7 days (usually 3 days)
Scarlet fever	1–4 days
Yellow fever	3–6 days

TABLE 17.16 Incubation Period Usually 1–3 Weeks

Brucellosis	7–21 days
Chickenpox	7–23 days (usually 14 days)
Lassa fever	3–16 days
Leptospirosis	2–21 days (usually 7–12 days)
Malaria (falciparum)	7–14 days (occasionally longer)
Malaria (vivax, malariae, ovale)	12–40 days (occasionally > 1 year)
Measles	10–18 days (rash usually 14–18 days)
Mumps	14–18 days
Pertussis (whooping cough)	5–14 days (usually 7–10 days)
Poliomyelitis	3–21 days (usually 7–10 days)
Rubella	14–21 days
Tetanus	1 day–3 months (usually 4–14 days)
Typhoid	8–21 days
Typhus	4–21 days

TABLE 17.17 Incubation Period Usually > 3 Weeks

Amoebiasis	2 weeks–many months
Hepatitis A	3–5 weeks (usually 4 weeks)
Hepatitis B, hepatitis C	6 weeks–6 months
HIV	3 weeks–3 months (anti-HIV appears)
Infectious mononucleosis	4–6 weeks
Rabies	4 days–2 years (usually 3–12 weeks)
Syphilis	10 days–10 weeks (usually 3 weeks)

TABLE 17.18 Duration of Infectivity of Infectious Diseases

Chickenpox	5 days before rash until last vesicle crusts
Hepatitis A	2 weeks before until 1 week after jaundice starts
Measles	From initial symptoms to 5 days after rash appears
Mumps	3 days before to 1 week after salivary swelling
Pertussis	3 days before to 3 weeks after start of symptoms (3 days if on erythromycin)
Rubella	1 week before to 5 days after onset of rash
Scarlet fever	10–21 days from onset of rash (1 day if on penicillin)

Index

Note: Page numbers followed by "*f*" and "*t*" refer to figures and tables, respectively.

INDEX